Cambridge Imperial and Post-Colonial Studies

Series Editors

Richard Drayton, Department of History, King's College London,
London, UK

Saul Dubow, Magdalene College, University of Cambridge, Cambridge,
UK

The Cambridge Imperial and Post-Colonial Studies series is a well-established collection of over 100 volumes focussing on empires in world history and on the societies and cultures that emerged from, and challenged, colonial rule. The collection includes transnational, comparative and connective studies, as well as works addressing the ways in which particular regions or nations interact with global forces. In its formative years, the series focused on the British Empire and Commonwealth, but there is now no imperial system, period of human history or part of the world that lies outside of its compass. While we particularly welcome the first monographs of young researchers, we also seek major studies by more senior scholars, and welcome collections of essays with a strong thematic focus that help to set new research agendas. As well as history, the series includes work on politics, economics, culture, archaeology, literature, science, art, medicine, and war. Our aim is to collect the most exciting new scholarship on world history and to make this available to a broad scholarly readership in a timely manner.

Linda Maria Ratschiller Nasim

Medical Missionaries and Colonial Knowledge in West Africa and Europe, 1885–1914

Purity, Health and Cleanliness

palgrave
macmillan

Linda Maria Ratschiller Nasim
Department of Contemporary
History
University of Fribourg
Fribourg, Switzerland

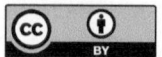

ISSN 2635-1633   ISSN 2635-1641   (electronic)
Cambridge Imperial and Post-Colonial Studies
ISBN 978-3-031-27127-4   ISBN 978-3-031-27128-1   (eBook)
https://doi.org/10.1007/978-3-031-27128-1

The open access publication of this book has been published with the support of the
Swiss National Science Foundation.

Cover Credit: Grosse Wäsche im Beremfluss (Kyebi), BMA QQ-30.027.0307, Basler
Missionsbuchhandlung, Basel, Switzerland / BM Archives

This Palgrave Macmillan imprint is published by the registered company Springer Nature
Switzerland AG
The registered company address is: Gewerbestrasse 11, 6330 Cham, Switzerland

In loving memory of Ida (1920–2022), who sparked my interest in history from a young age.

ACKNOWLEDGEMENTS

I would like to express my gratitude to all the people who have contributed to shaping the outcome of this intellectual journey. I am especially grateful to Siegfried Weichlein, Christina Späti, Richard Hölzl and Martina King for providing extended commentary on this book's original manuscript. Very much in line with the knowledge produced by the Basel Mission doctors, this book is a product of a protracted process of entanglements and negotiations between different people and places, networks and institutions.

Siegfried Weichlein continually supported the realisation of this endeavour by providing intellectual stimuli, securing funding and initiating conferences and book projects. His passion for history is truly contagious, never ceasing to spur my curiosity for new perspectives on the past. Together, we spun up networks with colleagues interested in the histories of mission, science and colonialism in Basel, Berlin, Cambridge, Göttingen and beyond. I particularly benefitted from exchanges with Rebekka Habermas, Patrick Harries, David Maxwell, Paul Jenkins, Jakob Zollmann, Svenja Goltermann and Bernhard C. Schär. I am especially thankful for the fruitful cooperation and enriching conversations with Karolin Wetjen.

My institutional affiliation at the Department of Contemporary History of the University of Fribourg continuously provided me with fresh perspectives thanks to my colleagues' wide range of expertise. I would like to thank them for their many informal and formal contributions to this project. Simone Rees and Barbara Miller, in particular, have offered valuable insights from their work on Swiss Catholic missionaries in twentieth century Zimbabwe. I share with them a passion for conveying new insights on Switzerland's colonial past to a wider public and I am grateful for their hard work in creating our website www.colonial-local.ch.

Damir Skenderovic, Christina Späti and Francesca Falk entrusted me with the coordination of the Doctoral Programme "Migration and Post-coloniality Meet Switzerland" at the University of Fribourg from 2014 to 2021. This role significantly contributed to my understanding of the research landscape and shaped the conceptual frameworks at the heart of this book. I would like to thank them for this valuable opportunity.

A large part of the original sources on which this study is built are held in the Basel Mission archives. My recognition goes to the team there who have supported my research ever since my first visit to their collection in 2009. I also thank the staff and librarians at the British Library, the Bundesarchiv Berlin-Lichterfelde, the School of Oriental and African Studies, the Staatsarchiv des Kantons Basel-Stadt and the Staatsbibliothek zu Berlin.

The many years of research that went into this book would not have been possible without generous funding from the Swiss National Science Foundation (SNSF). I am very grateful for their support of project number 153079 ("Hygiene Abroad and at Home: The Basel Mission Doctors and Spaces of Knowledge 1885–1914") and particularly the open-access grant number 218060 which allows for the book's wider distribution.

I count myself lucky for the network of family and friends in Switzerland, London, Cape Town and Berlin who have encouraged me, all in their own ways, from culinary inspirations to regular distractions during urban and rural discovery trips. I am most indebted to my devoted exploration companion, Faisal, who has provided knowledgeable feedback and emotional support throughout this journey. I dedicate this book to him in anticipation of the winding road ahead of us, and to our children Nahla and Djibril who have opened up a new chapter in the unexpected journey we call life.

COVER IMAGE

In analysing the cover image, we encounter a problem that often arises when working with mission archives. Despite their rich visual legacy, mission archives offer few clues about the creation of images and even less about the protagonists who feature in them. In this case, we also have no information on the number of copies printed or the channels in which they were distributed. However, this picture represents many of the themes woven into this book.

The cover image is a postcard produced by the Basel Mission between 1901 and 1917, showing people "doing the washing in the River Berem (Kyebi)", in modern-day Ghana. The Basel Mission used postcards for advertising and fundraising purposes and became one of the most important producers of colonial knowledge in Switzerland, Southern Germany and beyond. The fact that this postcard was reproduced in colour in the early twentieth century indicates that the Basel Mission spared no expense or effort in promoting their civilising mission.

The postcard shows a seemingly banal activity: women and children washing their clothes in a river. Yet it entails considerable ambiguity. For the Basel Mission, and other institutions involved with the civilising mission, an important argument in justifying their need for intervention was a lack of cleanliness among the people they wished to refine. Simultaneously, this image reveals that the concern for hygiene was a basic human need found around the world. The Basel Mission navigated between these two contradicting messages in their search for support.

By selling, buying, writing, sending and receiving this postcard, people communicated across social and geographical divides. Despite being clearly staged with the children staring at the camera's lens, it nourished colonial curiosity by offering seemingly rare insights into Africans' everyday lives. Europeans who set eyes on this postcard looked these children straight in the eyes. Their gazes crossed. This form of appeal for donations persists in the visual representation of Africans to this day.

Images from the colonial period are strikingly often characterised by their focus on bodily practices. They make clear that colonialism was always more than ideology, politics, military conflicts and economic exploitation. European missionaries set out to reform peoples' bodies, combining ideas of purity, health and cleanliness in their endeavour. This book focuses on six medical missionaries, who offer a fine example of how religious, scientific and colonial efforts for hygiene came together during High Imperialism.

CONTENTS

ABBREVIATIONS

BArch	Bundesarchiv Berlin-Lichterfelde—Federal Archives Berlin-Lichterfelde
BMA	Basel Mission Archives
BV	Brüderverzeichnis—Index of the Basel male missionaries
GGG	Gesellschaft für das Gute und Gemeinnützige
GStA PK	Geheimes Staatsarchiv Preussischer Kulturbesitz—Secret State Archives Prussian Cultural Heritage
SOAS	School of Oriental and African Studies
StABS	Staatsarchiv des Kantons Basel-Stadt—State Archives of the Canton Basel-Stadt
SV	Schwesternverzeichnis—Index of the Basel female missionaries

LIST OF FIGURES

CHAPTER 1

Introduction

1.1 THEMATIC INTRODUCTION

In 1881, the Evangelical Missionary Society in Basel advertised a scientific position for a medical research expedition to the Gold Coast.[1] Since the launch of missionary work in the area in 1828, more than 150 Basel missionaries had lost their lives prematurely, mostly due to what they identified as tropical fevers. The Basel Mission leadership, referred to as the Committee, chose Ernst Mähly, a practising doctor from Basel and devout Pietist, from 46 candidates to fill this position. His role involved researching the causes of disease and compiling facts about "the hygienic conditions of Europeans in the tropics" by considering their housing, clothing, diet and means of travel.[2] Mähly spent nearly two years in West Africa. Upon his return to Basel, he published his insights in a wide range of publications from scientific journals and missionary magazines to colonial periodicals.[3]

---

[1] The job advertisement appeared in the *Berliner klinischen Wochenschrift*, the *Correspondenzblatt für Schweizer Ärzte*, the *Allgemeine Schweizer Zeitung* and the Basel Mission's popular monthly magazine *Der Evangelische Heidenbote*.

[2] Committee report, 14.09.1881, BMA, Komitee-Protokoll 1881, §409.

[3] Ernst Mähly, Die Gesundheitsverhältnisse auf der Goldküste, in: Evangelisches Missionsmagazin 29 (1885) p. 396–417, 445–461; Ibid., Zur Geographie und Ethnographie der Goldküste, in: Verhandlungen der Naturforschenden Gesellschaft in Basel 7

© The Author(s) 2023
L. M. Ratschiller Nasim, *Medical Missionaries and Colonial Knowledge in West Africa and Europe, 1885–1914*,
Cambridge Imperial and Post-Colonial Studies,
https://doi.org/10.1007/978-3-031-27128-1_1

In 1885, Mähly contributed a piece to the *Proceedings of the Society for Natural Sciences in Basel*, dealing with the geography and ethnography of the Gold Coast:

> On this occasion it is worth considering the bad smell, which blacks are infamous for, mainly due to accounts of slave traders and holders; the same is extremely rare with the population on the Gold Coast, which meticulously observes bodily cleanliness and also washes light garments diligently, and if it is to be found with some individuals nonetheless, they are derided by their community.[4]

Mähly's depiction, which contradicted the negative characterisation of Africans disseminated by slave traders and holders, sheds light on the historical context in which the Basel Mission had emerged 70 years earlier. Created in 1815, during an evangelical revival on the European continent, the Basel Mission resulted from the synergy of the city's bourgeoisie and devout Pietists. The founding members of the mission seminary understood their evangelising aspirations as an atonement for the transatlantic slave trade initiated and controlled by Europeans, as was the case for most mission societies emerging around 1800.[5] The first young men to complete their training in Basel worked for British and Dutch mission societies, mainly the Church Missionary Society, which held close ties with the British abolition movement.[6]

(1885) 3, p. 809–852; Ibid., Über das sogenannte "Gallenfieber" an der Goldküste, in: Correspondenz-Blatt für Schweizer Ärzte 15 (1885), p. 73–79, 108–116; Ibid., Akklimatisation und Klimafieber, in: Deutsche Kolonialzeitung 3 (1886), p. 72–83; Ibid., Gesundheitszustand bzw. Sterblichkeit auf der Goldküste und in Westafrika überhaupt, in: Deutsche Kolonialzeitung 3 (1886), p. 555–559; Ibid., Akklimatisation und Klimafieber, in: Evangelisches Missionsmagazin 30 (1886), p. 129–147.

[4] Mähly, Zur Geographie und Ethnographie der Goldküste, p. 842.

[5] Karl Rennstich, The Understanding of Mission, Civilisation and Colonialism in the Basel Mission, in: Torben Christensen/William R. Hutchison (eds.), Missionary Ideologies in the Imperialist Era, 1880–1920, Aarhus 1983, p. 94–103; Brian Stanley, Christian Missions, Antislavery and the Claims of Humanity, c. 1813–1873, in: Sheridan Gilley/Brian Stanley (eds.), World Christianities c. 1815–c. 1914, Cambridge 2006, p. 443–457.

[6] Founding members of the Church Missionary Society established in 1799 included famous abolitionists such as William Wilberforce, Henry Thornton, John Benn and John Newton. See Elizabeth Elbourne, The Foundation of the Church Missionary Society. The Anglican Missionary Impulse, in: John Walsh/Colin Haydon/Stephen Taylor (eds.), The Church of England c. 1689–1833, Cambridge 1993, p. 247–264.

From 1821, the Basel Mission set up their own mission stations abroad, including on the Gold Coast in 1828 and in Cameroon from 1885. Over the course of the nineteenth century, the Basel Mission evolved into one of the most significant evangelical mission societies, involved in many different fields of activity such as trade, agriculture, education and medicine. Mähly's employment reflected a radical shift within the Committee regarding the significance of medical sciences for physical and spiritual healing. Whilst the Basel missionaries in West Africa had been requesting the presence of a mission doctor for decades, scientific medicine only became part and parcel of the Basel Mission in 1885. The Basel Mission became the first German-speaking evangelical mission society to launch a sustained medical mission with scientifically trained mission doctors by formulating theological arguments for the value of mission medicine.

The Basel Mission doctors operated as scientific field workers and intermediaries between remote regions in the colonial world and metropolitan interest groups. Their long-term observations and insights into health environments hitherto unknown to Europeans cemented their position as valuable medical experts. The fact that Mähly's findings appeared in several renowned scientific journals such as the *Proceedings of the Society for Natural Sciences in Basel* clearly identified him as part of the scientific establishment. Before his journey to the west coast of Africa in 1882, Mähly had attended the University of Munich, where he took classes with Max von Pettenkofer, Germany's most prominent figure in experimental hygiene at the time.[7] He further underlined his scientific expertise by drawing on medical terminology:

> I did not discover something specific in these cases; exactly the same excessive or abnormal perspiration along with rapid decomposition of fatty acids on the skin is to be found with Europeans. Where washing water is missing, the black and his dress principally smell of smoke caused by the constant fire burning by, or even in, the hut; and when he has eaten fish dried in the air, one can indeed tell; moreover, sick people, especially when they have daubed themselves with soil, do not spout pleasant fragrances. However, never has my nasal organ in an African hut been insulted by the sort of

---

[7] Martin Weyer-von Schoultz, Max von Pettenkofer, 1818–1901. Die Entstehung der modernen Hygiene aus den empirischen Studien menschlicher Lebensgrundlagen, Frankfurt a. M. 2006; Wolfgang G. Locher, Max von Pettenkofer: Pionier der wissenschaftlichen Hygiene, Regensburg 2018.

unqualifiable, infernal air so often blowing towards us from the housing of our proletariat.[8]

Mähly's anthropological account challenged common stereotypes about Africans and significantly differs from most colonial sources originating in the late nineteenth century. In contrast to widespread racial theories, he denied any fundamental physical differences between people on the Gold Coast and in Europe. He recorded that when Africans smelled, it was not because of natural but cultural and social reasons.[9] This distinction was central to the message of the Basel Mission since it meant that the status quo could be changed. Crucially, the Basel Mission's aspirations were not limited to converting Africans to Christianity but also to transforming entire societies economically, socially and medically.

By comparing the smell in huts on the Gold Coast to that found in proletarian flats in Europe, Mähly contributed to a colonial discourse that stressed the need to civilise both the people in the colonies and the working class in Europe.[10] The Basel Mission represented the outward expression of a welfare system initiated by awakened Pietists and Basel patricians in light of the increasingly pressing social question in nineteenth-century Basel. The home mission movement, known as *Innere Mission* in German, tackled the ostensible problem of de-Christianisation within Europe and fundamentally depended on voluntary work, especially by women and children. Welfare facilities such as poverty and medical relief, Bible circles, Sunday schools, youth associations and the Basel City Mission, founded in 1859, recruited personnel and funds from the same pool of resources as the Basel Mission.

On closer inspection, Mähly's clarifications contradicted a prominent narrative of the Basel Mission, which portrayed missionaries as operating

---

[8] Mähly, Zur Geographie und Ethnographie der Goldküste, p. 842–843.

[9] On the history of odour, see Alain Corbin, Le miasme et la jonquille. L'odorat et l'imaginaire sociale XVIIIe-XIXe siècles, Paris 1982; Jonathan Reinarz, Past Scents: Historical Perspectives on Smell, Urbana 2014.

[10] John Comaroff/Jean Comaroff, Home-Made Hegemony: Modernity, Domesticity, and Colonialism in South Africa, in: Karen Tranberg Hansen (ed.), African Encounters with Domesticity, New Brunswick 1992, p. 37–74; Susan Thorne, "The Conversion of Englishmen and the Conversion of the World Inseparable". Missionary Imperialism and the Language of Class in Early Industrial Britain, in: Frederick Cooper/Ann Laura Stoler (eds.), Tensions of Empire. Colonial Cultures in a Bourgeois World, Berkeley et al. 1997, p. 238–262.

on the frontier of hygiene, where people lived in dirt, ignorance and sin. His observation that people who smelled were "derided by their community" demonstrated that physical cleanliness played an important role in West African societies, despite official mission propaganda suggesting otherwise. Upon their arrival in West Africa, the Basel missionaries encountered existing bodily knowledge, engrained values and practices of purity, health and cleanliness, which they tried to understand and relate to their own experiences.[11]

This book moves beyond the dichotomy of dominance and resistance to examine how entanglements of hygiene between West Africa and Europe around 1900 shaped religious, scientific and colonial bodies of knowledge.[12]

By tracing the multiple interactions and negotiations of six Basel Mission doctors between West Africa and Europe from 1885 to 1914, it demonstrates how notions of religious purity, scientific health and colonial cleanliness came together in the making of hygiene around 1900.[13] The heyday of Protestant medical missions abroad coincided with the emergence of tropical medicine as a scientific discipline during what became known as the Scramble for Africa. The focus on medical missionaries reveals that these projects were intertwined in many ways and that

[11] On the importance of bodily cleanliness and ritual cleansing on the Gold Coast in pre-colonial times, see Thomas C. McCaskie, State and Society in Pre-Colonial Asante, Cambridge/New York 1995. See further, Timothy Burke, Lifebuoy Men, Lux Women. Commodification, Consumption and Cleanliness in Modern Zimbabwe, Durham/London 1996.

[12] This study employs "West Africa" and "Europe" as analytical categories while acknowledging that their exact meanings remained constantly in flux, despite historical actors suggesting otherwise and often using them as self-explanatory terms. In the source material, "West Africa" is frequently identified as a region by missionaries, colonial authorities and scientists, referring for instance to "British West Africa" and "German West Africa". The sheer diversity in languages and histories certainly made it difficult for commentators to differentiate between more specific regions within West Africa. At the same time, the region referred to as West Africa by both observers in the nineteenth century and historians today does share an extensive history, of trade and slavery for example.

[13] These six Basel Mission doctors were Rudolf Fisch, Alfred Eckhardt, Friedrich Hey, Hermann Vortisch, Arthur Häberlin and Theodor Müller. Ernst Mähly operated in West Africa before the start of the medical mission in 1885, and Karl Huppenbauer started working on the Gold Coast in 1914, when the outbreak of the First World War interrupted most of the Basel Mission's activities in West Africa. For further details, see the short biographies in the appendix.

hygiene played an important role in all three of them. How did religious notions of purity, scientific concepts of health and colonial views of cleanliness and civilisation combine with one another to constitute hygienic knowledge between 1885 and 1914?

1.2   RESEARCH REVIEW

This monograph focuses on six Basel Mission doctors who worked on the Gold Coast and in Cameroon, from 1885 to 1914, to analyse how knowledge of hygiene was negotiated and transformed through contact with places and people in West Africa. Hygiene constitutes one of the "magic words of modernity, a magic word with a turbulent history," as Philipp Sarasin has argued.[14] Today, the term is primarily used to describe germ-free cleanliness while the notion of "racial hygiene" still reminds us of the murderous connotation it adopted in the twentieth century. The knowledge of hygiene that emerged in the late nineteenth and early twentieth centuries, by contrast, proved to be both more comprehensive than present-day meanings of hygiene and more complex than the later usage of the word for totalitarian and eugenic projects of cleansing.

Studies on the historical genesis of hygiene, such as Sarasin's seminal history of the body, have identified hygiene as a distinctly bourgeois project taking root in eighteenth-century Europe.[15] The role of religious campaigners, however, in promoting new ideas and practices of health and cleanliness has been widely underrated. This is particularly true for the greater area around Basel, where the social question and public health issues were addressed by distinctly pious policy-makers and supported by

[14] Philipp Sarasin, Reizbare Maschinen. Eine Geschichte des Körpers, 1765–1914, Frankfurt a. M. 2003, p. 17.

[15] Beatrix Mesmer, Reinheit und Reinlichkeit. Bemerkungen zur Durchsetzung der häuslichen Hygiene in der Schweiz, in: Nicolai Bernard/Quirinus Reichen (eds.), Gesellschaft und Gesellschaften. Festschrift zum 65. Geburtstag von Professor Dr. Ulrich Im Hof, Bern 1982, p. 470–494; Gerd Göckenjan, Kurieren und Staat machen. Gesundheit und Medizin in der bürgerlichen Welt, Frankfurt a. M. 1985; Alfons Labisch, Homo Hygienicus. Gesundheit und Medizin in der Neuzeit, Frankfurt a. M. 1992; Barbara Koller, Gesundes Wohnen. Ein Konstrukt zur Vermittlung bürgerlicher Werte und Verhaltensnormen und seine praktische Umsetzung in der Deutschschweiz 1880–1940, Zürich 1995; Manuel Frey, Der reinliche Bürger. Entstehung und Verbreitung bürgerlicher Tugenden in Deutschland, 1760–1860, Göttingen 1997; Philipp Sarasin, The Body as Medium. Nineteenth-Century European Hygiene Discourse, in: Grey Room 29 (2007), p. 48–65.

a broad coalition of evangelical activists. Crucially, the people involved in the hygiene movement in Basel and the Alemannic surroundings did not limit themselves to their immediate vicinities but extended their efforts in propagating new values and behaviours of hygiene overseas, where their prominent mission society had established stations.

The history of hygiene remains incomplete without taking into account the knowledge that was acquired in imperial enterprises and colonial settings. Hygiene was a key dimension of colonialism, initially in allowing for imperial expansion and subsequently in bolstering what was conceived as the civilising mission.[16] Surprisingly little attention, however, has been paid in the history of hygiene and colonialism to the main protagonists of the civilising mission: Christian missionaries. Johannes Fabian's 1990 essay on *Religious and Secular Colonization* pointed to this shortcoming by arguing that there were "much older and deeper associations between physical hygiene and spiritual as well as political self-possession enabling colonial agents to take command over others."[17]

To trace the connected histories of evangelicalism, scientific medicine and colonialism in the making of hygiene in the late nineteenth and early twentieth centuries, this book combines three fields of research and their historiographies: mission history, particularly mission medicine; the history of science, with a focus on tropical medicine; and colonial history,

---

[16] Nancy Rose Hunt, Negotiated Colonialism: Domesticity, Hygiene and Birth Work in the Belgian Congo, Ph.D. diss., University of Wisconsin-Madison 1992; Andreas Eckert, Sauberkeit und "Zivilisation": Hygiene und Kolonialismus in Afrika, in: Sozialwissenschaftliche Informationen 26 (1997) 1, p. 16–19; Walter Bruchhausen, "Practising Hygiene and Fighting the Natives' Diseases". Public and Child Health in German East Africa and Tanganyika Territory, 1900–1960, in: Dynamis 23 (2003), p. 85–113; Ibid., Die "hygienische Eroberung" der Tropen. Gesundheitsschutz als europäischer Export in kolonialer und nachkolonialer Zeit, in: "Sei Sauber...!" Eine Geschichte der Hygiene und der öffentlichen Gesundheitsvorsorge in Europa, ed. by Musée d'Histoire de la Ville de Luxembourg, Köln 2004, p. 204–217; Alison Bashford, Imperial Hygiene. A Critical History of Colonialism, Nationalism and Public Health, Basingstoke/New York 2004; Warwick Anderson, Colonial Pathologies. American Tropical Medicine, Race, and Hygiene in the Philippines, Durham/London 2006; Robert Peckham/David M. Pomfret (eds.), Imperial Contagions. Medicine, Hygiene, and Cultures of Planning in Asia, Hong Kong 2013.

[17] Johannes Fabian, Time and the Work of Anthropology. Critical Essays 1971–1991, Chur et al. 1991, p. 163.

specifically the knowledge produced in colonial entanglements. By themselves, these topics have gained considerable scholarly attention, yet the interconnections between them remain underexposed.

1.2.1   Mission History and Medicine

Mission history offers fertile ground to examine how knowledge travelled between continents during the colonial period.[18] Through their far-reaching networks and extensive media, mission societies created long-lasting entanglements across the world. A wide range of actors both at home and abroad participated in forging and maintaining these connections, including missionaries and their wives, parishioners, donors, staff members, knowledge brokers, mission directors, members of missionary support groups, editors, itinerant preachers, traders and scientists as well as regional and colonial authorities. They communicated through a variety of channels and exchanged ideas, images and objects. The knowledge emerging from these exchanges had a bearing beyond individual mission societies, prompting large-scale debates about the body, religious principles, cultural identities, scientific assumptions, social issues and political questions, shaping material conditions in societies around the globe.[19]

---

[18] Sujit Sivasundaram, Nature and the Godly Empire. Science and Evangelical Mission in the Pacific, 1795–1850, Cambridge 2005; Patrick Harries, Butterflies and Barbarians. Swiss Missionaries and Systems of Knowledge in South-East Africa, Oxford 2007; Rebekka Habermas, Wissenstransfer und Mission. Sklavenhändler, Missionare und Religionswissenschaftler, in: Geschichte und Gesellschaft 36 (2010) 2, p. 257–284; Ulrich van der Heyden/Andreas Feldtkeller (eds.), Missionsgeschichte als Geschichte der Globalisierung von Wissen. Transkulturelle Wissensaneignung und -vermittlung durch christliche Missionare in Afrika und Asien im 17., 18. und 19. Jahrhundert, Stuttgart 2012; Patrick Harries/David Maxwell (eds.), The Spiritual in the Secular. Missionaries and Knowledge about Africa, Grand Rapids 2012; Linda Ratschiller/Siegfried Weichlein (eds.), Der schwarze Körper als Missionsgebiet. Medizin, Ethnologie, Theologie in Afrika und Europa 1880–1960, Köln/Weimar/Wien 2016; David Maxwell, Religious Entanglements. Central African Pentecostalism, The Creation of Cultural Knowledge and the Making of the Luba Katanga, Wisconsin 2022.

[19] Rebekka Habermas, Mission im 19. Jahrhundert. Globale Netze des Religiösen, in: Historische Zeitschrift 287 (2008) 3, p. 629–679; Helge Wendt, Mission transnational, trans-kolonial, global: Missionsgeschichtsschreibung als Beziehungsgeschichte, in: Schweizerische Zeitschrift für Religions- und Kulturgeschichte 105 (2011), p. 95–116; Rebekka Habermas/Richard Hölzl (eds.), Mission global. Eine Verflechtungsgeschichte seit dem 19. Jahrhundert, Köln/Weimar/Wien 2012; Christine Egger/Martina Gugglberger,

The rise of global and cultural perspectives has not only helped to lift mission history out of the disciplinary and historiographical isolation surrounding church history but also enlarged our understanding of the nineteenth-century religious landscape.[20] Instead of describing this landscape with generalising and mutually exclusive categories of analysis, assuming either the dawn of a secular age or a sweeping religious revival, scholars have started asking how knowledge of the secular and the religious have reciprocally constituted and shaped each other in this period.[21] Missionaries contributed to the making of secularism and religion on a global scale by categorising, for example, whether customs in Africa were part of the spiritual or worldly realm. Their reports and publications are

Editorial, in: ibid. (eds.), Missionsräume, in: Österreichische Zeitschrift für Geschichtswissenschaft 24 (2013) 2, p. 5–18; Tony Ballantyne, Entanglements of Empire. Missionaries, Māori, and the Question of the Body, Durham/London 2014; Julia Hauser, German Religious Women in Late Ottoman Beirut. Competing Missions, Leiden 2015; David Maxwell, The Missionary Movement in African and World History: Mission Sources and Religious Encounter, in: The Historical Journal 58 (2015) 4, p. 901–930; Elisabeth Engel, Encountering Empire. African American Missionaries in Colonial Africa, 1900–1939, Stuttgart 2015; Christine Egger, Transnationale Biographien. Die Missionsbenediktiner von St. Ottilien in Tanganjika 1922–1965, Köln/Weimar/Wien 2016; Linda Ratschiller/Karolin Wetjen (eds.), Verflochtene Mission. Perspektiven auf eine neue Missionsgeschichte, Köln/Weimar/Wien 2018; Jenna M. Gibbs (ed.), Global Protestant Missions. Politics, Reform, and Communication 1730s–1830s, New York 2019; Michael Eckardt (ed.), Mission Afrika: Geschichtsschreibung über Grenzen hinweg. Festschrift für Ulrich van der Heyden, Stuttgart 2019; Karolin Wetjen, Mission als theologisches Labor: Koloniale Aushandlungen des Religiösen in Ostafrika um 1900, Stuttgart 2020; Richard Hölzl, Gläubige Imperialisten: Katholische Mission in Deutschland und Ostafrika (1830–1960), Frankfurt a. M./ New York 2021.

[20] Christopher Alan Bayly, The Birth of the Modern World 1780–1914. Global Connections and Comparisons, Oxford 2004, p. 325–365; Sebastian Conrad, Religion in der globalen Welt, in: ibid./Jürgen Osterhammel (eds.), Geschichte der Welt. Wege zur modernen Welt, 1750–1870, München 2016, p. 559–625.

[21] Helmut Walser Smith (ed.), Protestants, Catholics and Jews in Germany, 1800–1914, Oxford 2001; Talal Asad (ed.), Formations of the Secular: Christianity, Islam, Modernity, Stanford 2003; Markus Dressler/Arvind-Pal S. Mandair, Secularism and Religion-Making, Oxford 2011; Monika Wohlrab-Sahr/Marian Burchardt, Multiple Secularities: Toward a Cultural Sociology of Secular Modernities, in: Comparative Sociology 11 (2012), p. 875–909; Rebekka Habermas (ed.), Negotiating the Secular and the Religious in the German Empire. Transnational Approaches, New York/Oxford 2019; Philip Nord/Katja Guenther/Max Weiss (eds.), Formations of Belief. Historical Approaches to Religion and the Secular, Princeton 2019.

important sources to question the notion of separate spheres in the nineteenth century, since they crucially participated in the formation of these religious, scientific and colonial spaces of knowledge.

Mission societies conveyed stories and images to a broad European public that for the first time in history developed detailed ideas of people and places around the globe. Drawing inspiration from New Imperial History and postcolonial studies, historians have highlighted the significance of mission societies for the production of imagery about the colonial world and their role in the creation of identities in Europe, not only in imperial metropolises but also in remote corners of rural societies.[22] Mission societies were rooted in specific regions within Europe with distinct denominational traditions, economic structures and social circumstances. At the same time, they operated in certain regions of Africa, Asia, America and Oceania, characterised by particular languages, histories and peoples.[23]

This study adopts an actor-based approach by focusing on medical missionaries, in order to trace the entanglements of religious, scientific and colonial knowledge in the making of hygiene. Nevertheless, it comprehends mission history as a transregional phenomenon. A transregional perspective is well suited to the empirical realities of missionary encounters and challenges the universal claim of the evangelical missionary movement.[24] The unique geographical, social, economic,

---

[22] Susan Thorne, Congregational Missions and the Making of an Imperial Culture in Nineteenth-Century England, Stanford 1999; Reinhard Wendt (ed.), Sammeln, Vernetzen, Auswerten. Missionare und ihr Beitrag zum Wandel europäischer Weltsicht, Tübingen 2001; Andreas Nehring, Orientalismus und Mission. Die Repräsentation der tamilischen Gesellschaft und Religion durch Leipziger Missionare 1840–1940, Wiesbaden 2003; Anna Johnston, Missionary Writing and Empire, 1800–1860, Cambridge 2003; Rebekka Habermas, Colonies in the Countryside: Doing Mission in Imperial Germany, in: Journal of Social History 50 (2017), p. 502–517.

[23] For actor-based and microhistorical approaches applied to mission history, see Harries, Butterflies and Barbarians; Helge Wendt, Die missionarische Gesellschaft. Mikrostrukturen einer kolonialen Globalisierung, Stuttgart 2011; Hauser, German Religious Women in Late Ottoman Beirut; Kirsten Rüther, Zugänge zur Missionsgeschichte: Plädoyer für eine akteurszentrierte Geschichte religiöser Veränderung, in: Zeitschrift für Missionswissenschaft und Religionswissenschaft 100 (2016), p. 211–219.

[24] Matthias Middell (ed.), The Routledge Handbook of Transregional Studies, London/New York 2019; Paul Jenkins, Württemberg als Hauptsäule der historischen Basler Mission—transregionale Erwägungen über Entwicklungen bis 1914, in: Blätter für württembergische Kirchengeschichte 116 (2016), p. 29–54; Ulrike Freitag/Achim

cultural, political and spiritual environments meant that there was not one Basel Mission experience but many different types of regional manifestation. While missionaries undoubtedly contributed to the increasing interdependence of the world and their knowledge had global significance, their fields of action were always confined to particular regions both abroad and at home, which shaped the knowledge they produced.[25]

Mission medicine became an important point of contact between Africans and Europeans, providing the ground for intimate physical and spiritual interactions. By focussing on the development of clinical medicine, for instance, recent studies have shown that mission hospitals were often the only place where people in colonial Africa would have experienced medical care provided by Europeans.[26] Africanists, anthropologists and historians have deepened our understanding of how medical missionaries adopted scientific practices and technologies to advance their religious agenda but ultimately saw themselves confronted with a persistent medical pluralism, which questioned the exclusivity of their healing and belief system. Thus, a more complex picture of medical missions has emerged than narratives of either colonial complicity or self-sacrificing benevolence.[27]

von Oppen (eds.), Translocality. The Study of Globalising Processes from a Southern Perspective, Leiden 2010.

[25] John Comaroff/Jean Comaroff, Of Revelation and Revolution, vol. 1: Christianity, Colonialism and Consciousness in South Africa, Chicago 1991; Ibid., Of Revelation and Revolution, vol. 2: The Dialectics of Modernity on a South African Frontier, Chicago 1997; Patricia Grimshaw/Andrew May (eds.), Missionaries, Indigenous Peoples and Cultural Exchange, Brighton/Portland/Toronto 2010; Hilde Nielssen/Inger Marie Okkenhaug/Karina Hestad Skeie (eds.), Protestant Missions and Local Encounters in the Nineteenth and Twentieth Centuries. Unto the Ends of the World, Leiden/Boston 2011.

[26] Walter Bruchhausen, Medicine Between Religious Worlds: The Mission Hospitals of South-East Tanzania During the Twentieth Century, in: Mark Harrison/Margaret Jones/Helen Sweet (eds.), From Western Medicine to Global Medicine. The Hospital Beyond the West, Hyderabad 2009, p. 172–192; David Hardiman, The Mission Hospital 1880–1960, in: Mark Harrison/Margaret Jones/Helen Sweet (eds.), From Western Medicine to Global Medicine. The Hospital Beyond the West, Hyderabad 2009, p. 198–220; Pascal Schmid, Medicine, Faith and Politics in Agogo: A History of Health Care Delivery in Rural Ghana, ca. 1925 to 1980, Wien/Zürich 2018.

[27] Megan Vaughan, Curing Their Ills. Colonial Power and African Illness, Cambridge 1991, ch. 3, p. 55–76; Terence O. Ranger, Godly Medicine. The Ambiguities of Medical Mission in Southeastern Tanzania 1900–1945, in: Steven Feierman/John M. Janzen (eds.), The Social Basis of Health and Healing in Africa, Berkley/Los Anegels/Oxford 1992, p. 256–282; Charles M. Good, The Steamer Parish. The Rise and Fall of Missionary

The question of how the Basel Mission doctors participated in the production of hygienic knowledge is interwoven with the histories of race, domesticity and gender. While these specific topics have been treated carefully by scholars studying mission societies and missionaries, the significance of hygiene for mission history remains a blind spot.[28] This is all the more regrettable since the subject of hygiene offers an excellent opportunity to link mission history to the histories of science and colonialism. The predominant representations of missionaries as living in the past, rejecting modernity and opposing scientific developments not only contradicted their self-image as people who controlled their natural and human environments with the help of technology and science, but also significantly contributed to excluding them from the history of science for

Medicine on an African Frontier, Chicago/London 2004; David Hardiman (ed.), Healing Bodies, Saving Souls. Medical Missions in Asia and Africa, Amsterdam/New York 2006; Markku Hokkanen, Medicine and Scottish Missionaries in the Northern Malawi Region 1875–1930. Quests for Health in a Colonial Society, Lewiston 2007; Patrick Harries/ Marcel Dreier, Medizin und Magie in Afrika. Eine Sozialgeschichte des Wissens, in: Nach Feierabend. Zürcher Jahrbuch für Wissensgeschichte 8, Zürich 2012, p. 85–104; Walima T. Kalusa, Christian Medical Discourse and Praxis on the Imperial Frontier. Explaining the Popularity of Missionary Medicine in Mwinilunga District, Zambia, 1906–1935, in: Patrick Harries/David Maxwell (eds.), The Spiritual in the Secular. Missionaries and Knowledge about Africa, Grand Rapids 2012, p. 245–266; Hines Mabika, Shaping Swiss Medical Practice in South Africa Before Apartheid (1873–1948), in: Schweizerische Zeitschrift für Geschichte 67 (2017) 3, p. 381–404.

[28] Comaroff/Comaroff, Home-made Hegemony; Mary Taylor Huber/Nancy C. Lutkehaus (eds.), Gendered Missions. Women and Men in Missionary Discourse and Practice, Ann Arbor 1999; Andreas Eckl, Grundzüge einer feministischen Missionsgeschichtsschreibung. Missionarsgattinnen, Diakonissen und Missionsschwestern in der deutschen kolonialen Frauenmission, in: Marianne Bechhaus-Gerst/Mechthild Leutner (eds.), Frauen in den deutschen Kolonien, Berlin 2009, p. 132–145; Rhonda Anne Semple, Missionary Women. Gender, Professionalism and the Victorian Idea of Christian Mission, Woodbridge/Rochester 2003; Esme Cleall, Missionary Discourses of Difference. Negotiating Otherness in the British Empire, Basingstoke 2012; Emily J. Manktelow, Missionary Families: Race, Gender and Generation on the Spiritual Frontier, Manchester/New York 2013; David Maxwell, The Missionary Home as a Site for Mission: Perspectives from Belgian Congo, in: Studies in Church History 50 (2014), p. 428–455; Kirsten Rüther/Angelika Schaser/Jacqueline van Gent, Gender and Conversion Narratives in the Nineteenth Century. German Mission at Home and Abroad, Surrey 2015.

many years. Yet the reciprocal connections between missionary endeavours and scientific activities constitute a significant chapter in the global history of science, as a new generation of researchers has demonstrated.[29]

1.2.2   History of Science and Tropical Medicine

In examining actors that were both evangelical missionaries and medical scientists operating in West African colonies, this study contributes to the ongoing re-evaluation of the role of religion in the history of science. The colonial period provided the setting for profound exchanges and delineations between religious and scientific knowledge across the globe. This resulted in the emergence of new religious values and customs on the one hand, and the development of new scientific ideas and practices on the other. A number of recent historiographical shifts in the history of science have helped to push back on residual resistance to bringing religion and science under the same analytic lens and thus reinvigorated interest in mission societies and missionaries as relevant actors in the production of scientific knowledge.[30]

The most important historiographical shift was that the dissemination of scientific knowledge was no longer seen as a one-way process

[29] John MacKenzie, Missionaries, Science and the Environment in Nineteenth-Century Africa, in: Andrew Porter (ed.), The Imperial Horizons of British Protestant Missions, 1880–1914, Grand Rapids/Cambridge 2003, p. 106–130; David N. Livingstone, Scientific Inquiry and the Missionary Enterprise, in: Ruth Finnegan (ed.), Participating in the Knowledge Society. Researchers Beyond the University Walls, Basingstoke 2005, p. 50–64; Sujit Sivasundaram, A Global History of Science and Religion, in: Thomas Dixon/Geoffrey Cantor/Stephen Pumfrey (eds.), Science and Religion. New Historical Perspectives, Cambridge 2010, p. 177–197; John Stenhouse, Missionary Science, in: Hugh Richard Slotten/Ronald L. Numbers/David N. Livingstone (eds.), The Cambridge History of Science, Vol. 8: Modern Science in National, Transnational, and Global Context, Cambridge 2020, p. 90–107.

[30] For general overviews of the history of science, see Richard Drayton, Science, Medicine and the British Empire, in: Robin W. Winks (ed.), The Oxford History of the British Empire, vol. 5: Historiography, Oxford 1999, p. 264–276; Jan Golinski, Making Natural Knowledge: Constructivism and the History of Science, Chicago 2005; Kostas Gavroglou/Jürgen Renn (eds.), Positioning the History of Science, Dordrecht 2007; Pratik Chakrabarti/Michael Worboys, Science and Imperialism since 1870, in: Hugh Richard Slotten/Ronald L. Numbers/David N. Livingstone (eds.), The Cambridge History of Science, vol. 8: Modern Science in National, Transnational, and Global Context, Cambridge 2020, p. 9–31.

of progress that inevitably led to the demise of other forms of knowledge. By looking at science as a form of practice, historians were able to trace the history of science in everyday social and public life.[31] Instead of assigning epistemic privilege to scientific knowledge, this allows one to examine the ways in which knowledge took on popular expertise in non-academic contexts. This more dynamic and fragmented account of knowledge focuses on the interactive creation of knowledge, rather than viewing it as already fully formed. Scholars now pay attention to the contexts of production, materiality, circulation, representation and transformation of knowledge and ask why certain knowledge was suppressed, lost or ignored while other knowledge obtained validity.[32]

Seeing science as socially constructed knowledge allowed scholars to question the Eurocentric narrative and analyse the complex histories of science around the world.[33] The notion of networks has proven particularly fruitful to trace the global circulation of ideas, practices and

---

[31] Pierre Bourdieu, Outline of a Theory of Practice, Cambridge 1977; Jakob Vogel, Von der Wissenschafts- zur Wissensgeschichte. Für eine Historisierung der "Wissensgesellschaft", in: Geschichte und Gesellschaft 30 (2004) 4, p. 639–660; Peter Burke, A Social History of Knowledge, vol. 1: From Gutenberg to Diderot, Cambridge 2000; Ibid., A Social History of Knowledge, vol. 2: From the Encyclopédie to Wikipedia, Cambridge 2012; Ibid., What is the History of Knowledge? Cambridge/Malden 2015; Philipp Sarasin, Was ist Wissensgeschichte? in: Internationales Archiv für Sozialgeschichte der deutschen Literatur 36 (2003), p. 159–172; Bozena Chołuj/Jan C. Joerden (eds.), Von der wissenschaftlichen Tatsache zur Wissensproduktion, Frankfurt a. M. 2007; Achim Landwehr, Wissensgeschichte, in: Rainer Schützeichel (ed.), Handbuch Wissenssoziologie und Wissensforschung, Konstanz 2007, p. 801–813; Wolfgang Kaschuba, Vorbemerkung. Wissensgeschichte als Gesellschaftsgeschichte, in: Geschichte und Gesellschaft 34 (2008) 4, p. 419–424; Daniel Speich-Chassé/David Gugerli, Wissensgeschichte. Eine Standortbestimmung, in: Traverse (2012) 1, p. 85–100; Johan Östling et al. (eds.), Circulation of Knowledge. Explorations in the History of Knowledge, Lund 2018.

[32] Jim Secord, Knowledge in Transit, in: Isis 95 (2004) 4, p. 654–672; Robert N. Proctor/Londa Schiebinger (eds.), Agnotology. The Making und Unmaking of Ignorance, Stanford 2008; Andreas Beer/Gesa Mackenthun (eds.), Fugitive Knowledge. The Loss and Preservation of Knowledge in Cultural Contact Zones, Münster/New York 2015.

[33] Bruno Latour, Science in Action: How to Follow Scientists and Engineers Through Society, Milton Keynes 1987; Ibid., Reassembling the Social. An Introduction to Actor-Network-Theory, Oxford 2005; Simon Schaffer/Lissa Roberts/Kapil Raj/James Delbourgo (eds.), The Brokered World: Go-Betweens and Global Intelligence, 1770–1820, Sagamore Beach 2009; Diarmid A. Finnegan/Jonathan Jeffrey Wright (eds.), Spaces of Global Knowledge. Exhibition, Encounter and Exchange in an Age of Empire, Farnham 2015; Kapil Raj, Go-Betweens, Travelers, and Cultural Translators, in: Bernard Lightman (ed.), A Companion to the History of Science, New York 2016, p. 39–57.

technologies during the colonial age. At the same time, the study of networks must be complemented with questions of privilege, power and inequality, especially when dealing with imperial networks. As cultural polyglots, the Basel Mission doctors positioned themselves at the interface of religious, scientific and colonial networks. Their knowledge production shows that the movement of ideas, practices and images between Europe and West Africa was a two-way process. However, their encounters were characterised by marked power imbalances and the flows of knowledge were neither qualitatively nor quantitatively equal.

The question as to what extent science, medicine and technology enabled imperial expansion and the consolidation of colonial rule remains a central bone of contention. Scholars who have created and endorsed the notion of colonial science have elaborated on the political role of knowledge produced during the colonial age and debunked the understanding of science as a universalist, disinterested form of knowledge driven by the organised scepticism of the involved scientists. To them we owe valuable insights into the ways in which scientists, including explorers, botanists, physicians, missionaries and their technologies, such as surveys, maps, microscopes and quinine advanced the colonial project. This scholarship has also demonstrated how knowledge acquired on imperial frontiers stimulated the formation of new scientific methods, disciplines and institutions in nineteenth-century Europe.[34]

Yet historians who have criticised the concept of colonial science point out that relying on science and technology to achieve political aims was no unique feature of colonial powers. Moreover, they have argued that reducing science to a tool of empire ignores the partially divergent interests between scientists and colonial states.[35] This critique has given rise

---

[34] Daniel R. Headrick, The Tools of Empire. Technology and European Imperialism in the Nineteenth Century, Oxford 1981; Ibid., Power Over Peoples: Technology, Environments, and Western Imperialism, 1400 to the Present, Princeton 2010; James E. McClellan, Colonialism and Science. Saint Domingue in the Old Regime, Baltimore 1992; Ibid./François Regourd, The Colonial Machine. French Science and Overseas Expansion in the Old Regime, Turnhout 2011; Richard Drayton, Nature's Government: Science, Imperial Britain, and the 'Improvement' of the World, New Haven 2000; Ibid., Knowledge and Empire, in: Peter James Marshall (ed.), The Oxford History of the British Empire, vol. 2: The Eighteenth Century, Oxford 2001, p. 231–251.

[35] Helen Tilley offered a comprehensive critique of colonial science in her 2011 publication *Africa as a Living Laboratory*, opposing any simplified polarisation between scientific and non-European knowledge in colonial settings and claiming that colonialism did not comprehensively destroy African forms of knowledge. She argued that knowledge emerged

to studies that analyse the diversity of scientific activities across the colonial world by paying attention to the natural, political, cultural and social circumstances of specific localities.[36] A major concern for much of current research is to overcome large-scale, generalising and mutually exclusive categories of analysis, such as "indigenous knowledge" or "Western science," since they are themselves products of colonial history. While it continues to be useful to consider science as an instrumental part of political control and economic exploitation in the colonies, focus now lies on detailed examinations of interactions between competing epistemologies in concrete places around the world.[37]

Interest in the relationship between scientific medicine and imperialism has produced a rich body of research, which has only gradually begun to examine more systematically the different ways knowledge systems around the world intersected during the colonial period.[38] For many years, the assumption that scientific medicine represented a coherent

---

in the field in Africa, based on local resources, and then travelled to Europe where it was canonised as authentic and objective. Helen Tilley, Africa as a Living Laboratory. Empire, Development, and the Problem of Scientific Knowledge, 1870–1950, Chicago 2011.

[36] Mark Harrison, Science and the British Empire, in: Isis 96 (2005) 1, p. 56–63; Kapil Raj, Relocating Modern Science. Circulation and the Construction of Knowledge in South Asia and Europe, New York 2007; William Beinart/Karen Brown/Daniel Gilfoyle, Experts and Expertise in Colonial Africa Reconsidered: Science and the Interpretation of Knowledge, in: African Affairs 108 (2009) 432, p. 413–433; Sujit Sivasundaram, Sciences and the Global. On Methods, Questions, and Theory, in: Isis 101 (2010) 1, p. 146–158; Jürgen Renn (ed.), The Globalization of Knowledge in History, Berlin 2012.

[37] David Wade Chambers/Richard Gillespie, Locality in the History of Science. Colonial Science, Technoscience, and Indigenous Knowledge, in: Osiris 15 (2000), p. 221–240; David N. Livingstone, Putting Science in Its Place: Geographies of Scientific Knowledge, Chicago/London 2003; Lissa Roberts, Situating Science in Global History: Local Exchanges and Networks of Circulation, in: Itinerario 33 (2009) 1, p. 9–27; Helen Tilley, Global Histories, Vernacular Science, and African Genealogies; or, Is the History of Science Ready for the World? in: Isis 101 (2010) 1, p. 110–119; Brett M. Bennett/Joseph M. Hodge (eds.), Science and Empire. Knowledge and Networks of Science across the British Empire, 1800–1970, Basingstoke/New York 2011; Sujit Sivasundaram, Science, Medicine and Technology, in: Philippa Levine/John Marriott (eds.), The Ashgate Research Companion to Modern Imperial Histories, London/New York 2012, p. 549–566; Martin Lengwiler/Nigel Penn/Patrick Harries (eds.), Science, Africa and Europe. Processing Information and Creating Knowledge, London/New York 2019.

[38] Roy MacLeod/Lewis Milton (eds.), Disease, Medicine, and Empire. Perspectives on Western Medicine and the Experience of European Expansion, London 1988; David Arnold (ed.), Imperial Medicine and Indigenous Societies, Manchester 1988; Maryinez Lyons, The Colonial Disease. A Social History of Sleeping Sickness in Northern Zaire,

body of knowledge and powerful tool of governance obscured the multi-faceted and often conflicting interpretations of disease. The encounter between the materialist and universalist worldview of scientific medicine and the complexity of the pre-colonial field of healing in Africa resulted in the application of the label "traditional African medicine" to a highly heterogeneous collection of old and novel concepts and practices. Medical traditions, however, even if invented, are inherently plural, contrary to the persistent unifying ambitions and intentions of scientific medicine.[39]

The contributions of the Basel Mission doctors to the field of tropical medicine and hygiene highlight the significance of religious actors to the development of the scientific discipline, challenging the hitherto dominant narratives focussing on prominent researchers, specific diseases, academic institutions and national borders.[40] In her 2012 study *Networks*

1900–1940, Cambridge/New York 1992; Shula Marks, What Is Colonial about Colonial Medicine? And What Happened to Imperialism and Health? in: Social History of Medicine 10 (1997) 2, p. 205–219; Wolfgang U. Eckart, Medizin und Kolonialimperialismus. Deutschland 1884–1945, Paderborn 1997; Kirk Arden Hoppe, Lords of the Fly. Colonial Visions and Revisions of African Sleeping-Sickness Environments on Ugandan Lake Victoria, 1906–1961, in: Africa 67 (1997) 1, p. 86–105; Robert Debusmann, Krankheit im kolonialen Alltag. Ärztliche Erfahrungen und Patientenverhalten in Kamerun, 1890–1930, in: Hans Peter Hahn (ed.), Afrika und die Globalisierung, Münster 1999, p. 217–225; Myron J. Echenberg, Black Death, White Medicine. Bubonic Plague and the Politics of Public Health in Colonial Senegal, 1914–1945, Portsmouth 2002; Margrit Davies, Public Health and Colonialism. The Case of New Guinea, 1884–1914, Wiesbaden 2002; Michael Worboys, Colonial and Imperial Medicine, in: Deborah Brunton (ed.), Medicine Transformed. Health, Disease and Society in Europe 1880–1930, Manchester/New York 2004, p. 211–238; Hiroyuki Isobe, Medizin und Kolonialgesellschaft. Die Bekämpfung der Schlafkrankheit in den deutschen "Schutzgebieten" vor dem Ersten Weltkrieg, Berlin 2009; Nancy Rose Hunt, A Nervous State: Violence, Remedies and Reverie in Colonial Congo, Durham 2016.

[39] Nancy Rose Hunt, A Colonial Lexicon of Birth Ritual, Medicalization and Mobility in the Congo, Durham 1999; Luise White, Speaking with Vampires. Rumor and History in Colonial Africa, Berkley 2000; Julie Livingston, Debility and the Modern Imagination in Botswana, Bloomington 2005; Walter Bruchhausen, Medizin zwischen den Welten. Geschichte und Gegenwart des medizinischen Pluralismus im südöstlichen Tansania, Göttingen 2006; Ibid., Medical Pluralism as a Historical Phenomenon: A Regional and Multi-Level Approach to Health Care in German, British and Independent East Africa, in: Anne Digby/Waltraud Ernst/Projit B. Mukharji (eds.), Crossing Colonial Historiographies. Histories of Colonial and Indigenous Medicines in Transnational Perspective, Newcastle 2010, p. 99–113.

[40] Gordon Harrison, Mosquitoes, Malaria and Man: A History of the Hostilities Since 1880, London 1978; Michael Worboys, Manson, Ross and Colonial Medical Policy: Tropical Medicine in London and Liverpool, 1899–1914, in: Roy MacLeod/Milton Lewis

in Tropical Medicine, Deborah J. Neill reassessed the history of tropical medicine by demonstrating that transnational networks were constitutive to the formation of the new medical speciality around 1900, even if they concurred and intersected with international rivalry.[41] Most recently, Manuela Bauche and Sarah Ehlers have presented innovative studies on the entanglements of disease control between Africa and Europe, spanning the history of tropical medicine across imperial boundaries.[42]

The Basel Mission doctors' sources constitute a valuable resource for historians seeking to reconstruct the interactions, exchanges and conflicts between European and African medical knowledge around 1900. In contrast to "imperial tropical medicine," which the historian John Farley characterised as a triad of "definition, imposition and non-involvement," the Basel Mission doctors had an interest in winning the African population over to their cause while heavily relying on the cooperation of local experts, assistants, informants and patients for their medical knowledge production.[43] Their evangelising agenda required negotiation skills and linguistic dexterity as well as a degree of sensitivity and flexibility, which is why their sources remain so useful for scholars interested in exchange processes and histories of entanglement during the colonial age.

(eds.), Disease, Medicine, and Empire. Perspectives on Western Medicine and the Experience of European Expansion, London/New York 1988, p. 21–37; David Arnold (ed.), Warm Climates and Western Medicine. The Emergence of Tropical Medicine 1500–1900, Amsterdam/Atlanta 1996; Gordon Charles Cook, Tropical Medicine. An Illustrated History of the Pioneers, Paris/London 2007; Douglas Melvin Haynes, Imperial Medicine. Patrick Manson and the Conquest of Tropical Disease, Philadelphia 2001; Lise Wilkinson/ Anne Hardy, Prevention and Cure: the London School of Hygiene and Tropical Medicine. A 20th Century Quest for Global Public Health, London/New York 2001; Nandini Bhattacharya, Contagion and Enclaves: Tropical Medicine in Colonial India, Liverpool 2012; Michael A. Osborne, The Emergence of Tropical Medicine in France, Chicago/London 2014.

[41] Deborah J. Neill, Networks in Tropical Medicine. Internationalism, Colonialism, and the Rise of a Medical Specialty, 1890–1930, Stanford 2012. Also see Myriam Mertens/ Guillaume Lachenal, The History of "Belgian" Tropical Medicine from a Cross-Border Perspective, in: Revue belge de philologie et d'histoire 90 (2012) 4, p. 1249–1271.

[42] Manuela Bauche, Medizin und Herrschaft. Malariabekämpfung in Kamerun, Ostafrika und Ostfriesland 1890–1919, Frankfurt a. M. 2017; Sarah Ehlers, Europa und die Schlafkrankheit. Koloniale Seuchenbekämpfung, europäische Identitäten und moderne Medizin 1890–1950, Göttingen 2019.

[43] John Farley, Bilharzia. A History of Imperial Tropical Medicine, Cambridge 1991, p. 293.

1.2.3 Colonial History and Knowledge

The Basel Mission doctors participated in networks that crossed imperial borders, which highlights that colonial history can never be fully understood in national terms. Recent studies have examined the role of transimperial networks, providing us with a more nuanced understanding of how empires were shaped by missionaries, mercenaries, scientists, families, guilds and other social groups that operated across political boundaries.[44] They have prompted a reconsideration of the relationship between centres and peripheries, devaluing the idea of empires as political entities tightly controlled by metropolitan elites. This fresh perspective is also reflected in the growing scholarship on Switzerland's colonial entanglements.[45] The hitherto dominant historiography, which has been

---

[44] Benedikt Stutchey (ed.), Science across the European Empires 1800–1950, Oxford 2005; Ulrike Lindner, Koloniale Begegnungen. Deutschland und Grossbritannien als Imperialmächte in Afrika 1880–1914, Frankfurt a. M. 2011; Volker Barth/Roland Cvetkovski (eds.), Imperial Co-Operation and Transfer, 1870–1930: Empires and Encounters, London 2015; Tanja Bührer/Flavio Eichmann/Stig Förster/Benedikt Stuchtey (eds), Cooperation and Empire. Local Realities of Global Processes, New York/Oxford 2017; Bernhard C. Schär, Introduction. The Dutch East Indies and Europe, ca. 1800–1930. An Empire of Demands and Opportunities, in: BMGN—Low Countries Historical Review 134 (2019) 3, p. 4–20; Ibid., From Batticaloa via Basel to Berlin. Transimperial Science in Ceylon and Beyond around 1900, in: The Journal of Imperial and Commonwealth History 48 (2020) 2, p. 230–262, https://doi.org/10.1080/03086534.2019.1638620; Moritz von Brescius, German Science in the Age of Empire. Enterprise, Opportunity and the Schlagintweit Brothers, Cambridge 2019.

[45] Andreas Zangger, Koloniale Schweiz. Ein Stück Globalgeschichte zwischen Europa und Südostasien (1860–1930), Bielefeld 2011; Patricia Purtschert/Barbara Lüthi/Francesca Falk (eds.), Postkoloniale Schweiz. Formen und Folgen eines Kolonialismus ohne Kolonien, Bielefeld 2012; Lukas Zürcher, Die Schweiz in Ruanda: Mission, Entwicklungshilfe und nationale Selbstbestätigung (1900–1975), Zürich 2014; Christof Dejung, Jenseits der Exzentrik. Aussereuropäische Geschichte in der Schweiz. Einleitung zum Themenschwerpunkt, in: Schweizerische Zeitschrift für Geschichte 64 (2014) 2, p. 195–209; Patricia Purtschert/Harald Fischer-Tiné (eds.), Colonial Switzerland. Rethinking Colonialism from the Margins, Basingstoke 2015; Bernhard C. Schär, Tropenliebe. Schweizer Naturforscher und niederländischer Imperialismus in Südostasien um 1900, Frankfurt a. M./New York 2015; Patricia Purtschert/Francesca Falk/Barbara Lüthi, Switzerland and 'Colonialism without Colonies'. Reflections on the Status of Colonial Outsiders, in: Interventions 18 (2016) 2, p. 286–302; Barbara Lüthi/Francesca Falk/Patricia Purtschert, Colonialism without Colonies: Examining Blank Spaces in Colonial Studies, in: National Identities 18 (2016) 1, p. 1–9; Pierre Eichenberger/Thomas David/Lea Haller/Matthieu Leimgruber/Bernhard C. Schär/Christa Wirth, Beyond Switzerland. Reframing the Swiss Historical Narrative in Light of Transnational History, in: Traverse

devoted to a predominantly national narrative and largely ignored colonialism and migration as formative forces of Swiss history, is facing headwinds.[46]

The Basel Mission stood at the heart of transregional networks, maintained mission stations in British and German colonies, such as the Gold Coast and Cameroon, and acted as a knowledge broker across the imperial world, adding to the ongoing debates about Switzerland's colonial involvements. By producing and propagating knowledge of hygiene, the Basel Mission doctors created lasting views and practices of purity, health and cleanliness that affected not only the colonies but also the very conception of Europe itself.[47] Influenced by anthropology, literary and cultural studies, scholars have analysed knowledge as a central feature of colonialism for over four decades.[48] An ever growing body of colonial knowledge, including texts, photographs and objects, provided people in nineteenth-century Europe with a unique foil on which to draw up and contrast images of the colonial other and themselves.[49]

(2017) 1, p. 137–152; Patricia Purtschert, Kolonialität und Geschlecht im 20. Jahrhundert. Eine Geschichte der weissen Schweiz, Bielefeld 2019; Simone Bleuer/Barbara Miller, Verkörpern—verfestigen—verflechten. Resonanz missionarischer Kulturkontakte in der katholischen Schweiz der 1950er- und 1960er-Jahre, in: Traverse (2019) 1, p. 94–108.

[46] On migration as a constitutive factor of Swiss history, see Francesca Falk, Gender Innovation and Migration in Switzerland, Cham 2018; André Holenstein/Patrick Kury/Kristina Schulz, Schweizer Migrationsgeschichte. Von den Anfängen bis zur Gegenwart, Baden 2018; Barbara Lüthi/Damir Skenderovic (eds.), Switzerland and Migration. Historical and Current Perspectives on a Changing Landscape, Cham 2019.

[47] Recent studies on the impact of European colonialism on the making of Europe itself include Wolfgang Reinhard, Die Unterwerfung der Welt: Globalgeschichte der europäischen Expansion 1415–2015, München 2016; Christof Dejung/Martin Lengwiler (eds.), Ränder der Moderne. Neue Perspektiven auf die Europäische Geschichte (1800–1930), Köln/Weimar/Wien 2016.

[48] The classic studies include Edward Said, Orientalism, New York 1978; Ronald Inden, Imagining India, Oxford 1990; Bernard Cohn, Colonialism and Its Forms of Knowledge: The British in India, Princeton 1996; Nicholas Dirks, Castes of Mind: Colonialism and the Making of Modern India, Princeton 2001.

[49] For Switzerland, see Harries, Butterflies and Barbarians; Patrick Minder, La Suisse coloniale. Les représentations de l'Afrique et des Africains en Suisse au temps des colonies (1880–1939), Berne 2011; Bernhard C. Schär, Bauern und Hirten *reconsidered*. Umrisse der "erfundenen" Schweiz im imperialen Raum, in: Patricia Purtschert/Barbara Lüthi/Francesca Falk (eds.), Postkoloniale Schweiz. Formen und Folgen eines Kolonialismus ohne Kolonien, Bielefeld 2012, p. 315–331. For Germany, Susanne Zantop, Colonial Fantasies: Conquest, Family, and Nation in Precolonial Germany, 1770–1870, Durham

Recent years have seen the emergence of a lively debate over the nature of colonial knowledge. Critics have pointed out that the notion of colonial knowledge is a problematic one, since it bundles together a range of highly diverse historical actors, places and moments in which knowledge emerged that were not linked to colonial rule or not intended to produce knowledge for imperial objectives. In a broad and critical sense, however, colonial knowledge is not merely knowledge produced to serve concrete colonial aims, but the ensemble of those European bodies of knowledge that dealt with the non-European world and could therefore not elude the internal logic and hegemonic discourses of the colonial period.[50]

In his 2014 publication *Entanglements of Empire*, Tony Ballantyne showed that British missionaries were pivotal in entangling the Māori in the webs of empire despite their objection to formal colonisation. They produced knowledge about the conditions on the ground, denouncing the physical suffering inflicted by Europeans on the Māori, which ultimately provided a powerful rationale for the British colonisation of New Zealand, portrayed as an act of protection.[51] The knowledge produced by missionaries, as well-intended or not as it might have been, was part of a growing body of knowledge, which implicitly or explicitly assumed the inherent superiority of Christian religion and European civilisation. While they did not necessarily support colonial rule or imperial domination, they were inevitably interwoven in uneven, hierarchical power relations between imperial Europe and the colonial world.

1997; Birthe Kundrus (ed.), Phantasiereiche. Zur Kulturgeschichte des deutschen Kolonialismus, Frankfurt a. M./New York 2003; Alexander Honold/Klaus R. Scherpe (eds.), Mit Deutschland um die Welt. Eine Kulturgeschichte des Fremden in der Kolonialzeit, Stuttgart 2004; Wolfgang Struck, Die Eroberung der Phantasie. Kolonialismus, Literatur und Film zwischen deutschem Kaiserreich und Weimarer Republik, Göttingen 2010; Dirk van Laak, Die deutsche Kolonialgeschichte als Fantasiegeschichte, in: Marianne Bechhaus-Gerst/Joachim Zeller (eds.), Deutschland postkolonial? Die Gegenwart der imperialen Vergangenheit, Berlin 2018, p. 123–142. For the British Empire, Catherine Hall (ed.), Cultures of Empire. A Reader: Colonizers in Britain and the Empire in the Nineteenth and Twentieth Centuries, New York 2000; Ibid., Civilising Subjects. Metropole and Colony in the English Imagination 1830–1867, Chicago 2002; Ibid./Sonya O. Rose (eds.), At Home with the Empire: Metropolitan Culture and the Imperial World, Cambridge 2006.

[50] Frederick Cooper, Colonialism in Question. Theory, Knowledge, History, Berkeley 2005; Tony Ballantyne, Colonial Knowledge, in: Sarah Stockwell (ed.), The British Empire. Themes and Perspectives, Malden 2008, p. 177–198.

[51] Ballantyne, Entanglements of Empire.

Postcolonial scholarship has emphasised the long-term impact of colonial knowledge on categories of analysis and academic concepts, and offered innovative ways of eluding Eurocentric perspectives in historical writing.[52] At the same time, the idea that colonial knowledge was a homogenous, omnipotent force suggests that sources in colonial archives are useless to critical histories of colonialism, since they only contain European preconceptions and misrepresentations. Colonial knowledge, however, emerged from situated bodily encounters that were unforeseen and unpredictable, and thus conceals considerable complexity.[53]

Colonialism must be examined as a decidedly fractured phenomenon, which left considerable space for anxiety, subversion and vulnerability. Despite the centrality of knowledge to colonialism, there was no straightforward correlation between knowledge and power. Much of the historiography of colonialism "has taken the categories of 'colonizer' and 'colonized' as givens, rather than as constructions that need to be explained," as Ann Laura Stoler observed.[54] It is necessary, therefore, as Sujit Sivasundaram emphasised, "to think beyond categories of colonized and colonial and to fragment traditions of knowledge on all sides."[55] To expose colonial archives as sites of contested knowledge, Stoler has proposed the method of reading along the archival grain, rather than

[52] Dipesh Chakrabarty, Provincializing Europe: Postcolonial Thought and Historical Difference, Princeton 2000; Ann Laura Stoler/Frederick Cooper, Beetween Metropole and Colony: Rethinking a Research Agenda, in: ibid. (eds.), Tensions of Empire. Colonial Cultures in the Bourgeois World, Berkeley et al. 1997, p. 1–56; Sebastian Conrad/Shalini Randeria, Einleitung: Geteilte Geschichten—Europa in einer postkolonialen Welt, in: ibid./Regina Römhild (eds.), Jenseits des Eurozentrismus. Postkoloniale Perspektiven in den Geschichts- und Kulturwissenschaften, 2nd ed., Frankfurt a. M./New York 2013, p. 32–70.

[53] Ricardo Roque/Kim A. Wagner (eds.), Engaging Colonial Knowledge. Reading European Archives in World History, Basingstoke/New York 2012; Klaus Hock/Gesa Mackenthun (eds.), Entangled Knowledge. Scientific Discourses and Cultural Difference, Münster et al. 2012; Rebekka Habermas/Alexandra Przyrembel (eds.), Von Käfern, Märkten und Menschen. Kolonialismus und Wissen in der Moderne, Göttingen 2013; Harald Fischer-Tiné, Pidgin Knowledge. Wissen und Kolonialismus, Zürich 2013; Sebastian Dorsch, Translokale Wissensakteure: Ein Debattenvorschlag zu Wissens- und Globalgeschichtsschreibung, in: Zeitschrift für Geschichtswissenschaft 64 (2016) 9, p. 778–795.

[54] Ann Laura Stoler, Cultivating Bourgeois Bodies and Racial Selves, in: Catherine Hall (ed.), Cultures of Empire. A Reader: Colonizers in Britain and the Empire in the Nineteenth and Twentieth Centuries, New York 2000, p. 87–119, here p. 89.

[55] Sivasundaram, Sciences and the Global, p. 155.

simply against it. There is no grand narrative to explain the nature of colonialism, and scholars who make that assumption, according to Stoler, ignore the true nature of the archival record. We must therefore work with rather than against the contents of colonial accounts.[56]

This study adds to this strand of research by analysing the construction and conflictual relationship between different spaces of knowledge. The Basel missionaries not only closely examined non-European knowledge systems and crucially relied on intermediaries in their quest for evangelisation, but were also brokers of knowledge in many directions. The disparate knowledge they produced makes it possible to think beyond dichotomous colonial categories and reveals that colonialism was a highly fragile and contradictory project. A core concern of this book, therefore, is to examine the multi-layered and varied ways in which the Basel Mission doctors and their contributions to the making of hygiene supported, justified and at times challenged the colonial project.

For many years, historians focused on the question of how Christianity offered justification for imperial expansion and to what extent missionaries served as promoters of colonialism. It is clear by now that the role of missions, and religion more generally, in supporting the colonial project cannot be reduced to mere ideological justification or pragmatic collaboration. Numerous studies demonstrated the complex entanglements between missions and colonialism around the world but these detailed accounts also highlight the need for synthesising approaches. Hygiene offers one such synthesising approach to the colonial period, allowing one to scrutinise how religious, scientific and colonial spaces of knowledge interacted with one another.

1.3 RESEARCH AIMS AND METHODOLOGICAL REFLECTIONS

The aim of this study is to extend the history of nineteenth-century hygiene: firstly, beyond scientific and secular narratives by showing that religious stakeholders crucially participated in producing and promoting hygienic knowledge between 1885 and 1914; and secondly, by analysing how hygiene was shaped by colonial entanglements. The Basel Mission

---

[56] Ann Laura Stoler, Along the Archival Grain. Epistemic Anxieties and Colonial Common Sense, Princeton 2009.

doctors form a stimulating point of entry to examine these different layers of hygiene. They were socialised in European societies in which hygiene had become a crucial dimension of private and public life by the late nineteenth century. More precisely, the Basel Mission doctors were Pietist missionaries, who had completed a five-year course in the mission seminary in Basel. They held firm religious views about purity and the body, which were rooted in biblical narratives about sin and disease.

In addition to their missionary training, the Basel Mission doctors also qualified as physicians at European universities with renowned teachers, such as Max von Pettenkofer, Robert Koch and Rudolf Virchow. They moved in transnational academic circles and participated in the scientific debates of the time, dealing for instance with what many scientists of the period saw as the all-important problem of European acclimatisation—the viability and functioning of the "white race" in the tropics. The Basel Mission doctors became recognised experts, most notably in the field of tropical medicine and hygiene, which emerged as an institutionalised discipline around 1900.

The formation of a medical speciality devoted to health conditions in tropical colonies exclusively highlights that the age of hygiene was also the age of High Imperialism. Metropolitan policy-makers attached more and more importance to the physical value of their colonial subjects and recognised that medical missions presented a valuable resource for the implementation of hygienic norms in tropical colonies.[57] The tropics provided a setting in which the Basel Mission doctors not only gained scientific reputation but also political authority. Their studies on hygiene produced colonial knowledge, which served European imperial interests in Africa on the one hand, and shaped the colonial imagination of Africa on the other. At the same time, their position as authorities on tropical hygiene indicates that hygienic knowledge around 1900 was infused with pious notions of purity.

How did the Basel Mission doctors generate, systematise and disseminate knowledge on hygiene between West Africa and Europe from

---

[57] On the meaning of the body in colonial contexts, see David Arnold, Colonizing the Body. State Medicine and Epidemic Disease in Nineteenth-Century India, Berkeley/Los Angeles/London 1993; Anne McClintock, Imperial Leather. Race, Gender and Sexuality in the Colonial Contest, New York 1995; Ann Laura Stoler, Carnal Knowledge and Imperial Power. Race and the Intimate in Colonial Rule, Berkeley/Los Angeles/London 2002; Tony Ballantyne/Antoinette Burton (eds.), Bodies in Contact. Rethinking Colonial Encounters in World History, Durham 2005.

1885 to 1914? Their knowledge emerged in protracted and contentious exchange processes on the ground in the specific locations in which they lived. This study goes beyond these local production contexts, however, by investigating how these situated negotiations of hygiene circulated and influenced religious, scientific and colonial bodies of knowledge.[58] Hygiene was not only a relational discourse of difference that intersected with other discourses of difference on gender, race and class but also a structuring concept of difference that produced inequality. It thus offers a vantage point from which to question the development of these intersecting colonial concepts of difference in the late nineteenth and early twentieth centuries.

1.3.1   Spaces of Knowledge

This study traces various meanings of hygiene emerging over the nineteenth century and their reciprocal interactions between 1885 and 1914. Spaces of knowledge offer an analytical lens through which to examine the interactive and contested nature of knowledge and allow us to analyse how different discourses and practices of hygiene overlapped, differed and influenced each other. The Basel Mission doctors participated in the making of hygiene in a number of ways. It is necessary, therefore, to dissect this amalgam. The concept of spaces of knowledge makes it possible to identify competing epistemologies and to examine how people navigated between multiple systems of knowledge. A basic assumption thereby is that the Basel Mission doctors themselves contributed to the construction, consolidation and perpetuation of these spaces of knowledge, thereby stabilising the illusion of separate spheres.

The book is structured around three distinct, yet interwoven, spaces of knowledge, in which the Basel Mission doctors and their knowledge of hygiene played a pivotal role. Spaces of knowledge describe the appearance of social and cognitive structures between actors, institutions and networks. They contain worlds of meanings by which humans come to understand and make sense of the world. Spaces of knowledge transport assumptions, norms and values but also constantly generate new stories,

---

[58] Helen Tilley has argued that the circulation of knowledge between different localities was more relevant than the context of origin, since European and African forms of knowledge often only loosely interacted and co-existed in incommensurable fields. Tilley, Africa as a Living Laboratory.

meanings and connections. Knowledge is conceived here as a cognitive and social process, which transforms information and data into discourses and practices and thus enables individuals, institutions and whole societies to act and plan ahead. This includes academic and scientific knowledge but also various forms of public and popular knowledge, which circulates within and between spaces of knowledge.

Spaces of knowledge are characterised by hierarchical and hegemonial aspirations as well as collective and individual negotiation processes that determine which information is integrated, adapted or disqualified from the dominant body of knowledge. People contributing to a space of knowledge design certain criteria, categories and principles to generate and order their body of thought. Yet different actors possess more or less power in a specific space of knowledge depending on their position and reputation as laypeople, informants or experts, which influences whether their opinions are accepted as knowledge. The same people, such as the Basel Mission doctors, adopt different roles in different spaces of knowledge depending on whether they are complying with the according epistemology, modes of expression and models of truth.

Spaces of knowledge are dynamic and have a porous but tangible external border. Although one space may dominate, many spaces can and do exist simultaneously. There are personal, institutional and thematic overlaps between them, which create in-between spaces and border areas. Mobility between them, however, should not be stressed to the extent that immobility, disjuncture and ignorance are forgotten. Actors, institutions and networks from the religious, scientific and colonial spaces of knowledge interacted more or less between 1885 and 1914, and thus changed the substance of hygiene. The knowledge resulting from this interplay shaped conceptions of the colonial other and triggered the reordering of various bodies of knowledge and identities in European societies.

The Basel Mission doctors, and their influence on hygienic knowledge around 1900, are evidence that there were no insurmountable boundaries between religious, scientific and political domains of society. Au contraire, their sources reveal that hygiene absorbed highly diverse meanings of spiritual purity, physical health and civilisational cleanliness. To use a term coined by Bruno Latour, "practices of purification"—describing processes of secularisation and differentiation—have obscured the common origin as well as the ensuing convergences and mutual influences between religious, scientific and colonial knowledge.[59] On a methodological level, however, spaces of knowledge prove highly useful to disentangle this complexity and reconstruct the diverging forces that came together in the making of hygiene around 1900.

1.3.2   Source Material

The Basel Mission doctors left a rich and diverse body of sources ranging from scientific treatises and medical guidebooks to devotional writings and popular travelogues. The core of the source material consists of reports, private letters, journal articles and monographs written from 1885, when the first Basel Mission doctor Rudolf Fisch arrived on the Gold Coast, to 1914, when the Basel Mission was forced to interrupt their operations in West Africa due to the outbreak of the First World War. This period of research opens up a unique historical configuration, which stimulated the creation and circulation of hygienic knowledge. By focusing on six main protagonists and adopting a transregional perspective, this study hopes to break through the seemingly abstract process of knowledge production and do justice to the individuals and localities, in which hygienic knowledge emerged.

Hygiene was interactive and contested knowledge. Various forms of bodily knowledge on the Gold Coast and in Cameroon, Christian beliefs, scientific concepts and colonial views differed and partly contradicted each other. The bulk of published source material, however, conceals this complexity because it was composed and ordered for European readers, revealing very different ends of knowledge-making abroad and at home. The reports, studies and letters written by the Basel missionaries in West Africa were condensed, edited and substantially reworked, as editors of missionary magazines, scientific journals and colonial periodicals prepared texts with the expectations and sensibilities of their metropolitan readers in mind. Not surprisingly, the routine trials and anxieties of life in tropical colonies or the uncertain self-reflections rarely made it into publications designed to educate, entertain and solicit funds and support.

One of this book's major challenges thus consists of breaking through superficial narratives and exposing the multiple interactions that created

---

[59] Bruno Latour, We Have Never Been Modern, Cambridge MA 1993.

the bodies of knowledge accredited to the Basel Mission doctors. This study addresses this challenge in four ways. Firstly, the comprehensive written records are examined in a way that exposes their porousness. The Basel Mission doctors utilised a wide range of literary genres to reach out to different readers from evangelical circles and colonial enthusiasts to scientific communities. They adapted their cognitive models, strategies of persuasion and plausibility procedures, in order to position themselves as experts in the respective space of knowledge. Their written sources, therefore, are not consistent, which provides a methodological entry point to contrast differing accounts and expose the social interactions behind the fashioning of hygienic knowledge.

The Basel Mission archives hold a significant number of confidential reports, personal letters and diaries that contain intimate and revealing details. Of course, these documents are still authored from a European point of view, including a sense of inherent superiority, but they do not speak in just one single voice. They are multivocal, fractured and contradictory, and thus call into question the prevailing canon of knowledge. Testimonies written by missionaries are products of prolonged and personal exchanges with the resident population in specific regions of the colonial world, and thus differ sharply from the majority of sources composed by colonial officials, traders and scientists. They thus offer a promising starting point to question established historical master narratives.[60]

Secondly, this study illuminates how Africans, women and other hidden contributors dialogically shaped missionary texts, images and collections. The Basel Mission doctors' stories are impossible to understand without considering the open and silent protest but also the cooperation and support of the inhabitants in the places they called home in West Africa. In the end, it was Africans' desire for contact with Europeans, their interest in agriculture, literacy, medicine and technology, and the support of certain rulers that enabled the foundation of mission stations. Regional authorities, medical assistants, translators and teachers enabled the Basel Mission to gain and broaden their influence on the Gold Coast and in Cameroon. It is crucial therefore to visualise these exchange processes,

---

[60] Kirsten Rüther, Through the Eyes of Missionaries and the Archives They Created: The Interwoven Histories of Power and Authority in the Nineteenth-Century Transvaal, in: Journal of Southern African Studies, 38 (2012) 2, p. 369–384, here p. 384.

mostly hidden between the lines, without simultaneously neglecting the existing power disparities in the production of knowledge.

By examining developments in parts of West Africa and the Alemannic region in the same analytical framework, this book offers an entangled and dialectic history of hygiene. It is clear, however, that an asymmetrical body of sources complicates this undertaking. While we have access to plenty of source material in Basel, we are confronted with very few direct sources from the communities in West Africa. Scholars have shown, however, that it is possible through critical reading of colonial sources to retrieve the voices of people from whom we mostly lack text sources.[61] When historians take into account protagonists who commonly did not leave written testimonies, such as Africans, women and people from the lower social strata, as active shapers of social interactions and historical sources, they can no longer write them out of the history of these entanglements or simply reduce them to being objects of colonial discourse.

Thirdly, the practicality and materiality of hygienic knowledge offers an effective method to fragment simplifying assumptions. Hygiene was always more than a unified discourse, it was a heterogeneous practice that had to be put to everyday use by African parishioners, missionary wives, city missionaries, maids, porters, school children, medical assistants, abstainers, travellers, traders, colonial officials and many more both abroad and at home.[62] The rich non-written body of sources in the Basel Mission archives highlights that hygiene cannot be reduced to deconstructionist language games and provides an opportunity to trace the material entanglements between West Africa and Europe. Photographs, commodities and objects testify to the lasting and close exchanges between the Basel Mission doctors and the people with whom they lived and worked.

---

[61] Ann Laura Stoler, "In Cold Blood": Hierarchies of Credibility and the Politics of Colonial Narratives, in: Representations 37 (1992), p. 151–189; Ibid., Colonial Archives and the Arts of Governance, in: Archival Science 2 (2002), p. 87–109; Sivasundaram, Sciences and the Global; Ricardo Roque/Kim A. Wagner, Introduction: Engaging Colonial Knowledge, in: ibid. (eds.), Engaging Colonial Knowledge. Reading European Archives in World History, Basingstoke/New York 2012, p. 1–32; Ballantyne, Entanglements of Empire; Schär, Tropenliebe.

[62] On the historiography of writing about everyday life in African history and beyond, see Andreas Eckert/Adam Jones, Introduction: Historical Writing about Everyday Life, in: Journal of African Cultural Studies 15 (2002) 1, p. 5–16.

Fourthly, this study contrasts the source material in the Basel Mission archives with additional evangelical, scientific and colonial collections and publications. These holdings make it possible to reconstruct the different spaces of knowledge in which the mission doctors operated and add an important external perspective to question their influence. Their knowledge has to be contextualised in order to understand the particularity of their contributions and to assess what impact they had on the formation of hygiene. This approach not only discloses alliances, interdependencies and rivalries between different individuals, groups and institutions but also highlights correlations and tensions between developments abroad and at home. When consulting various archives, it becomes clear that knowledge about hygiene around 1900 was rife with contradictions and inconsistencies.

1.3.3   Structure of the Book

This book is divided into three main parts. The first one starts by reconstructing the broader social frameworks and historical contexts in which the Basel Mission doctors were socialised to gain an understanding of the nature of their knowledge of hygiene before they moved overseas. Their sources contain many blind spots, covering the significant participation of women and children for example, which is why it is particularly important to examine the communities of origin and historical circumstances in which the Basel Mission emerged. This perspective prevents a simplifying juxtaposition between the Basel Mission doctors as uprooted global protagonists and the seemingly immobile local actors in West Africa. Once we have turned the historical gaze onto the mental and material world of the Basel Mission doctors at home, we are better equipped to deal with their perceptions of Africa.

The first part contains three chapters that trace the formation of the religious, scientific and colonial spaces of knowledge respectively and examine how knowledge of purity, health and cleanliness evolved over the nineteenth century. The focus on the Basel Mission doctors shows that hygiene had the capacity to absorb multiple layers of meaning. Hygiene held an interdiscursive capacity around 1900, meaning it had the ability to connect different discursive fields. It stood at the centre of a vast semantic field of notions such as purity, health and cleanliness, and their opposites: impurity, disease and filth. Very different moral leaders including religious protagonists, social reformers, medical scientists and colonial masterminds used hygiene narratives to promote their own concepts of order, create distinct notions of normality and assert a shared, yet delimited, identity. The making of hygiene between 1885 and 1914 cannot be understood without a detailed map of prior meanings.

The second part includes three chapters that focus on negotiations of purity, health and cleanliness on the alleged margins of hygiene in West Africa from 1885 to 1914. These chapters analyse how the Basel Mission doctors resorted to hygiene in their mission in West Africa, highlighting that in order to be effective, their knowledge needed to be constantly reframed and amended to the conditions on the ground. Their encounters with people in West Africa were dynamic, yet conflictual, processes of mutual entanglement, which included both appropriation and rejection. This part reveals misunderstandings, controversies and trade-offs within the missionary community and the resident population as well as between them. Crucially, it shows that the hygiene mission in West Africa was not about the transfer of knowledge from Europe to Africa but about the very creation of hygiene on the supposed periphery of civilisation.

The third part comprises three chapters that explore how the knowledge of hygiene emerging from these complex interactions reverberated and affected religious, scientific and colonial debates and practices between 1885 and 1914. The obsession with hygiene in the tropics correlated with a fundamental change of attitudes towards hygiene in late nineteenth-century Europe. How did trials of purity, health and cleanliness in West Africa alter or endorse existing assumptions about hygiene? Hygiene not only produced lasting perceptions about race, gender and class but also had profound practical and material consequences for people around the world. What impact did the Basel Mission doctors and their transregional negotiations of hygiene have on scientific theories, segregation policies, bodily practices, commodity culture, social interactions, political developments, cultural norms, religious values and colonial identities both abroad and at home?

REFERENCES

Warwick Anderson, Colonial Pathologies. American Tropical Medicine, Race, and Hygiene in the Philippines, Durham/London 2006.
David Arnold (ed.), Imperial Medicine and Indigenous Societies, Manchester 1988.

David Arnold, Colonizing the Body. State Medicine and Epidemic Disease in Nineteenth-Century India, Berkeley/Los Angeles/London 1993.

David Arnold (ed.), Warm Climates and Western Medicine. The Emergence of Tropical Medicine 1500–1900, Amsterdam/Atlanta 1996.

Talal Asad (ed.), Formations of the Secular: Christianity, Islam, Modernity, Stanford 2003.

Tony Ballantyne, Colonial Knowledge, in: Sarah Stockwell (ed.), The British Empire. Themes and Perspectives, Malden 2008, p. 177–198.

Tony Ballantyne, Entanglements of Empire. Missionaries, Māori, and the Question of the Body, Durham/London 2014.

Tony Ballantyne/Antoinette Burton (eds.), Bodies in Contact. Rethinking Colonial Encounters in World History, Durham 2005.

Volker Barth/Roland Cvetkovski (eds.), Imperial Co-Operation and Transfer, 1870–1930: Empires and Encounters, London 2015.

Alison Bashford, Imperial Hygiene. A Critical History of Colonialism, Nationalism and Public Health, Basingstoke/New York 2004.

Manuela Bauche, Medizin und Herrschaft. Malariabekämpfung in Kamerun, Ostafrika und Ostfriesland 1890–1919, Frankfurt a. M. 2017.

Christopher Alan Bayly, The Birth of the Modern World 1780–1914. Global Connections and Comparisons, Oxford 2004, p. 325–365.

Andreas Beer/Gesa Mackenthun (eds.), Fugitive Knowledge. The Loss and Preservation of Knowledge in Cultural Contact Zones, Münster/New York 2015.

William Beinart/Karen Brown/Daniel Gilfoyle, Experts and Expertise in Colonial Africa Reconsidered: Science and the Interpretation of Knowledge, in: African Affairs 108 (2009) 432, p. 413–433.

Brett M. Bennett/Joseph M. Hodge (eds.), Science and Empire. Knowledge and Networks of Science across the British Empire, 1800–1970, Basingstoke/New York 2011.

Nandini Bhattacharya, Contagion and Enclaves: Tropical Medicine in Colonial India, Liverpool 2012.

Simone Bleuer/Barbara Miller, Verkörpern—verfestigen—verflechten. Resonanz missionarischer Kulturkontakte in der katholischen Schweiz der 1950er- und 1960er-Jahre, in: Traverse (2019) 1, p. 94–108.

Pierre Bourdieu, Outline of a Theory of Practice, Cambridge 1977.

Walter Bruchhausen, "Practising Hygiene and Fighting the Natives' Diseases". Public and Child Health in German East Africa and Tanganyika Territory, 1900–1960, in: Dynamis 23 (2003), p. 85–113.

Walter Bruchhausen, Die "hygienische Eroberung" der Tropen. Gesundheitsschutz als europäischer Export in kolonialer und nachkolonialer Zeit, in:

"Sei Sauber...!" Eine Geschichte der Hygiene und der öffentlichen Gesundheitsvorsorge in Europa, ed. by Musée d'Histoire de la Ville de Luxembourg, Köln 2004, p. 204–217.

Walter Bruchhausen, Medizin zwischen den Welten. Geschichte und Gegenwart des medizinischen Pluralismus im südöstlichen Tansania, Göttingen 2006.

Walter Bruchhausen, Medicine Between Religious Worlds: The Mission Hospitals of South-East Tanzania During the Twentieth Century, in: Mark Harrison/ Margaret Jones/Helen Sweet (eds.), From Western Medicine to Global Medicine. The Hospital Beyond the West, Hyderabad 2009, p. 172–192.

Walter Bruchhausen, Medical Pluralism as a Historical Phenomenon: A Regional and Multi-Level Approach to Health Care in German, British and Independent East Africa, in: Anne Digby/Waltraud Ernst/Projit B. Mukharji (eds.), Crossing Colonial Historiographies. Histories of Colonial and Indigenous Medicines in Transnational Perspective, Newcastle 2010, p. 99–113.

Tanja Bührer/Flavio Eichmann/Stig Förster/Benedikt Stuchtey (eds.), Cooperation and Empire. Local Realities of Global Processes, New York/Oxford 2017.

Peter Burke, A Social History of Knowledge, vol. 1: From Gutenberg to Diderot, Cambridge 2000.

Peter Burke, A Social History of Knowledge, vol. 2: From the Encyclopédie to Wikipedia, Cambridge 2012.

Peter Burke, What is the History of Knowledge? Cambridge/Malden 2015.

Timothy Burke, Lifebuoy Men, Lux Women. Commodification, Consumption and Cleanliness in Modern Zimbabwe, Durham/London 1996.

Pratik Chakrabarti/Michael Worboys, Science and Imperialism since 1870, in: Hugh Richard Slotten/Ronald L. Numbers/David N. Livingstone (eds.), The Cambridge History of Science, vol. 8: Modern Science in National, Transnational, and Global Context, Cambridge 2020, p. 9–31.

Dipesh Chakrabarty, Provincializing Europe: Postcolonial Thought and Historical Difference, Princeton 2000.

David Wade Chambers/Richard Gillespie, Locality in the History of Science. Colonial Science, Technoscience, and Indigenous Knowledge, in: Osiris 15 (2000), p. 221–240.

Bozena Chołuj/Jan C. Joerden (eds.), Von der wissenschaftlichen Tatsache zur Wissensproduktion, Frankfurt a. M. 2007.

Bernard Cohn, Colonialism and Its Forms of Knowledge: The British in India, Princeton 1996.

John Comaroff/Jean Comaroff, Of Revelation and Revolution, vol. 1: Christianity, Colonialism and Consciousness in South Africa, Chicago 1991.

John Comaroff/Jean Comaroff, Home-Made Hegemony: Modernity, Domesticity, and Colonialism in South Africa, in: Karen Tranberg Hansen (ed.), African Encounters with Domesticity, New Brunswick 1992, p. 37–74.

John Comaroff/Jean Comaroff, Of Revelation and Revolution, vol. 2: The Dialectics of Modernity on a South African Frontier, Chicago 1997.

Sebastian Conrad, Religion in der globalen Welt, in: ibid./Jürgen Osterhammel (eds.), Geschichte der Welt. Wege zur modernen Welt, 1750–1870, München 2016, p. 559–625.

Sebastian Conrad/Shalini Randeria, Einleitung: Geteilte Geschichten—Europa in einer postkolonialen Welt, in: ibid./Regina Römhild (eds.), Jenseits des Eurozentrismus. Postkoloniale Perspektiven in den Geschichts- und Kulturwissenschaften, 2nd ed., Frankfurt a. M./New York 2013, p. 32–70.

Gordon Charles Cook, Tropical Medicine. An Illustrated History of the Pioneers, Paris/London 2007.

Frederick Cooper, Colonialism in Question. Theory, Knowledge, History, Berkeley 2005.

Alain Corbin, Le miasme et la jonquille. L'odorat et l'imaginaire sociale XVIIIe-XIXe siècles, Paris 1982.

Margrit Davies, Public Health and Colonialism. The Case of New Guinea, 1884–1914, Wiesbaden 2002.

Robert Debusmann, Krankheit im kolonialen Alltag. Ärztliche Erfahrungen und Patientenverhalten in Kamerun, 1890–1930, in: Hans Peter Hahn (ed.), Afrika und die Globalisierung, Münster 1999, p. 217–225.

Christof Dejung, Jenseits der Exzentrik. Aussereuropäische Geschichte in der Schweiz. Einleitung zum Themenschwerpunkt, in: Schweizerische Zeitschrift für Geschichte 64 (2014) 2, p. 195–209.

Christof Dejung/Martin Lengwiler (eds.), Ränder der Moderne. Neue Perspektiven auf die Europäische Geschichte (1800–1930), Köln/Weimar/Wien 2016.

Nicholas Dirks, Castes of Mind: Colonialism and the Making of Modern India, Princeton 2001.

Sebastian Dorsch, Translokale Wissensakteure: Ein Debattenvorschlag zu Wissens- und Globalgeschichtsschreibung, in: Zeitschrift für Geschichtswissenschaft 64 (2016) 9, p. 778–795.

Richard Drayton, Science, Medicine and the British Empire, in: Robin W. Winks (ed.), The Oxford History of the British Empire, vol. 5: Historiography, Oxford 1999, p. 264–276.

Richard Drayton, Nature's Government: Science, Imperial Britain, and the 'Improvement' of the World, New Haven 2000.

Richard Drayton, Knowledge and Empire, in: Peter James Marshall (ed.), The Oxford History of the British Empire, vol. 2: The Eighteenth Century, Oxford 2001, p. 231–251.

Markus Dressler/Arvind-Pal S. Mandair, Secularism and Religion-Making, Oxford 2011.

Myron J. Echenberg, Black Death, White Medicine. Bubonic Plague and the Politics of Public Health in Colonial Senegal, 1914–1945, Portsmouth 2002.

Michael Eckardt (ed.), Mission Afrika: Geschichtsschreibung über Grenzen hinweg. Festschrift für Ulrich van der Heyden, Stuttgart 2019.

Wolfgang U. Eckart, Medizin und Kolonialimperialismus. Deutschland 1884–1945, Paderborn 1997.

Andreas Eckert, Sauberkeit und "Zivilisation": Hygiene und Kolonialismus in Afrika, in: Sozialwissenschaftliche Informationen 26 (1997) 1, p. 16–19.

Andreas Eckert/Adam Jones, Introduction: Historical Writing about Everyday Life, in: Journal of African Cultural Studies 15 (2002) 1, p. 5–16.

Andreas Eckl, Grundzüge einer feministischen Missionsgeschichtsschreibung. Missionarsgattinnen, Diakonissen und Missionsschwestern in der deutschen kolonialen Frauenmission, in: Marianne Bechhaus-Gerst/Mechthild Leutner (eds.), Frauen in den deutschen Kolonien, Berlin 2009, p. 132–145.

Christine Egger, Transnationale Biographien. Die Missionsbenediktiner von St. Ottilien in Tanganjika 1922–1965, Köln/Weimar/Wien 2016.

Christine Egger/Martina Gugglberger, Editorial, in: ibid. (eds.), Missionsräume, in: Österreichische Zeitschrift für Geschichtswissenschaft 24 (2013) 2, p. 5–18.

Sarah Ehlers, Europa und die Schlafkrankheit. Koloniale Seuchenbekämpfung, europäische Identitäten und moderne Medizin 1890–1950, Göttingen 2019.

Pierre Eichenberger/Thomas David/Lea Haller/Matthieu Leimgruber/Bernhard C. Schär/Christa Wirth, Beyond Switzerland. Reframing the Swiss Historical Narrative in Light of Transnational History, in: Traverse (2017) 1, p. 137–152.

Elizabeth Elbourne, The Foundation of the Church Missionary Society. The Anglican Missionary Impulse, in: John Walsh/Colin Haydon/Stephen Taylor (eds.), The Church of England c. 1689–1833, Cambridge 1993, p. 247–264.

Elisabeth Engel, Encountering Empire. African American Missionaries in Colonial Africa, 1900–1939, Stuttgart 2015.

Johannes Fabian, Time and the Work of Anthropology. Critical Essays 1971–1991, Chur et al. 1991.

Francesca Falk, Gender Innovation and Migration in Switzerland, Cham 2018.

John Farley, Bilharzia. A History of Imperial Tropical Medicine, Cambridge 1991.

Diarmid A. Finnegan/Jonathan Jeffrey Wright (eds.), Spaces of Global Knowledge. Exhibition, Encounter and Exchange in an Age of Empire, Farnham 2015.

Harald Fischer-Tiné, Pidgin Knowledge. Wissen und Kolonialismus, Zürich 2013.

Ulrike Freitag/Achim von Oppen (eds.), Translocality. The Study of Globalising Processes from a Southern Perspective, Leiden 2010.

Manuel Frey, Der reinliche Bürger. Entstehung und Verbreitung bürgerlicher Tugenden in Deutschland, 1760–1860, Göttingen 1997.

Kostas Gavroglou/Jürgen Renn (eds.), Positioning the History of Science, Dordrecht 2007.

Jenna M. Gibbs (ed.), Global Protestant Missions. Politics, Reform, and Communication 1730s–1830s, New York 2019.

Gerd Göckenjan, Kurieren und Staat machen. Gesundheit und Medizin in der bürgerlichen Welt, Frankfurt a. M. 1985.

Jan Golinski, Making Natural Knowledge: Constructivism and the History of Science, Chicago 2005.

Charles M. Good, The Steamer Parish. The Rise and Fall of Missionary Medicine on an African Frontier, Chicago/London 2004.

Patricia Grimshaw/Andrew May (eds.), Missionaries, Indigenous Peoples and Cultural Exchange, Brighton/Portland/Toronto 2010.

Rebekka Habermas, Mission im 19. Jahrhundert. Globale Netze des Religiösen, in: Historische Zeitschrift 287 (2008) 3, p. 629–679.

Rebekka Habermas, Wissenstransfer und Mission. Sklavenhändler, Missionare und Religionswissenschaftler, in: Geschichte und Gesellschaft 36 (2010) 2, p. 257–284.

Rebekka Habermas (ed.), Negotiating the Secular and the Religious in the German Empire. Transnational Approaches, New York/Oxford 2019.

Rebekka Habermas/Richard Hölzl (eds.), Mission global. Eine Verflechtungsgeschichte seit dem 19. Jahrhundert, Köln/Weimar/Wien 2012.

Rebekka Habermas/Alexandra Przyrembel (eds.), Von Käfern, Märkten und Menschen. Kolonialismus und Wissen in der Moderne, Göttingen 2013.

Catherine Hall (ed.), Cultures of Empire. A Reader: Colonizers in Britain and the Empire in the Nineteenth and Twentieth Centuries, New York 2000.

Catherine Hall, Civilising Subjects. Metropole and Colony in the English Imagination 1830–1867, Chicago 2002.

Catherine Hall/Sonya O. Rose (eds.), At Home with the Empire: Metropolitan Culture and the Imperial World, Cambridge 2006.

David Hardiman (ed.), Healing Bodies, Saving Souls. Medical Missions in Asia and Africa, Amsterdam/New York 2006.

David Hardiman, The Mission Hospital 1880–1960, in: Mark Harrison/Margaret Jones/Helen Sweet (eds.), From Western Medicine to Global Medicine. The Hospital Beyond the West, Hyderabad 2009, p. 198–220.

Patrick Harries, Butterflies and Barbarians. Swiss Missionaries and Systems of Knowledge in South-East Africa, Oxford 2007.

Patrick Harries/Marcel Dreier, Medizin und Magie in Afrika. Eine Sozialgeschichte des Wissens, in: Nach Feierabend. Zürcher Jahrbuch für Wissensgeschichte 8, Zürich 2012, p. 85–104.

Patrick Harries/David Maxwell (eds.), The Spiritual in the Secular. Missionaries and Knowledge about Africa, Grand Rapids 2012.

Gordon Harrison, Mosquitoes, Malaria and Man: A History of the Hostilities Since 1880, London 1978.

Mark Harrison, Science and the British Empire, in: Isis 96 (2005) 1, p. 56–63.

Julia Hauser, German Religious Women in Late Ottoman Beirut. Competing Missions, Leiden 2015.

Douglas Melvin Haynes, Imperial Medicine. Patrick Manson and the Conquest of Tropical Disease, Philadelphia 2001.

Daniel R. Headrick, The Tools of Empire. Technology and European Imperialism in the Nineteenth Century, Oxford 1981.

Daniel R. Headrick, Power Over Peoples: Technology, Environments, and Western Imperialism, 1400 to the Present, Princeton 2010.

Klaus Hock/Gesa Mackenthun (eds.), Entangled Knowledge. Scientific Discourses and Cultural Difference, Münster et al. 2012.

Markku Hokkanen, Medicine and Scottish Missionaries in the Northern Malawi Region 1875–1930. Quests for Health in a Colonial Society, Lewiston 2007.

André Holenstein/Patrick Kury/Kristina Schulz, Schweizer Migrationsgeschichte. Von den Anfängen bis zur Gegenwart, Baden 2018.

Richard Hölzl, Gläubige Imperialisten: Katholische Mission in Deutschland und Ostafrika (1830–1960), Frankfurt a. M./New York 2021.

Alexander Honold/Klaus R. Scherpe (eds.), Mit Deutschland um die Welt. Eine Kulturgeschichte des Fremden in der Kolonialzeit, Stuttgart 2004.

Kirk Arden Hoppe, Lords of the Fly. Colonial Visions and Revisions of African Sleeping-Sickness Environments on Ugandan Lake Victoria, 1906–1961, in: Africa 67 (1997) 1, p. 86–105.

Mary Taylor Huber/Nancy C. Lutkehaus (eds.), Gendered Missions. Women and Men in Missionary Discourse and Practice, Ann Arbor 1999.

Nancy Rose Hunt, Negotiated Colonialism: Domesticity, Hygiene and Birth Work in the Belgian Congo, Ph.D. diss., University of Wisconsin-Madison 1992.

Nancy Rose Hunt, A Colonial Lexicon of Birth Ritual, Medicalization and Mobility in the Congo, Durham 1999.

Nancy Rose Hunt, A Nervous State: Violence, Remedies and Reverie in Colonial Congo, Durham 2016.

Ronald Inden, Imagining India, Oxford 1990.

Hiroyuki Isobe, Medizin und Kolonialgesellschaft. Die Bekämpfung der Schlafkrankheit in den deutschen "Schutzgebieten" vor dem Ersten Weltkrieg, Berlin 2009.

Paul Jenkins, Württemberg als Hauptsäule der historischen Basler Mission—transregionale Erwägungen über Entwicklungen bis 1914, in: Blätter für württembergische Kirchengeschichte 116 (2016), p. 29–54.

Anna Johnston, Missionary Writing and Empire, 1800–1860, Cambridge 2003; Rebekka Habermas, Colonies in the Countryside: Doing Mission in Imperial Germany, in: Journal of Social History 50 (2017), p. 502–517.

Walima T. Kalusa, Christian Medical Discourse and Praxis on the Imperial Frontier. Explaining the Popularity of Missionary Medicine in Mwinilunga District, Zambia, 1906–1935, in: Patrick Harries/David Maxwell (eds.), The Spiritual in the Secular. Missionaries and Knowledge about Africa, Grand Rapids 2012, p. 245–266.

Wolfgang Kaschuba, Vorbemerkung. Wissensgeschichte als Gesellschaftsgeschichte, in: Geschichte und Gesellschaft 34 (2008) 4, p. 419–424.

Barbara Koller, Gesundes Wohnen. Ein Konstrukt zur Vermittlung bürgerlicher Werte und Verhaltensnormen und seine praktische Umsetzung in der Deutschschweiz 1880–1940, Zürich 1995.

Birthe Kundrus (ed.), Phantasiereiche. Zur Kulturgeschichte des deutschen Kolonialismus, Frankfurt a. M./New York 2003.

Alfons Labisch, Homo Hygienicus. Gesundheit und Medizin in der Neuzeit, Frankfurt a. M. 1992.

Achim Landwehr, Wissensgeschichte, in: Rainer Schützeichel (ed.), Handbuch Wissenssoziologie und Wissensforschung, Konstanz 2007, p. 801–813.

Bruno Latour, Science in Action: How to Follow Scientists and Engineers Through Society, Milton Keynes 1987.

Bruno Latour, We Have Never Been Modern, Cambridge MA 1993.

Bruno Latour, Reassembling the Social. An Introduction to Actor-Network-Theory, Oxford 2005.

Martin Lengwiler/Nigel Penn/Patrick Harries (eds.), Science, Africa and Europe. Processing Information and Creating Knowledge, London/New York 2019.

Ulrike Lindner, Koloniale Begegnungen. Deutschland und Grossbritannien als Imperialmächte in Afrika 1880–1914, Frankfurt a. M. 2011.

Julie Livingston, Debility and the Modern Imagination in Botswana, Bloomington 2005.

David N. Livingstone, Putting Science in Its Place: Geographies of Scientific Knowledge, Chicago/London 2003.

David N. Livingstone, Scientific Inquiry and the Missionary Enterprise, in: Ruth Finnegan (ed.), Participating in the Knowledge Society. Researchers Beyond the University Walls, Basingstoke 2005, p. 50–64.

Wolfgang G. Locher, Max von Pettenkofer: Pionier der wissenschaftlichen Hygiene, Regensburg 2018.

Barbara Lüthi/Damir Skenderovic (eds.), Switzerland and Migration. Historical and Current Perspectives on a Changing Landscape, Cham 2019.

Barbara Lüthi/Francesca Falk/Patricia Purtschert, Colonialism without Colonies: Examining Blank Spaces in Colonial Studies, in: National Identities 18 (2016) 1, p. 1–9.

Maryinez Lyons, The Colonial Disease. A Social History of Sleeping Sickness in Northern Zaire, 1900–1940, Cambridge/New York 1992.

Hines Mabika, Shaping Swiss Medical Practice in South Africa Before Apartheid (1873–1948), in: Schweizerische Zeitschrift für Geschichte 67 (2017) 3, p. 381–404.

John MacKenzie, Missionaries, Science and the Environment in Nineteenth-Century Africa, in: Andrew Porter (ed.), The Imperial Horizons of British Protestant Missions, 1880–1914, Grand Rapids/Cambridge 2003, p. 106–130.

Roy MacLeod/Lewis Milton (eds.), Disease, Medicine, and Empire. Perspectives on Western Medicine and the Experience of European Expansion, London 1988.

Ernst Mähly, Die Gesundheitsverhältnisse auf der Goldküste, in: Evangelisches Missionsmagazin 29 (1885) p. 396–417, 445–461.

Ernst Mähly, Zur Geographie und Ethnographie der Goldküste, in: Verhandlungen der Naturforschenden Gesellschaft in Basel 7 (1885) 3, p. 809–852.

Ernst Mähly, Über das sogenannte "Gallenfieber" an der Goldküste, in: Correspondenz-Blatt für Schweizer Ärzte 15 (1885), p. 73–79, 108–116.

Ernst Mähly, Akklimatisation und Klimafieber, in: Deutsche Kolonialzeitung 3 (1886), p. 72–83.

Ernst Mähly, Gesundheitszustand bzw. Sterblichkeit auf der Goldküste und in Westafrika überhaupt, in: Deutsche Kolonialzeitung 3 (1886), p. 555–559.

Ernst Mähly, Akklimatisation und Klimafieber, in: Evangelisches Missionsmagazin 30 (1886), p. 129–147.

Emily J. Manktelow, Missionary Families: Race, Gender and Generation on the Spiritual Frontier, Manchester/New York 2013.

Shula Marks, What Is Colonial about Colonial Medicine? And What Happened to Imperialism and Health? in: Social History of Medicine 10 (1997) 2, p. 205–219.

David Maxwell, The Missionary Home as a Site for Mission: Perspectives from Belgian Congo, in: Studies in Church History 50 (2014), p. 428–455.

David Maxwell, The Missionary Movement in African and World History: Mission Sources and Religious Encounter, in: The Historical Journal 58 (2015) 4, p. 901–930.

Thomas C. McCaskie, State and Society in Pre-Colonial Asante, Cambridge/New York 1995.

James E. McClellan, Colonialism and Science. Saint Domingue in the Old Regime, Baltimore 1992.

James E. McClellan/François Regourd, The Colonial Machine. French Science and Overseas Expansion in the Old Regime, Turnhout 2011.

Anne McClintock, Imperial Leather. Race, Gender and Sexuality in the Colonial Contest, New York 1995.

Myriam Mertens/Guillaume Lachenal, The History of "Belgian" Tropical Medicine from a Cross-Border Perspective, in: Revue belge de philologie et d'histoire 90 (2012) 4, p. 1249–1271.

Beatrix Mesmer, Reinheit und Reinlichkeit. Bemerkungen zur Durchsetzung der häuslichen Hygiene in der Schweiz, in: Nicolai Bernard/Quirinus Reichen (eds.), Gesellschaft und Gesellschaften. Festschrift zum 65. Geburtstag von Professor Dr. Ulrich Im Hof, Bern 1982, p. 470–494.

Matthias Middell (ed.), The Routledge Handbook of Transregional Studies, London/New York 2019.

Patrick Minder, La Suisse coloniale. Les représentations de l'Afrique et des Africains en Suisse au temps des colonies (1880–1939), Berne 2011.

Andreas Nehring, Orientalismus und Mission. Die Repräsentation der tamilischen Gesellschaft und Religion durch Leipziger Missionare 1840–1940, Wiesbaden 2003.

Deborah J. Neill, Networks in Tropical Medicine. Internationalism, Colonialism, and the Rise of a Medical Specialty, 1890–1930, Stanford 2012.

Hilde Nielssen/Inger Marie Okkenhaug/Karina Hestad Skeie (eds.), Protestant Missions and Local Encounters in the Nineteenth and Twentieth Centuries. Unto the Ends of the World, Leiden/Boston 2011.

Philip Nord/Katja Guenther/Max Weiss, Formations of Belief. Historical Approaches to Religion and the Secular, Princeton 2019.

Johan Östling et al. (eds.), Circulation of Knowledge. Explorations in the History of Knowledge, Lund 2018.

Michael A. Osborne, The Emergence of Tropical Medicine in France, Chicago/London 2014.

Robert Peckham/David M. Pomfret (eds.), Imperial Contagions. Medicine, Hygiene, and Cultures of Planning in Asia, Hong Kong 2013.

Robert N. Proctor/Londa Schiebinger (eds.), Agnotology. The Making und Unmaking of Ignorance, Stanford 2008.

Patricia Purtschert, Kolonialität und Geschlecht im 20. Jahrhundert. Eine Geschichte der weissen Schweiz, Bielefeld 2019.

Patricia Purtschert/Harald Fischer-Tiné (eds.), Colonial Switzerland. Rethinking Colonialism from the Margins, Basingstoke 2015.

Patricia Purtschert/Barbara Lüthi/Francesca Falk (eds.), Postkoloniale Schweiz. Formen und Folgen eines Kolonialismus ohne Kolonien, Bielefeld 2012.

Patricia Purtschert/Francesca Falk/Barbara Lüthi, Switzerland and 'Colonialism without Colonies'. Reflections on the Status of Colonial Outsiders, in: Interventions 18 (2016) 2, p. 286–302.

Kapil Raj, Relocating Modern Science. Circulation and the Construction of Knowledge in South Asia and Europe, New York 2007.

Kapil Raj, Go-Betweens, Travelers, and Cultural Translators, in: Bernard Lightman (ed.), A Companion to the History of Science, New York 2016, p. 39–57.

Terence O. Ranger, Godly Medicine. The Ambiguities of Medical Mission in Southeastern Tanzania 1900–1945, in: Steven Feierman/John M. Janzen (eds.), The Social Basis of Health and Healing in Africa, Berkley/Los Anegels/Oxford 1992, p. 256–282.

Linda Ratschiller/Siegfried Weichlein (eds.), Der schwarze Körper als Missionsgebiet. Medizin, Ethnologie, Theologie in Afrika und Europa 1880–1960, Köln/Weimar/Wien 2016.

Linda Ratschiller/Karolin Wetjen (eds.), Verflochtene Mission. Perspektiven auf eine neue Missionsgeschichte, Köln/Weimar/Wien 2018.

Jonathan Reinarz, Past Scents: Historical Perspectives on Smell, Urbana 2014.

Wolfgang Reinhard, Die Unterwerfung der Welt: Globalgeschichte der europäischen Expansion 1415–2015, München 2016.

Jürgen Renn (ed.), The Globalization of Knowledge in History, Berlin 2012.

Karl Rennstich, The Understanding of Mission, Civilisation and Colonialism in the Basel Mission, in: Torben Christensen/William R. Hutchison (eds.), Missionary Ideologies in the Imperialist Era, 1880–1920, Aarhus 1983, p. 94–103.

Lissa Roberts, Situating Science in Global History: Local Exchanges and Networks of Circulation, in: Itinerario 33 (2009) 1, p. 9–27.

Ricardo Roque/Kim A. Wagner, Introduction: Engaging Colonial Knowledge, in: ibid. (eds.), Engaging Colonial Knowledge. Reading European Archives in World History, Basingstoke/New York 2012, p. 1–32.

Ricardo Roque/Kim A. Wagner (eds.), Engaging Colonial Knowledge. Reading European Archives in World History, Basingstoke/New York 2012.

Kirsten Rüther, Through the Eyes of Missionaries and the Archives They Created: The Interwoven Histories of Power and Authority in the Nineteenth-Century Transvaal, in: Journal of Southern African Studies, 38 (2012) 2, p. 369–384.

Kirsten Rüther, Zugänge zur Missionsgeschichte: Plädoyer für eine akteurszentrierte Geschichte religiöser Veränderung, in: Zeitschrift für Missionswissenschaft und Religionswissenschaft 100 (2016), p. 211–219.

Kirsten Rüther/Angelika Schaser/Jacqueline van Gent, Gender and Conversion Narratives in the Nineteenth Century. German Mission at Home and Abroad, Surrey 2015.

Edward Said, Orientalism, New York 1978.

Philipp Sarasin, Reizbare Maschinen. Eine Geschichte des Körpers, 1765–1914, Frankfurt a. M. 2003.

Philipp Sarasin, Was ist Wissensgeschichte? in: Internationales Archiv für Sozialgeschichte der deutschen Literatur 36 (2003), p. 159–172.

Philipp Sarasin, The Body as Medium. Nineteenth-Century European Hygiene Discourse, in: Grey Room 29 (2007), p. 48–65.

Simon Schaffer/Lissa Roberts/Kapil Raj/James Delbourgo (eds.), The Brokered World: Go-Betweens and Global Intelligence, 1770–1820, Sagamore Beach 2009.

Bernhard C. Schär, Bauern und Hirten *reconsidered.* Umrisse der "erfundenen" Schweiz im imperialen Raum, in: Patricia Purtschert/Barbara Lüthi/Francesca Falk (eds.), Postkoloniale Schweiz. Formen und Folgen eines Kolonialismus ohne Kolonien, Bielefeld 2012, p. 315–331.

Bernhard C. Schär, Tropenliebe. Schweizer Naturforscher und niederländischer Imperialismus in Südostasien um 1900, Frankfurt a. M./New York 2015.

Bernhard C. Schär, Introduction. The Dutch East Indies and Europe, ca. 1800–1930. An Empire of Demands and Opportunities, in: BMGN—Low Countries Historical Review 134 (2019) 3, p. 4–20.

Bernhard C. Schär, From Batticaloa via Basel to Berlin. Transimperial Science in Ceylon and Beyond around 1900, in: The Journal of Imperial and Commonwealth History 48 (2020) 2, p. 230–262, DOI: https://doi.org/10.1080/03086534.2019.1638620.

Pascal Schmid, Medicine, Faith and Politics in Agogo: A History of Health Care Delivery in Rural Ghana, ca. 1925 to 1980, Wien/Zürich 2018.

Jim Secord, Knowledge in Transit, in: Isis 95 (2004) 4, p. 654–672.

Rhonda Anne Semple, Missionary Women. Gender, Professionalism and the Victorian Idea of Christian Mission, Woodbridge/Rochester 2003.

Sujit Sivasundaram, Nature and the Godly Empire. Science and Evangelical Mission in the Pacific, 1795–1850, Cambridge 2005.

Sujit Sivasundaram, Sciences and the Global. On Methods, Questions, and Theory, in: Isis 101 (2010) 1, p. 146–158.

Sujit Sivasundaram, A Global History of Science and Religion, in: Thomas Dixon/Geoffrey Cantor/Stephen Pumfrey (eds.), Science and Religion. New Historical Perspectives, Cambridge 2010, p. 177–197.

Sujit Sivasundaram, Science, Medicine and Technology, in: Philippa Levine/John Marriott (eds.), The Ashgate Research Companion to Modern Imperial Histories, London/New York 2012, p. 549–566.

Helmut Walser Smith (ed.), Protestants, Catholics and Jews in Germany, 1800–1914, Oxford 2001.

Daniel Speich-Chassé/David Gugerli, Wissensgeschichte. Eine Standortbestimmung, in: Traverse (2012) 1, p. 85–100.

Brian Stanley, Christian Missions, Antislavery and the Claims of Humanity, c. 1813–1873, in: Sheridan Gilley/Brian Stanley (eds.), World Christianities c. 1815–c. 1914, Cambridge 2006, p. 443–457.

John Stenhouse, Missionary Science, in: Hugh Richard Slotten/Ronald L. Numbers/David N. Livingstone (eds.), The Cambridge History of Science, vol. 8: Modern Science in National, Transnational, and Global Context, Cambridge 2020, p. 90–107.

Ann Laura Stoler, "In Cold Blood": Hierarchies of Credibility and the Politics of Colonial Narratives, in: Representations 37 (1992), p. 151–189.

Ann Laura Stoler, Cultivating Bourgeois Bodies and Racial Selves, in: Catherine Hall (ed.), Cultures of Empire. A Reader: Colonizers in Britain and the Empire in the Nineteenth and Twentieth Centuries, New York 2000, p. 87–119.

Ann Laura Stoler, Carnal Knowledge and Imperial Power. Race and the Intimate in Colonial Rule, Berkeley/Los Angeles/London 2002.

Ann Laura Stoler, Colonial Archives and the Arts of Governance, in: Archival Science 2 (2002), p. 87–109.

Ann Laura Stoler, Along the Archival Grain. Epistemic Anxieties and Colonial Common Sense, Princeton 2009.

Ann Laura Stoler/Frederick Cooper, Beetween Metropole and Colony: Rethinking a Research Agenda, in: ibid. (eds.), Tensions of Empire. Colonial Cultures in the Bourgeois World, Berkeley et al. 1997, p. 1–56.

Wolfgang Struck, Die Eroberung der Phantasie. Kolonialismus, Literatur und Film zwischen deutschem Kaiserreich und Weimarer Republik, Göttingen 2010.

Benedikt Stutchey (ed.), Science across the European Empires 1800–1950, Oxford 2005.

Susan Thorne, "The Conversion of Englishmen and the Conversion of the World Inseparable". Missionary Imperialism and the Language of Class in Early Industrial Britain, in: Frederick Cooper/Ann Laura Stoler (eds.), Tensions of Empire. Colonial Cultures in a Bourgeois World, Berkeley et al. 1997, p. 238–262.

Susan Thorne, Congregational Missions and the Making of an Imperial Culture in Nineteenth-Century England, Stanford 1999.

Helen Tilley, Global Histories, Vernacular Science, and African Genealogies; or, Is the History of Science Ready for the World? in: Isis 101 (2010) 1, p. 110–119.

Helen Tilley, Africa as a Living Laboratory. Empire, Development, and the Problem of Scientific Knowledge, 1870–1950, Chicago 2011.

Ulrich van der Heyden/Andreas Feldtkeller (eds.), Missionsgeschichte als Geschichte der Globalisierung von Wissen. Transkulturelle Wissensaneignung und -vermittlung durch christliche Missionare in Afrika und Asien im 17., 18. und 19. Jahrhundert, Stuttgart 2012.

Dirk van Laak, Die deutsche Kolonialgeschichte als Fantasiegeschichte, in: Marianne Bechhaus-Gerst/Joachim Zeller (eds.), Deutschland postkolonial? Die Gegenwart der imperialen Vergangenheit, Berlin 2018, p. 123–142.

Megan Vaughan, Curing Their Ills. Colonial Power and African Illness, Cambridge 1991.

Jakob Vogel, Von der Wissenschafts- zur Wissensgeschichte. Für eine Historisierung der "Wissensgesellschaft", in: Geschichte und Gesellschaft 30 (2004) 4, p. 639–660.

Moritz von Brescius, German Science in the Age of Empire. Enterprise, Opportunity and the Schlagintweit Brothers, Cambridge 2019.

Helge Wendt, Die missionarische Gesellschaft. Mikrostrukturen einer kolonialen Globalisierung, Stuttgart 2011.

Helge Wendt, Mission transnational, trans-kolonial, global: Missionsgeschichtsschreibung als Beziehungsgeschichte, in: Schweizerische Zeitschrift für Religions- und Kulturgeschichte 105 (2011), p. 95–116.

Reinhard Wendt (ed.), Sammeln, Vernetzen, Auswerten. Missionare und ihr Beitrag zum Wandel europäischer Weltsicht, Tübingen 2001.

Karolin Wetjen, Mission als theologisches Labor: Koloniale Aushandlungen des Religiösen in Ostafrika um 1900, Stuttgart 2020.

Martin Weyer-von Schoultz, Max von Pettenkofer, 1818–1901. Die Entstehung der modernen Hygiene aus den empirischen Studien menschlicher Lebensgrundlagen, Frankfurt a. M. 2006.

Luise White, Speaking with Vampires. Rumor and History in Colonial Africa, Berkley 2000.

Lise Wilkinson/Anne Hardy, Prevention and Cure: The London School of Hygiene and Tropical Medicine. A 20th Century Quest for Global Public Health, London/New York 2001.

Monika Wohlrab-Sahr/Marian Burchardt, Multiple Secularities: Toward a Cultural Sociology of Secular Modernities, in: Comparative Sociology 11 (2012), p. 875–909.

Michael Worboys, Manson, Ross and Colonial Medical Policy: Tropical Medicine in London and Liverpool, 1899–1914, in: Roy MacLeod/Milton Lewis (eds.), Disease, Medicine, and Empire. Perspectives on Western Medicine and the Experience of European Expansion, London/New York 1988, p. 21–37.

Michael Worboys, Colonial and Imperial Medicine, in: Deborah Brunton (ed.), Medicine Transformed. Health, Disease and Society in Europe 1880–1930, Manchester/New York 2004, p. 211–238.

Andreas Zangger, Koloniale Schweiz. Ein Stück Globalgeschichte zwischen Europa und Südostasien (1860–1930), Bielefeld 2011.

Susanne Zantop, Colonial Fantasies: Conquest, Family, and Nation in Precolonial Germany, 1770–1870, Durham 1997.

Lukas Zürcher, Die Schweiz in Ruanda: Mission, Entwicklungshilfe und nationale Selbstbestätigung (1900–1975), Zürich 2014.

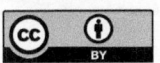

PART I

Spaces of Knowledge and Meanings of Hygiene in the Nineteenth Century

CHAPTER 2

The Religious Space of Knowledge: The Basel Mission, Worldwide Webs and Pietist Purity

2.1 PIETISTS, PATRICIANS AND THE SOCIAL QUESTION IN BASEL

The religious space of knowledge, in which the Basel Mission doctors were socialised, was rooted in the tradition of Pietism, which, alongside Anglo-American puritanism, formed the most significant Protestant revival since the Reformation. Pietists believed in the necessity of a spiritual rebirth and intense Bible-study as well as bodily asceticism and discipline. They strongly supported education and literacy, and focused on the individual's emotional connection with God. At the same time, Pietism brought people together in circles that not only became places of mutual edification but also initiated social change. Founded in the wake of the so-called *Erweckung*—the early nineteenth-century evangelical awakening on the European continent—the Basel Mission drew upon the support of wealthy and powerful bourgeois families from Basel and far-flung Pietist networks reaching across Europe and beyond.[1]

---

[1] For an overview of the scholarship on the *Erweckung*, see Andrew Kloes, The German Awakening: Protestant Renewal after the Enlightenment, 1815–1848, Oxford 2020.

© The Author(s) 2023   49
L. M. Ratschiller Nasim, *Medical Missionaries and Colonial Knowledge in West Africa and Europe, 1885–1914*,
Cambridge Imperial and Post-Colonial Studies,
https://doi.org/10.1007/978-3-031-27128-1_2

2.1.1   Wurttemberg Pietism

Pietism was a significant religious movement within Protestantism that emerged at the end of the seventeenth century and reached full blossom in the eighteenth century. Pietists called for an end to denominational strife and promoted a practical form of Christianity marked by personal piety, programmes for social betterment and efforts to spread Christ's Kingdom on earth. Originating in present-day Germany, Pietism had a lasting impact on Protestantism worldwide, particularly in Europe and North America. Far from being a homogenous movement however, Pietism changed considerably over time and adopted different forms according to regional, structural and political conditions.[2] The version of Pietism that was most influential in Basel and the Alemannic-speaking areas of Germany and Switzerland around 1800 is called "Wurttemberg Pietism," after the region where it originated.[3]

Wurttemberg was a Duchy in southwest Germany until it was enlarged and raised to the status of a Kingdom in a loose German Confederation during the Napoleonic period. Pietists often found themselves at the heart of controversies with governments whose authority they challenged. Therefore, they constantly had to look for places where they could practise their faith without persecution. In 1743, the Government of Wurttemberg passed the "Pietist Rescript," a law which guaranteed Pietists freedom from persecution if they stayed within certain limits. The Pietist population subsequently grew in Wurttemberg and became very influential in the life of the Protestant community there. In 1871,

---

[2] Martin Brecht/Klaus Deppermann/Ulrich Gäbler/Hartmut Lehmann (eds.), Geschichte des Pietismus, 4 vol., Göttingen 1993–2004; Hartmut Lehmann, Engerer, weiterer und erweiterter Pietismusbegriff, in: Pietismus und Neuzeit 29 (2003), p. 18–37; Douglas H. Shantz, An Introduction to German Pietism: Protestant Renewal at the Dawn of Modern Europe, Baltimore 2013; Christian T. Collins Winn et al. (eds.), The Pietist Impulse in Christianity, Eugene 2011; Justin A. Davis, Pietism and the Foundations of the Modern World, Eugene 2019.

[3] Wurttemberg Pietism is well documented. See Ulrike Gleixner, Pietismus und Bürgertum. Eine historische Anthropologie der Frömmigkeit, Göttingen 2005; Andreas Gestrich, Pietismus und ländliche Frömmigkeit in Württemberg im 18. und frühen 19. Jahrhundert, in: Norbert Haag/Sabine Holtz/Wolfgang Zimmermann/Dieter R. Bauer (eds.), Ländliche Frömmigkeit. Konfessionskulturen und Lebenswelten, Stuttgart 2002, p. 343–357; Hartmut Lehmann, Pietismus und weltliche Ordnung in Württemberg vom 17. bis zum 20. Jahrhundert, Stuttgart 1969.

Wurttemberg joined the new and more strongly unified German Empire, headed by the Kaiser and King of Prussia Otto von Bismarck.[4]

The city of Basel became a focal point of Wurttemberg Pietism and the subsequent transnational missionary movement that arose from the religious revival in both European and American churches in the first half of the nineteenth century.[5] The main focus of this renewal lay in the creation of a more practical and active approach to Christianity, including evangelising and welfare work both abroad and at home.[6] Pietists felt that the epochal political conflicts following the French Revolution and the subsequent economic and social transformations had led to the disintegration of traditional communities. They interpreted these changes as signs of de-Christianisation and thus the approaching end of the world, the second coming of Christ and the imminent establishment of the Kingdom of God. This perception energised the missionary movement, which promised to expand God's Kingdom by human effort.[7]

Although the connections between Pietism and the nineteenth-century evangelical awakening within German-speaking Protestantism are discussed controversially in research, most historians agree that they shared a focus on personal belief and subjective religious experience.[8]

[4] Wurttemberg had a population of 1.3 million in 1812, rising to about 2 million by the end of the century. See Jenkins, Württemberg als Hauptsäule der historischen Basler Mission.

[5] Erika Hebeisen, Leidenschaftlich fromm. Die pietistische Bewegung in Basel 1750–1830, Köln/Weimar/Wien 2005; Thomas K. Kuhn/Martin Sallmann (eds.), Das "fromme Basel". Religion in einer Stadt des 19. Jahrhunderts, Basel 2002.

[6] Karl Rennstich, Mission—Geschichte der protestantischen Mission in Deutschland, in: Ulrich Gäbler (ed.), Geschichte des Pietismus, vol. 3: Der Pietismus im neunzehnten und zwanzigsten Jahrhundert, Göttingen 2000, p. 308–319; Lucian Hölscher, Geschichte der protestantischen Frömmigkeit in Deutschland, München 2005, p. 347–351.

[7] Judith Becker, Zukunftserwartungen und Missionsimpetus bei Missionsgesellschaften in der ersten Hälfte des 19. Jahrhunderts, in: Wolfgang Breul/Jan Carsten Schnurr (eds.), Geschichtsbewusstsein und Zukunftserwartungen in Pietismus und Erweckungsbewegung, Göttingen 2013, p. 244–270; Ibid., "Gehet hin in alle Welt...". Sendungsbewusstsein in der evangelischen Missionsbewegung der ersten Hälfte des 19. Jahrhunderts, in: Evangelische Theologie 72 (2012) 2, p. 134–154.

[8] Thomas K. Kuhn/Veronika Albrecht-Birkner (eds.), Zwischen Aufklärung und Moderne: Erweckungsbewegungen als historiographische Herausforderung, Berlin 2017; Gustav Adolf Benrath, Die Erweckung innerhalb der deutschen Landeskirchen, in: Ulrich Gäbler (ed.), Geschichte des Pietismus, vol. 3: Der Pietismus im neunzehnten und zwanzigsten Jahrhundert, Göttingen 2000, p. 150–271.

The *Erweckung* transformed Christian mission from being a concern of rulers and church leaders to an initiative to be supported and upheld by every committed Christian. Born-again laypeople, many of them women, became agents of their own spirituality, meeting in non-church settings to pray, read and discuss the Bible, and to encourage each another in their faith. Tract and missionary societies emerged, which had no organic connection with a specific church and set out to enlist backing from congregations elsewhere, regardless of territorial church jurisdictions.[9]

Inspired by English writers of religious tracts, a group of Protestants from Basel's surrounding area adopted the renewed interest in the Bible and the missionary cause.[10] The indifference of Pietism towards confessional tenets facilitated coalitions between different denominations and allowed for Swabian Lutherans and Swiss Calvinists to take Christian action together. In 1780, they founded the "German Society for the Promotion of Pure Instruction and True Piety" in Basel, commonly referred to as the *Deutsche Christentumsgesellschaft*—German Society for Christianity. The Bible study and discussion group brought together prominent clergymen, politicians, business owners and theologians from the Alemannic region, who identified themselves with the Pietist movement and wanted to establish visible, outward expression of their religious beliefs.[11]

The society's primary objectives were to build networks with other evangelical groups across Europe and to disseminate Christian literature. From about 1800, the *Deutsche Christentumsgesellschaft* started publishing German translations of reports, tracts and other publications produced by the burgeoning British missionary societies, such as the Baptist Missionary Society. Due to the increasingly strong missionary

[9] By 1800, the Kingdom of Wurttemberg alone counted more than fifty of these voluntary societies.

[10] On the renewed interest in the Bible in Basel, see Hans Hauzenberger, Basel und die Bibel. Die Bibel als Quelle ökumenischer, missionarischer, sozialer und pädagogischer Impulse in der ersten Hälfte des 19. Jahrhunderts, Basel 1996.

[11] Martin Brecht/Friedrich de Boor/Klaus Deppermann/Harmut Lehmann/Andreas Lindt/Johannes Wallmann (eds.), Die Basler Christentumsgesellschaft, Göttingen 1982.

element in their thinking, members of the *Deutsche Christentumsge-sellschaft* initiated a seminary for the education of overseas evangelists in Basel in 1815.[12]

2.1.2   The Basel Patricians

The inception of the Basel Evangelical Missionary Society in 1815 drew on long-standing religious, commercial and political networks rooted in the city on the Rhine. Located in the heartland of an interregional triangle between Switzerland, Alsace and the Kingdom of Wurttemberg, Basel was home to one of the few ancient bridges across the Rhine, which made it an economic hub long before its industries had fully matured. The ruling elite, the patricians, not only fostered important trade ties across Europe but also paid special attention to religious issues.[13] They organised their own Reformation in 1529 and displayed particular sympathy for revivalist movements such as Pietism and the evangelical awakening over the next centuries. These Protestant merchants and manufacturers, who dominated politics in the city-state well into twentieth century, provided the necessary financial, organisational and political support for the establishment of a mission society in Basel.[14]

From the late seventeenth century, the patricians occupied most political offices and regularly sent representatives from their ranks to the so-called *Tagsatzung*—the Federal Diet of Switzerland.[15] Growing

---

[12] Horst Weigelt, Die Diasporaarbeit der Herrnhuter Brüdergemeine und die Wirksamkeit der Deutschen Christentumsgesellschaft im 19. Jahrhundert, in: Ulrich Gäbler (ed.), Geschichte des Pietismus, vol. 3: Der Pietismus im neunzehnten und zwanzigsten Jahrhundert, Göttingen 2000, p. 113–148.

[13] On the term "patrician" in the Basel context, see Schär, Tropenliebe, p. 42; Philipp Sarasin, Stadt der Bürger. Bürgerliche Macht und städtische Gesellschaft, Basel 1846–1914, Göttingen 1997, p. 13. For a critical view on the use of the term, see Sara Janner, Zwischen Machtanspruch und Autoritätsverlust. Zur Funktion von Religion und Kirchlichkeit in Politik und Selbstverständnis des konservativen alten Bürgertums im Basel des 19. Jahrhunderts, Basel 2012, p. 30–31.

[14] Basel's upper class was composed of old as well as new money generated by global trade and industries such as silk, cotton and tobacco.

[15] This legislative and executive council of the Swiss Confederacy was a meeting of delegates of the individual cantons and existed in various forms since the beginnings of Swiss independence until the formation of the Swiss Federal State in 1848. See Andreas Würgler, Die Tagsatzung der Eidgenossen: Politik, Kommunikation und Symbolik einer repräsentativen Institution im europäischen Kontext, Epfendorf 2010.

religious and political conflicts between liberal and conservative forces dominated Swiss society from the late eighteenth century, as was the case across Europe. The end of the Old Confederacy began with the invasion of Napoleon's troops in Basel in 1798. The cantons subsequently experienced a temporary loss of their independence and the Napoleonic wars threatened more than once to engulf the city on the Rhine.[16]

Basel, the largest and wealthiest town in German-speaking Switzerland at this time, had become a byword for political conservatism by the 1830s. Alone among the major Protestant cantons, it withstood the Revolution of 1830 and resisted the liberalisation of the *Ratsherrenregiment*—the rule of the merchant elite. Increasing tensions between the relatively disenfranchised countryside surrounding Basel and the urban elite led to a short civil war and the separation of the territory into two new half-cantons in 1833, *Basel-Stadt* and *Basel-Landschaft*. The patricians subsequently had to concede their territory south of the city, where their silk ribbon factories and summer residences stood. The split of the canton of Basel also meant that the patricians lost considerable influence in the Confederacy and steadily alienated themselves from federal matters.[17]

The liberal forces dominating the majority of the other cantons had supported the insurgency against the conservative elite in Basel. The city's wealth and independence, together with its orientation to the outside world, had long made it an object of envy and resentment among the other cantons. On the other side, most voices in the city of Basel opposed liberal centralisation plans, such as the proposed transformation of Switzerland from a *Staatenbund*, a confederation of states, into a *Bundesstaat*, a federal state. Basel remained loyal to the Confederation during the civil war of 1847 but there were many patricians who sympathised with the conservative cause of maximum cantonal independence. The *Bundesverfassung*—Federal Constitution—of 1848 was passed

---

[16] Matthias   Manz,   Basel.   Von   der   Helvetik   bis   zur   Kantonstrennung   (1798–1833),   in: Historisches   Lexikon   der   Schweiz, https://hls-dhs-dss.ch/de/articles/007387/2016-01-13/#HVonderHelvetikbiszur Kantonstrennung 28 17 98–183,329, version 13.01.2016 (last access: 22.07.2022).

[17] Claudia Opitz, Von der Aufklärung zur Kantonstrennung, in: Georg Kreis/Beat von Wartburg (eds.), Basel. Geschichte einer städtischen Gesellschaft, Basel 2000, p. 150–185.

in Basel in a similar grudging spirit with many *Ratsherren* simply not voting.[18]

The foundation of the Swiss Federal State in 1848 led to the implementation of political reforms. The new Federal Constitution was based on the democratic participation of all men, yet without fundamentally affecting the sovereignty of the cantons. Basel thus remained a city-state ruled by Patrician councilmen, who held exclusive decision-making authority over municipal and religious matters, despite the development of a more democratic Swiss Federal State. They dominated the economic life of the region, controlled the government of the canton and held leading positions in the local churches.[19]

Religion and politics were closely linked in the city on the Rhine. Most Basel patricians were devout Protestants who believed in liberal trade and business but supported conservative values and policies. This combination of worldly activism, energetic pursuit of trade and profit, devotion to political conservatism and the religious piety that dominated the city gave observers the impression of an oppressively pious, duplicitous society.[20] For a long time, patrician families could be certain of their influence in both the political and religious domain. Only in the second half of the nineteenth century did religious as well as political liberalism gain momentum. A new church constitution was passed in 1874 guaranteeing the Protestant cantonal church more independence from the city-state, and 1875 saw the adoption of a liberal cantonal constitution based on the model of other cantons.[21]

For many patricians, while the cantonal separation of 1833 had been a life changing and humiliating experience, it had also served as a wake-up call to redefine their place in the world. Many of them subsequently turned towards evangelicalism.[22] The Basel Mission's leadership

---

[18] Lionel Gossman, Basel in the Age of Burckhardt: A Study in Unseasonable Ideas, Chicago 2000, p. 17.

[19] Sarasin, Stadt der Bürger, p. 91–119; Schär, Tropenliebe, p. 38–78; Janner, Zwischen Machtanspruch und Autoritätsverlust, p. 73–160.

[20] Gossman, Basel in the Age of Burckhardt, p. 59.

[21] Regina Wecker, 1833 bis 1910. Die Entwicklung zur Grossstadt, in: Georg Kreis/ Beat von Wartburg (eds.), Basel. Geschichte einer städtischen Gesellschaft, Basel 2000, p. 196–224.

[22] Martin W. Pernet, Nietzsche und das "fromme" Basel, Basel 2014, p. 41–64; Janner, Zwischen Machtanspruch und Autoritätsverlust, p. 161–293.

consisted of a self-perpetuating circle of men, called the Committee, that usually had about twelve members, mostly academics, politicians, jurists, merchants, bankers and manufacturers originating from patrician families.[23] While they prevailed numerically, representatives of the Pietist theological elite of Wurttemberg, especially from Tubingen University, also held key policymaking positions. The Inspector, for example, who was in charge of daily administration, was usually a German theologian.[24]

By 1821, the Committee members had decided to establish their own mission stations abroad and subsequently tried to take root in Russia, China, India and Africa, most notably on the Gold Coast in 1828 and in Cameroon in 1885. Officially, this move assured that the distinctive Pietist worldview was brought to regions that were still labouring in "unchristian darkness," as the Committee expounded.[25] Most Committee members, however, also had strong economic incentives in expanding their sphere of influence overseas. Some of Basel's most prominent merchants sat on the Basel Mission's board of directors and on the mission's trade commission. The Basel Mission's trade commission gave rise to the Basel Mission Trading Company, founded in 1859. The corporation, which remained under direct Basel Mission management until 1917, supplied mission stations in West Africa and South India with European goods and traded cacao, palm oil, rubber and cotton on a global scale.[26]

---

[23] Thirty-three of the forty men who served on the Committee between 1815 and 1900 had relatives in positions of responsibility in the Basel Mission. The admission and re-election of a Committee member had to be decided unanimously by all other members to avoid disagreements. On the social makeup of the Basel Mission Committee, see Jon Miller, Missionary Zeal and Institutional Control. Organizational Contradictions in the Basel Mission on the Gold Coast, 1828–1917, London/New York 2003, p. 38–45.

[24] The Inspector was chosen from the existing Committee members and had to be elected unanimously. See Tobias Eiselen, "Zur Erziehung einer zuverlässigen, wohld-isziplinierten Streiterschar für den Missionskrieg". Basler Missionarsausbildung im 19. Jahrhundert, in: Werner Ustorf (ed.), Mission im Kontext. Beiträge zur Sozialgeschichte der Norddeutschen Missionsgesellschaft im 19. Jahrhundert, Bremen 1986, p. 47–120, here p. 48–49.

[25] Wilhelm Schlatter, Geschichte der Basler Mission 1815–1915, vol. 1, Basel 1916, p. 93.

[26] Gustav Wanner, Die Basler Handels-Gesellschaft A.G. 1859–1959, Basel 1959; Giorgio Miescher, Hermann Ludwig Rottmann. Zu den Anfängen der Basler Missions-Handels-Gesellschaft in Christiansborg (Ghana), in: Lilo Roost Vischer/Anne Mayor/Dag Henrichsen (eds.), Werkschau Afrikastudien, vol. 2: Brücken und Grenzen, Münster 1999, p. 345–362; Andrea Franc, Wie die Schweiz zur Schokolade kam. Der Kakaohandel der

The Basel Mission was materialised, and their leadership provided, by the representatives of a visible and stable religious, political and economic elite. The Basel Mission Trading Company was created to provide a Christian commercial alternative to colonial traders, who, the Committee members argued, often exploited and corrupted the people in their sphere of influence. Basel Mission traders were the first to ship cacao from the Gold Coast overseas in 1893, turning the British colony into the world's largest cocoa exporter over the next few years. The success of the trading company was much welcomed by its shareholders, mostly Basel patricians, who received six per cent of revenue as a dividend. By 1914, the number of traders trained at the mission seminary in Basel exceeded that of common missionaries in West Africa.[27] This illustrates the converging interests between worldwide evangelicalism and trade.

The Basel patricians benefitted from the rise of industrial modes of production, the establishment of large-scale factories and the expansion of the world economy. The new mechanical engineering, metal and chemical industries created an increasing demand for labour while the old silk industry survived the industrial transition by sourcing raw materials overseas and establishing a significant export market in the United States. At the same time, these fundamental economic transformations also triggered serious social consequences. In the "old city of faith," as contemporaries referred to Basel, the radical economic changes and social upheavals were feared to diminish the influence of Pietism Basel's ruling elite responded to these challenges by building an extensive welfare network. Voluntary service and honorary work were the driving forces of this system, which was built on the tenets of Christian charity.[28]

Basler Handelsgesellschaft mit der Kolonie Goldküste (1893–1960), Basel 2008; Heinrich Christ, Zwischen Religion und Geschäft. Die Basler Missions-Handlungs-Gesellschaft und ihre Unternehmensethik, 1859–1917, Basel 2015.

[27] Heinrich Christ, Mission und Geld. Die Missions-Handlungs-Gesellschaft, in: Christine Christ-von Wedel/Thomas K. Kuhn (eds.), Basler Mission. Menschen, Geschichte, Perspektiven 1815–2015, Basel 2015, p. 93–98.

[28] Urs Hofmann, "Nur das Evangelium vermag die soziale Frage zu lösen". Die reformierte Kirche und die Armenpolitik im 19. und frühen 20. Jahrhundert, in: Josef Mooser/Simon Wenger (eds.), Armut und Fürsorge in Basel. Armutspolitik vom 13. Jahrhundert bis heute, Basel 2011, p. 134–142.

2.1.3   The Social Question

In a global trading town like Basel, industrial paternalism and private charity were believed to be the best options for alleviating the social question. Significantly, it was a private society, the *Freiwillige Armenpflege*—Voluntary Poor Relief—that coordinated welfare work in Basel without any state supervision until 1897. This approach found its earliest and strongest expression in the *Gesellschaft zur Aufmunterung und Beförderung des Guten und Gemeinnützigen (GGG)*—Society for the Encouragement and Promotion of Works of Public Benefit and Utility—founded in 1777. Initiated by the philosopher, historian and educator Isaak Iselin, and supported by a large number of conservative merchant families, this society brought together humanitarian and Pietist circles to address socio-political issues, such as poor relief and education policy.[29]

Trade and industry flourished rapidly in Basel over the nineteenth century, as a result of the improvement of Rhine navigation in the 1820s, the arrival of the railways in 1845 and the expansion of global markets.[30] The population of 22,000 inhabitants in the 1830s had almost doubled by 1860 and by 1900 Basel was the second Swiss city after Zurich to count over 100,000 inhabitants. Child labour, long working hours and an overall underpaid and undernourished working class were part of the cityscape. The majority of Basel's inhabitants were neither wealthy nor clean and healthy at this time. Overcrowded and unsanitary housing facilities, together with an insufficient sewer system and poor water supply, resulted in frequent typhus and cholera epidemics.[31] For the Basel patricians, the greatest threat to the social order, to a compliant, well-regulated labour force, and to their own ascendancy, was a population living in poverty.

[29] Sara Janner, GGG 1777–1914. Basler Stadtgeschichte im Spiegel der "Gesellschaft für das Gute und Gemeinnützige", Basel 2015; Beatrice Schumacher, Braucht es uns? Selbstbilder, Arbeitsweisen und organisatorische Strukturen der Schweizerischen Gemeinnützigen Gesellschaft (1810–1970), in: ibid. (ed.), Freiwillig verpflichtet. Gemeinnütziges Denken und Handeln in der Schweiz seit 1800, Zürich 2010, p. 37–69.

[30] Basel was the first Swiss city to be connected to the railways and became the leading commercial city in the Swiss Confederation. See Wecker, 1833 bis 1910. Die Entwicklung zur Grossstadt.

[31] Martin Schaffner, Die Basler Arbeiterbevölkerung im 19. Jahrhundert. Beiträge zur Geschichte ihrer Lebensformen, Basel/Stuttgart 1972; Luca Trevisan, Das Wohnungselend der Basler Arbeiterbevölkerung in der zweiten Hälfte des 19. Jahrhunderts, Basel 1989.

The *GGG* formed a commission to investigate the conditions of factory workers in the early 1840s and subsequently introduced a broad range of measures to address these hygienic and social shortcomings.[32] These included the foundation of retail cooperatives, the promotion of health insurance and assistance funds as well as the construction of social housing estates and public bath and laundry facilities from the 1860s. Educational programmes directed at the working class such as reading circles, choir societies and gymnastic clubs complemented these practical measures.[33] The ever-increasing misery, however, radically contradicted the idea that private philanthropy and Christian charity would put an end to the social question. The social precariousness of the growing population triggered upheavals, waves of strikes and demands for political reforms throughout Europe in the 1860s and 1870s.

The Basel patricians used their welfare system based on private donations as a political instrument to argue against the need for the state to intervene in welfare work, opposing the legal right to state care. In light of ever-stronger working-class and democratic movements, however, they conceded limited state regulations to improve the conditions of factory workers, thereby hoping to increase social stability and protect their dominant position. In the wake of industrial regulations implemented by the governments in the cantons of Glarus and Zurich, they too introduced factory laws in November of 1869 and supported the implementation of the Swiss Factory Act eight years later.[34]

Nevertheless, public welfare in Basel still crucially depended on the benevolence of the conservative elite. According to a survey prompted by the first social democrat in the cantonal Parliament, Eugen Wullschleger,

---

[32] In 1843, the *GGG* published an extensive study on the working conditions in Basel's silk ribbon factories: Gesellschaft für das Gute und Gemeinnützige (ed.), Über die Fabrikarbeiter-Verhältnisse der Baseler Industrie. Berichterstattung einer von der Baselerischen Abteilung der Schweizerischen Gemeinnützigen Gesellschaft aufgestellten Kommission, Basel 1843. See further William O. Shanahan, Der deutsche Protestantismus vor der sozialen Frage 1815–1871, München 1962, p. 378; Sarasin, Stadt der Bürger, p. 51.

[33] Martin Lengwiler, Wissenschaft und Sozialpolitik. Der Einfluss der Gelehrtengesellschaften und Experten auf die Sozialpolitik im 19. Jahrhundert, in: Josef Mooser/ Simon Wenger (des.), Armut und Fürsorge in Basel. Armutspolitik vom 13. Jahrhundert bis heute, Basel 2011, p. 111–122, here p. 116–117.

[34] Basel's factory laws were the first of their kind resulting from Protestant initiative in the German-speaking world. See Shanahan, Der deutsche Protestantismus, p. 382.

Basel housed over one hundred societies and institutions dedicated to poverty relief and health care in 1903.[35] Forty-eight were run privately, eighteen belonged to the *GGG*, sixteen to the reformed church, fourteen were state-owned facilities and six belonged to the so-called *Bürgergemeinde*—civil community. The Basel patricians, who dominated the *Bürgergemeinde*, the reformed church, the *GGG* and the majority of the private societies, controlled more than four-fifths of these organisations. Their financial contributions also amounted to four-fifths of the total funds employed for poverty alleviation, a total of 4.2 million Swiss francs in 1903.[36]

The patricians' charitable commitment highlights that the civilising offensive both abroad and at home was not only about the poor and their needs but the rich and their motives. By calling on the fundamental Christian pillar of charity and emphasising the moral importance of honorary work, Basel's ruling class succeeded for many years to hold their position against democratic, radical and liberal forces. Evidently, their conservative social policy fundamentally depended on unpaid work carried out by people from less fortunate backgrounds. A myriad of community workers, deaconesses, pastors, city missionaries, fundraisers and members of voluntary societies, charitable organisations and women's associations performed non-remunerated community service on a daily basis and thus implemented the patricians' welfare system.

2.1.4   The Basel City Mission

Basel's conservative leaders assessed the social question from a moral viewpoint and considered sin, filth and impurity to be at the root of human misery.[37] Like other protagonists of the Protestant religious revival, they

---

[35] Karl Stückelberger, Die Armen- und Krankenfürsorge in Basel, Basel 1906, p. 9–13, 29–55.

[36] Sara Janner, Korporative und private Wohltätigkeit. "Stadtgemeinde" und Stadtbürgertum als Träger der Armenpflege im 19. Jahrhundert, in: Josef Mooser/Simon Wenger (eds.), Armut und Fürsorge in Basel. Armutspolitik vom 13. Jahrhundert bis heute, Basel 2011, p. 101–109, here p. 101.

[37] Shanahan, Der deutsche Protestantismus, p. 373–388; Arnd Götzelmann, Die Soziale Frage, in: Ulrich Gäbler (ed.), Geschichte des Pietismus, vol. 3: Der Pietismus im neunzehnten und zwanzigsten Jahrhundert, Göttingen 2000, p. 272–307.

identified two main causes for the social problems of the time: a religious decline, on the one hand, and the erosion of family life in the lower classes, on the other, both of which they sought to counteract by charity.[38] Therefore, their answer to the social question consisted in a reinvigoration of faith and family values, in contrast to the revolutionaries of 1848–1849. Crucially, the majority of the charitable societies they supported thus not only promised material but also moral improvement. Bible circles, Sunday schools, youth associations, orphanages, nurseries and sewing workshops addressed the social question by seeking to (re-) Christianise the growing population.[39]

The clearest manifestation of the coupling of welfare with evangelising work was the establishment of the Evangelical Society for City Mission in Basel in 1859.[40] The Basel City Mission was but one manifestation of a pan-European movement that mushroomed in the mid-nineteenth century. Emanating from Glasgow and London, the idea of a home mission had reached Hamburg in 1848, where Johann Hinrich Wichern established the first German city mission.[41] The *Innere Mission*, as the movement was known in Germany, sought to reinvigorate Christian faith among European societies by the spread of "brotherly love," which included charitable work and education. During a stay at a health resort in Baden-Baden in the summer of 1857, an "eager" member of the

---

[38] Norbert Friedrich/Traugott Jähnichen, Geschichte der sozialen Ideen im deutschen Protestantismus, in: Helga Grebing (ed.), Geschichte der sozialen Ideen in Deutschland. Sozialismus—katholische Soziallehre—protestantische Sozialethik. Ein Handbuch, 2nd ed., Wiesbaden 2005, p. 867–1102, here p. 877–888, 895–903.

[39] Thomas K. Kuhn, Religion und neuzeitliche Gesellschaft. Studien zum sozialen und diakonischen Handeln in Pietismus, Aufklärung und Erweckungsbewegung, Tübingen 2003.

[40] Hans Anstein, Fünfzig Jahre Stadt-Mission in Basel. Rückblick auf die Tätigkeit der Evangelischen Gesellschaft für Stadt-Mission in Basel in den Jahren 1859 bis 1909, Basel 1909; Ernst Hauri, Die Evangelische Gesellschaft für Stadtmission in Basel. Kurze Darstellung ihrer Entwicklung von 1859–1959, Basel 1959; Irina Bossart, "Wuchern mit dem anvertrauten Pfunde" oder Krisenbewältigung durch Evangelisierung. Die Basler Stadtmission in der zweiten Hälfte des 19. Jahrhunderts, Doctoral Thesis, University of Basel, 2009.

[41] Alexandra Przyrembel, Der Missionar Johann Hinrich Wichern, die Sünde und das unabänderliche Elend der städtischen Unterschichten um 1850, in: WerkstattGeschichte 57 (2011), p. 53–67.

Hamburg City Mission convinced the Basel merchant Emanuel Herzog to establish a city mission in Basel.[42]

Herzog rallied a group of laypeople and pastors who like him perceived political and religious liberalism as well as rapid urban changes to be a threat to their hometown. The founders of the Basel City Mission classified the social changes brought about by industrialism, urbanisation and liberalism as pathologies—"cancer," "freedom dizziness," "pleasure and indulgence addiction"—and believed that proclaiming the gospel was the only way of healing these "diseases" of the time. The president of the Basel City Mission Albert Ostertag expounded in his annual account for 1868: "Only the gospel, the gospel alone, is capable of solving the important social question—everything else, as well-intentioned as it might be, leaves the heart unimproved and thus exposed to all influences."[43]

Basel had seen an upsurge in immigration since 1848, particularly from other regions in Switzerland, southern Germany, Alsace and Italy.[44] This led to a rapid growth of workers' districts and the demolition of the old town walls. By 1860, one-fourth of the city's population were Catholics.[45] The City Mission's declared goal was to religiously assimilate these immigrants into the Protestant population of the city.[46] The activities they pursued included systematic house visits, the distribution of the Bible and other religious tracts, public preaching, community care and practical support for people in need.[47] Pietists believed that their charitable involvement would exemplify the benefits of Christianity to people

---

[42] Anstein, Fünfzig Jahre Stadt-Mission in Basel, p. 13.

[43] Albert Ostertag, Jahresbericht der Stadtmission vom 1. April 1868, Basel 1869, p. 13.

[44] Basel counted 47,000 inhabitants in 1870, 112,227 in 1900 and 135,918 in 1910. See Josef Mooser, Armenpflege zwischen Freiwilligkeit und Verstaatlichung. Träger und Reformen der Armenpolitik im Umbruch zur Grossstadt um 1900, in: ibid./Simon Wenger (eds.), Armut und Fürsorge in Basel. Armutspolitik vom 13. Jahrhundert bis heute, Basel 2011, p. 177–204, here p. 179.

[45] Irina Bossart, 150 Jahre Basler Stadtmission. "… hervorgerufen durch den Ernst der Zeit", in: Basler Stadtbuch 130 (2009), ed. by Christoph Merian Stiftung, p. 143–145, here p. 143.

[46] Anstein, Fünfzig Jahre Stadt-Mission in Basel, p. 16. On the attempts to evangelise Italian immigrants in Zurich, see Ernst Matthias Rüsch, "Conversation über das Eine, was not tut". Evangelisch-reformierte Italienerseelsorge im Kanton Zürich im 19. und 20. Jahrhundert, Zürich 2010.

[47] Schaffner, Die Basler Arbeiterbevölkerung im 19. Jahrhundert, p. 103–105.

who, in their eyes, led profane lives. However, just as importantly, social deeds were essential for the salvation of Pietists themselves.[48]

The evangelising efforts abroad, which clearly predated the home mission movement, alerted many evangelicals to the perceived problem of de-Christianisation in Europe. They started to feel the need to promulgate a proper sense of morality, decency and hygiene among the people in their vicinity. The stories of successful missions in Africa served as an example and justification for the civilising mission of workers' districts in European cities. Historians have demonstrated the discursive and organisational connections between home and foreign missions in the British and German contexts, where metropolitan lower classes were perceived as the heathens of Europe.[49] It is instructive to view the welfare system in Basel and the missionary activities abroad in the same analytical framework, since they were both genuine acts of Pietism. Most people involved with the Basel Mission participated directly or held strong personal and financial ties with Christian charities at home, most prominently the Basel City MissionCity mission.[50]

2.2   THE WEB OF MISSION

Mission societies held key positions in the increasing interdependence of the world, creating durable entanglements between people and places near and far. In Europe, the nineteenth century saw the rise of an evangelical grassroots movement that was made up of countless missionaries, itinerant preachers, donors and members of support groups, among them a surprising number of women and children. Devotion to the evangelising cause brought people together across the divide of social, gender, confessional and regional differences. While Pietism relied on politically

---

[48] Rennstich, Mission—Geschichte der protestantischen Mission in Deutschland, p. 311–312.

[49] Alexa Geisthövel/Ute Siebert/Sonja Finkbeiner, "Menschenfischer". Über die Parallelen von äusserer und innerer Mission um 1900, in: Rolf Lindner (ed.), "Wer in den Osten geht, geht in ein anderes Land". Die Settlementbewegung in Berlin zwischen Kaiserreich und Weimarer Republik, Berlin 1997, p. 27–50; Thorne, "The Conversion of Englishmen and the Conversion of the World Inseparable"; Habermas, Mission im 19. Jahrhundert, p. 664–671; Comaroff/Comaroff, Of Revelation and Revolution, vol. 2.

[50] Evangelische Gesellschaft für Stadtmission Basel, BMA, U.15; Korrespondenz zwischen der Basler Mission und der Basler Stadtmission sowie Stadtmissionsgesellschaften in Deutschland und im Elsass, 1913–1952, BMA, QH-10.16.

influential personalities, most supporters of the Basel Mission came from politically and socially less influential strata. Evangelicalism was a socially broad-based, globally designed project, carried out in manifold ways in different parts of the world. This web of mission facilitated the worldwide exchange of ideas, images and objects.

2.2.1   Worldwide Webs

The Basel Mission was never an organisation of merely one denomination or church. From the beginning, it drew support from the more Reformed tradition of the Swiss Protestant churches and the Lutheran tradition of many South German Protestant churches, like the one in Wurttemberg. The founders of the mission seminary in Basel invoked the scriptural injunction to go into the world and share the gospel of Jesus Christ. The global ambitions of awakened evangelicals fuelled the emergence of an informal spiritual realm, a network of formal bodies that connected believers across increasingly distinct national boundaries. This coopera-tion was facilitated by a shared vision about the oncoming Kingdom of God, which devout Christians considered to be their true homeland.[51]

Support associations for the Basel Mission thrived across Switzer-land and Germany over the nineteenth century, some of which evolved into independent mission societies. They included the Berlin Mission founded in 1824, the Rheinische Mission created in 1828 and the *Norddeutsche Missionsgesellschaft* established in 1836. These organisations remained in close contact with Basel and contributed to the good connec-tions of the mission society in Germany.[52] The men in charge in Basel also maintained close relations with the *Mission de Paris* and British missionary circles. More than one hundred missionaries from the Anglican Church Missionary Society received their training in the seminary in Basel

---

[51] Habermas, Mission im 19. Jahrhundert, p. 656–657; Dana L. Robert, Christian Mission: How Christianity Became a World Religion, Chichester 2009, p. 1; Michael Gladwin, Mission and Colonialism, in: Joel D. S. Rasmussen/Judith Wolfe/Johannes Zachhuber (eds.), The Oxford Handbook of Nineteenth-Century Christian Thought, Oxford 2017, p. 282–304, here p. 282.

[52] The missionaries of the *Norddeutsche Missionsgesellschaft* even trained at the seminary in Basel from 1850, when their own society was unable to sustain its own training facility. See Eiselen, "Zur Erziehung einer zuverlässigen, wohldisziplinierten Streiterschar", p. 47.

between 1819 and 1858; among them a future consecrated Bishop of Jerusalem.[53]

Building on their Pietist origins, the Basel Mission was firmly established in evangelical networks. The Inspector—the mission's director—and the Committee members regularly corresponded with colleagues in other countries, mutually published articles in their respective mission magazines and met at international mission conferences. Evangelical culture and theology were always multifaceted and from the early twentieth century onwards were becoming ever more so as interdenominational connections and cooperation rapidly increased. The first World Mission Conference in Edinburgh in 1910, at which the International Mission Council was created, included an important Basel Mission delegation with a significant number of missionaries on furlough.[54]

The Basel Mission's global aspirations were also apparent in the way it conceptualised the diverse places in which it operated—in West Africa, Europe and Asia—as one conceptual space. The popular monthly magazine, *Der Evangelische Heidenbote*, blended stories, pictures and maps from these diverse regions on every page. The most tangible expression of this universalising agenda came in the architectural form of a world community under one roof, on display in the Basel Mission's collection and touring exhibition. Models, mannequins and artefacts from all corners of the world were brought together and displayed next to each other. These items—held at the *Museum der Kulturen* in Basel today—served as material evidence for the mission's global outreach. The back cover of the museum guide for what the Basel Mission advertised as an "Ethnographic Exhibition" in 1908 exemplifies how the visitors were directed to view the world as one, held together by the mission's worldwide webs and the understanding of the gospel of Jesus Christ as a universal message (Fig. 2.1).[55]

Beyond and beneath this spiritual and symbolic dimension, the Basel Mission materialised their global ambitions by participating in

---

[53] Paul Jenkins, Short History of the Basel Mission, Basel 1989, p. 13.

[54] Matthäus Feigk, Von Edinburgh nach Oegstgeest. Die transnationalen missionarischen Netzwerke Europas am Beispiel der Basler Mission 1910–1920, in: Linda Ratschiller/Karolin Wetjen (eds.), Verflochtene Mission. Perspektiven auf eine neue Missionsgeschichte, Köln/Weimar/Wien 2018, p. 45–64.

[55] Die Basler Missionsgebiete, in: Führer durch die Völkerkundliche Ausstellung der Basler Mission, Basel 1908, BMA, Box "Missionsmuseum", without signature.

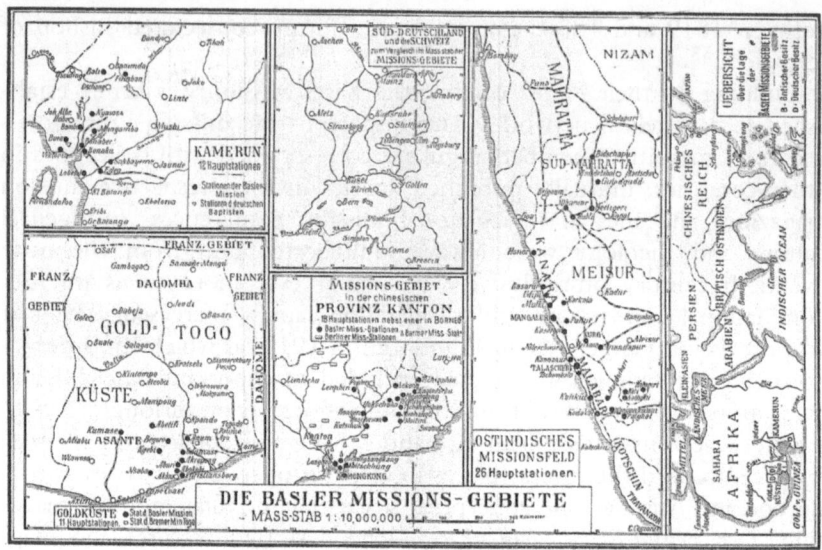

Fig. 2.1 Die Basler Missionsgebiete, in: Führer durch die Völkerkundliche Ausstellung der Basler Mission, Basel 1908, BMA, Box "Missionsmuseum", without signature

the expanding commodity trade. The Basel Mission Trading Company exported European goods to their trading posts overseas, introduced weaving workshops in Cameroon, printing plants on the Gold Coast, tile and brick factories in India and participated in the worldwide cash crop trade with coffee and cacao from West Africa. A distinctive feature of the Basel Mission, one that was not shared by most other mission societies, was their emphasis on practical industries. By building farms, roads, houses, hospitals and churches, the Basel missionaries fundamentally changed the material environments in which they lived and interwove disparate regions of the world in their unifying endeavours. By aspiring to global significance, the Basel Mission naturally competed with other forces. This was true not only for the economic realm but also the religious space.

For all the commitment of missionaries to a common Christianity, the history of missions forcefully illustrates the volatility of global evangelicalism. Theological disagreements and the increasing enmity between

Germany and Britain eventually broke the Basel Mission's special relationship with the Church Missionary Society. Frictions also emerged with the creation of purely Lutheran missions in Northern Germany, such as the Leipzig Mission in 1836. Differing views on the appropriate interaction with colonial authorities, conflicting notions of ecclesiastical order and theological disputes about questions such as baptism and salvation demonstrate the existence of profound divisions within the Protestant missionary movement. Ambiguous relations, and at times serious conflicts, between rival mission societies were a perennial feature of evangelical expansion and multiplied in the manifold areas where missionaries operated.[56]

In West Africa, the Basel missionaries always operated in a complex setting, obliged to deal with religious competitors, regional authorities, various colonial agencies and military bodies, European planters, African traders, their own trading company and the highly diversified population, who were sometimes helpful but just as often indifferent or actively hostile to their efforts. These groups had a decisive impact on the way missionary strategies and evangelical ideals were enacted on a daily basis.[57] While it is impossible to follow all of these trajectories in depth, they must be taken into account in order to even comprehend that missionary policy and knowledge was a product of negotiations on the ground. A transregional perspective redirects our attention to the fact that globalisation is a much more complex and contradictory process than is often assumed.[58]

Notwithstanding the competitive nature of missionary endeavours, missionaries operated as brokers of knowledge in multiple directions between different physical localities as well as conceptual spaces that

---

[56] Andrew Porter, 'Cultural Imperialism' and Protestant Missionary Enterprise, 1780–1914, in: The Journal of Imperial and Commonwealth History 25 (1997) 3, p. 367–391, here p. 380.

[57] See for instance the insightful microhistory study by John Middleton, One Hundred and Fifty Years of Christianity in a Ghanaian Town, in: Africa 53 (1983) 3, p. 2–19.

[58] Ulrike Freitag and Achim von Oppen have put forward the concept of translocality to account for the diversity of Asian and African experiences and agency in the transformatory process often subsumed under the blanket term of globalisation. Translocality very consciously attempts to transcend the elitist focus of much of global history. Ulrike Freitag/Achim von Oppen, Introduction: 'Translocality'. An Approach to Connection and Transfer in Area Studies, in: ibid. (eds.), Translocality. The Study of Globalising Processes from a Southern Perspective, Leiden 2010, p. 1–24.

reached beyond religious frameworks.[59] The Basel Mission generated and circulated knowledge across the globe, increased transregional connectivity and promoted globalised concepts of belonging through their diverse media. The expansion in print culture, the movement of people and the rise of civil society broadened the evangelical public sphere, allowing for evangelicalism to become a genuine but unstable global community.[60] Since globality is very much a mediated experience, it is crucial to keep in mind that a whole string of people, some of them almost invisible, contributed to the laborious fashioning of global narratives.[61]

2.2.2   Grassroots Movement

Soon after the founding of the Basel Mission in 1815, the Committee members decided to diversify the society's financial basis beyond their own class. The strategy was to reach down the social strata to tap the zeal and steady generosity of ordinary believers by opening regional bureaus. These auxiliary societies, called *Hilfsvereine*, were to organise reading circles and propagate mission literature such as the Basel Mission's official publications *Der Evangelische Heidenbote* and *Evangelisches Missionsmagazin*. They also took on sponsorships for mission contenders and collected money for their education at the seminary in Basel. Originating from the Wurttemberg area, these *Hilfsvereine* rapidly spread across the Swiss and German Confederations.[62]

By the end of the nineteenth century, auxiliary societies for the Basel Mission had emerged in Baden, Alsace, Strasbourg, the Rhineland and every major Swiss town. These official societies, closely related to the

---

[59] Abigail Green/Vincent Viaene, Rethinking Religion and Globalization, in: ibid. (eds.), Religious Internationals in the Modern World. Globalization and Faith Communities since 1750, Basingstoke 2012, p. 1–19; Egger/Gugglberger, Editorial.

[60] Christopher Clark/Michael Ledger-Lomas, The Protestant International, in: Abigail Green/Vincent Viaene (eds.), Religious Internationals in the Modern World. Globalization and Faith Communities since 1750, Basingstoke 2012, p. 23–52.

[61] Richard Hölzl has introduced the concept of "imperial communication work" to analyse the complex processes through which missionary narratives were created. See Richard Hölzl, Imperiale Kommunikationsarbeit. Zur medialen Rahmung von Mission im 19. und 20. Jahrhundert, in: medien&zeit 31 (2016) 2, p. 3–17.

[62] By 1819, the Basel Mission could count on the backing of 15 societies, which not only pledged their general support but also guaranteed the training costs of 28 pupils. See Eiselen, "Zur Erziehung einer zuverlässigen, wohldisziplinierten Streiterschar", p. 50.

headquarters in Basel, however, were only one type of organisation among many groups engaged in securing moral and financial support for the mission overseas. Numerous other less formal associations, clubs and societies existed next to the officially recognised support groups.[63] The term "*Vereine*"—associations—referred to subordinate auxiliaries of the Basel Mission as well as organisationally independent societies. Tens of thousands of devout Christians—many of them women—performed evangelical grassroots work by distributing missionary magazines, raising funds and organising mission services.[64]

Donations by Basel's economic elite and financial pledges by the London Missionary Society had guaranteed the Basel Mission's early years but, as time went on, they did not continue to be the society's principal source of financing. Of course, Committee members and their families sometimes contributed large sums to the Basel Mission. They backed the creation of an imposing mission house in Basel, which still serves as the society's headquarters today, by funding the purchase of a plot of land and the erection of buildings. Other wealthy and well-placed individuals, who remained outside the immediate leadership group, often supported specific causes and activities, such as the establishment of mission stations in certain areas that were of interest to them. These donations, however, did not constitute a steady and diversified source of income, which is why the Committee members were desperately looking for an alternative.[65]

For this purpose, Karl Sarasin, a silk manufacturer, member of the City Council, the *GGG*, the City Mission and the Basel Mission Committee, initiated the so-called *Halbbatzen-Kollekte*—halfpenny collection—in the early 1850s.[66] He started collecting five Swiss centimes—a *halben Batzen*—from his domestic staff and workers in his silk factories as a

---

[63] Schlatter, Die Geschichte der Basler Mission, vol. 1, p. 38–57.

[64] Simone Prodolliet, Wider die Schamlosigkeit und das Elend der heidnischen Weiber. Die Basler Frauenmission und der Export des europäischen Frauenideals in die Kolonien, Zürich 1987, p. 14–15.

[65] Miller, Missionary Zeal, p. 43–45.

[66] On Karl Sarasin, see Josef Mooser, Der "christliche Unternehmer" Karl Sarasin. Sozialer Protestantismus in der Schweiz und in Deutschland, 1860–1880, in: Thomas K. Kuhn/Martin Sallmann (eds.), Das "fromme Basel". Religion in einer Stadt des 19. Jahrhunderts, Basel 2002, p. 73–92; Marcel Köppli, Protestantische Unternehmer in der Schweiz des 19. Jahrhunderts. Christlicher Patriarchalismus im Zeitalter der Industrialisierung, Zürich 2012, p. 111–158; Schär, Tropenliebe, p. 66–78.

donation to the Basel Mission on a weekly basis.[67] Soon after Sarasin's initiative, the Committee founded a specialised society for the *Halbbatzen-Kollekte* with district treasurers who supervised the collectors. In adopting this strategy, the Basel Mission followed earlier experiences by British missions, such as the Church Missionary Society in London. The halfpenny collection turned out to be a highly profitable financial tool: over 40,000 people donated a total of 68,583 Swiss francs in the first year in 1855.[68]

The *Halbbatzen-Kollekte* rapidly expanded beyond the city of Basel into the Alemannic countryside and became one of the main financing sources for the Mission. By 1880, the annual revenue summed up to 268,271 Swiss francs and in 1905 it reached 450,000 Swiss francs, generating more than fourteen million Swiss francs in the first fifty years of its existence. The number of individual people donating to the halfpenny collection grew from around 75,000 in the 1860s to over 165,000 donors in 1905.[69] In 1913, it raised 602,021 Swiss francs, outperforming the revenue of the Basel Mission Trading Company by 60,000 Swiss francs, despite the concurrent cacao boom. It was so successful that the generated surpluses could be invested at interest and held in reserve against future needs.[70]

More importantly, the *Halbbatzen-Kollekte* illustrates that the Basel Mission fostered social entanglements and emotional ties that reached beyond institutional networks. By contributing five centimes weekly, donors in Europe—among them many women and children from the lower strata of society—actively participated in the mission in West Africa. In return, they received the *Kollekteblättli*, a booklet that offered vivid depictions of missionary work abroad. They also witnessed the impact of their regular contributions by listening to itinerant preachers or missionaries on home leave, by watching a magic lantern show or by visiting a mission exhibition. The halfpenny collection "provided an opportunity

---

[67] On the history of the Halbbatzen-Kollekte, see Beatrice Tschudi-Barbatti, Die Halbbatzen-Kollekte. Ein Kapitel aus der Finanzgeschichte der Basler Mission, Licentiate Thesis, University of Zurich, 1992.

[68] Schlatter, Geschichte der Basler Mission, vol. 1, p. 224.

[69] Tschudi-Barbatti, Die Halbbatzen-Kollekte, p. 112–119.

[70] Schlatter, Geschichte der Basler Mission, vol. 1, p. 335; Miller, Missionary Zeal, p. 44; Eiselen, "Zur Erziehung einer zuverlässigen, wohldisziplinierten Streiterschar", p. 53–54.

for the poor to achieve great things by giving regular, small bounties," as Wilhelm Schlatter phrased it in the official chronicle of the Basel Mission in 1916.[71]

The Basel Mission, and indeed the nineteenth-century missionary movement more generally, enjoyed social approval and financial support across many levels of European societies.[72] Studies about the Wurttemberg region have shown that the Pietist movement did not claim a majority of the members of any class as adherents but actually appealed to individuals from all social backgrounds.[73] Despite securing support across society, the actual mode of participation in the Basel Mission by people from different classes was quite disparate. While the leadership consisted of members from privileged families, most missionaries carrying out the day-to-day work of evangelism came from modest backgrounds. The majority of the pupils, who entered the Basel Mission seminary, were craftsmen, peasants and tradesmen, and had no university training, in contrast to the bourgeois and academic Committee members. This social disparity was believed to strengthen the hierarchical discipline at the heart of the organisation.[74]

Although the leaders and the rank and file of the Basel Mission occupied widely different positions in the social hierarchies of the time, they shared a common Pietist culture, in which mission was defined as a male enterprise, dominated by paternal authority at its core, with the expectation that male missionaries would duplicate that authority in the Christian communities they established abroad. Women were not included in seminary training and ordination, and those single women and wives who became involved in missionary work in West Africa were from a slightly higher social level than the ordinary male evangelists.[75] Over the course

[71] Schlatter, Geschichte der Basler Mission, vol. 1, p. 223.

[72] Lionel Gossman argued that the Basel Mission "was the expression of religious fervor of wide pietistic circles throughout Germany and Switzerland and it enjoyed broad support among all classes in Basel." Gossman, Basel in the Age of Burckhardt, p. 57.

[73] Martin Scharfe, Die Religion des Volkes. Kleine Kultur- und Sozialgeschichte des Pietismus, Gütersloh 1980, p. 136; Mary Fulbrook, Piety and Politics: Religion and the Rise of Absolutism in England, Württemberg and Prussia, Cambridge 1984, p. 36–40.

[74] Miller, Missionary Zeal, p. 35–45.

[75] Line Nyhagen Predelli/Jon Miller, Piety and Patriarchy: Contested Gender Regimes in Nineteenth-Century Evangelical Missions, in: Mary Taylor Huber/Nancy C. Lutkehaus

of the nineteenth century, however, women came to assume unprecedented importance for the Basel Mission and the missionary movement more broadly, as both protagonists and targets of evangelical missionary efforts.

2.2.3   Women and Children on a Mission

The Basel Mission held on to the ideal of the male celibate missionary until 1837, when it permitted employees to marry, yet continued to be reluctant towards female agency in the field. Despite the fact that piety and patriarchy remained interwoven principles in the governance of the Basel Mission, the attempts to preserve patriarchal domination were always limited by the material indispensability of women's participation. The great majority of the people collecting the weekly contributions for the *Halbbatzen-Kollekte* were women and girls from modest backgrounds, whose commitment was acknowledged anonymously in the Basel Mission's popular publications.[76] On the occasion of the 50th jubilee of the halfpenny collection, the editor of *Der Evangelische Heidenbote* wrote:

> And who names them all, the diligent contributors and tens of thousands of faithful female collectors in the city and in the countryside, some of which toured tirelessly for decades, often in deep snow for hours, from farm to farm, in order to beamingly bring the collected contributions to the district treasurer! Poor girls, who often lacked basic necessities themselves, have thereby over the years scraped together hundreds of francs for the mission.[77]

Women formed the backbone of the Basel Mission. The Committee considered collecting donations to be an intensely personal affair in which

---

(eds.), Gendered Missions. Women and Men in Missionary Discourse and Practice, Ann Arbor 1999, p. 67–112, here p. 73.

[76] Bernhard C. Schär, Philanthropie postkolonial. Macht und Mitleid zwischen der Schweiz und Indien, 1850–1900, in: Alix Heiniger/Sonja Matter/Stéphanie Ginalski (eds.), Die Schweiz und die Philanthropie. Reform, soziale Vulnerabilität und Macht (1850–1930), Basel 2017, p. 127–140.

[77] Hans Anstein, Das Jubiläum der Halbbatzenkollekte, in: Der Evangelische Heidenbote 78 (1905), p. 9.

women's maternal powers of persuasion over society's weaker beings—children, other women, and especially the lower classes—were believed to stand them in good stead. Approximately 28 per cent of the Basel Mission's yearly income was generated through the halfpenny collection throughout the second half of the nineteenth century.[78] The fact that women's involvement was largely confined to the more behind-the-scenes tasks, such as collecting subscriptions door-to-door or sewing goods for sale at missionary bazaars, has obscured just how important their financial and moral support was for the evangelical missionary movement.[79]

Women had taken on an active role in the Pietist movement since the eighteenth century by organising and attending *Erbauungsstunden*—edification or devotional hours—and by participating in Bible societies and support groups for mission societies. The *Deutsche Christentumsgesellschaft*, which gave birth to the Basel Mission, was an organisation of laypeople that was open to both men and women from the onset in 1780. While organised female voluntary work was a relatively recent phenomenon within Protestantism around 1800, Catholic female congregations had attended to the indigent and ill for centuries. Protestant activists, from the Napoleonic wars onwards, began to see them as a model to emulate, best exemplified by the resurgence of the deaconessate ministry model.[80]

The German Lutheran pastor Theodor Fliedner, one of the leading figures of the nineteenth-century Protestant awakening, who was in contact with evangelicals throughout Europe, created the first Order and

---

[78] Anke Schürer-Ries, Die Sammlerinnen und Sammler für die Balser Mission, in: Christine Christ-von Wedel/Thomas K. Kuhn (eds.), Basler Mission. Menschen, Geschichte, Perspektiven 1815–2015, Basel 2015, p. 99–100, here p. 99.

[79] For Britain, historians such as Susan Thorne and Jeffrey Cox have assessed that "the foreign mission cause was very probably the largest mass movement of women" and that "the missionary enterprise was predominantly female." Thorne, Congregational Missions and the Making of an Imperial Culture in Nineteenth-Century England, p. 94; Jeffrey Cox, Global Christianity in the Contact Zone, in: Judith Becker (ed.), European Missions in Contact Zones: Transformation Through Interaction in a (Post-)Colonial World, Göttingen 2015, p. 27–44, here p. 31.

[80] Karen Nolte, "Local Missionaries". Community Deaconesses in Early 19th Century Health Care, in: Martin Dinges/Robert Jütte (eds.), The Transmission of Health Practices (c. 1500 to 2000), Stuttgart 2011, p. 105–116; Catherine M. Prelinger, The Nineteenth-Century Deaconessate in Germany. The Efficacy of a Family Model, in: Ruth Ellen B. Joeres/Mary Jo Manyes (eds.), Germany Women in the Eighteenth and Nineteenth Centuries, Bloomington 1986, p. 215–229.

Institute of Deaconesses in Kaiserswerth, Prussia, in 1836, together with his wife Friederike. In the spirit of "motherhood as a profession," the idea was to train single women in either nursing or education as a means of re-Christianising society. The Kaiserswerth deaconessate, however, did not remain an institution of the *Innere Mission* exclusively. From the 1840s, it started sending out single women overseas who could act with relatively little male interference. It was via the home mission, therefore, that evangelical women in German-speaking areas carved out a space for themselves in mission-related work. Over the second half of nineteenth century, more and more women actively and publicly participated in institutions of Christian charity, health care and mission.[81]

The first women to get involved in the Basel Mission abroad were missionary wives who worked alongside their missionary husbands.[82] The Committee released a marriage statute in 1837, which stipulated that missionaries were allowed to request permission to marry once they had spent two years in their mission fields.[83] They could either suggest a suitable candidate themselves or ask the Committee to find a potential wife. Approximately 300 women married a Basel missionary overseas between 1837 and 1914.[84] Most of them did not know their future husbands personally—apart from a single photograph—when they left the European continent and embarked on the journey to join and marry them in India, China or West Africa.

Officially, missionary wives were helpers of their husbands. In reality, however, their tasks went far beyond that of a housewife and mother.

---

[81] In her insightful study on the work and life of Kaiserswerth deaconesses in late Ottoman Beirut, Julia Hauser has shown that "the concept of spiritual motherhood allowed them to transgress the sphere of domesticity even while remaining within its boundaries on a metaphoric level." Hauser, German Religious Women in Late Ottoman Beirut, p. 325.

[82] Dagmar Konrad, Missionsbräute. Pietistinnen des 19. Jahrhunderts in der Basler Mission, Münster 2001.

[83] Waltraud Haas, Erlitten und erstritten. Der Befreiungsweg von Frauen in der Basler Mission 1816–1966, Basel 1994, p. 25; Judith Becker, Frauen in der Mission und Mädchenschulen, in: Christine Christ-von Wedel/Thomas K. Kuhn (eds.), Basler Mission. Menschen, Geschichte, Perspektiven 1815–2015, Basel 2015, p. 57–62, here p. 57; Konrad, Missionsbräute, p. 34.

[84] Dagmar Konrad, Im Dienst des Herrn: Schweizer Missionarsfamilien des 19. Jahrhunderts in Übersee, in: Christine Christ-von Wedel/Thomas K. Kuhn (eds.), Basler Mission. Menschen, Geschichte, Perspektiven 1815–2015, Basel 2015, p. 63–68, here p. 64.

They were deeply involved in the health care of the mission community, in itself a stressful and time-consuming activity. Furthermore, they directed the girls' schools, taught home economics and handiwork classes, and visited women in surrounding villages, together with African Bible women, to introduce them to the gospel.[85] It was increasingly difficult for them to practically fulfil all of these duties. When their husbands became fully aware of their burden, they asked the leadership in Basel to send out single women to share their labour and, in particular, to focus on the education and religious instruction of African women.[86]

Gender was central to the Basel Mission in West Africa, for women were believed to hold the key to opening heathen hearts to the civilising influence of Christian love.[87] Basel was the first Protestant mission society in continental Europe to explicitly engage in the project of a women's mission in 1841, followed by Berlin a year later.[88] In contrast to the burgeoning British women's missions, however, the Basel women's mission proceeded at a very slow pace. For most of the nineteenth century, the leadership in Basel considered single female missionaries to be more of a challenge than a solution. Eventually, their number slowly increased from the 1880s, leading to the foundation of the Association for Women's Mission—*Verein für Frauenmission*—in 1901.[89] The Committee for Women's Mission consisted of ten female members, all related to male Committee members.[90]

In the early twentieth century, 151 missionary wives and only 11 single women worked as teachers and nurses for the Basel Mission

---

[85] On the role of Bible women in the Basel Mission in India, see Mrinalini Sebastian, Reading Archives from a Postcolonial Feminist Perspective: "Native" Bible Women and the Missionary Ideal, in: Journal of Feminist Studies in Religion 19 (2003) 1, p. 5–25.

[86] Predelli/Miller, Piety and Patriarchy, p. 81.

[87] Prodolliet, Wider die Schamlosigkeit; Ulrike Sill, Encounters in Quest of Christian Womanhood: The Basel Mission in Pre- and Early Colonial Ghana, Leiden/Boston 2010.

[88] Inspired by initiatives in England, the Basel Mission's second Inspector Friedrich Wilhelm Hoffmann founded the *Frauenverein zur Erziehung des weiblichen Geschlechts in den Heidenländern*—Society for the Education of the Female Gender in the Heathen Lands—in 1841.

[89] Schlatter, Geschichte der Basler Mission, vol. 1, p. 384. For further developments, see Christine Keim, Frauenmission und Frauenemanzipation. Eine Diskussion in der Basler Mission im Kontext der frühen ökumenischen Bewegung (1901–1928), Münster 2005.

[90] Haas, Erlitten und Erstritten, p. 58.

abroad.[91] Despite Basel's early attempts to send out unmarried female missionaries, the Pietist family model ultimately formed the core of the civilising project. Considered to be the most important place of religious socialisation or "the true Church," the Pietist family served as a role model located at the interface of private and public life, which ought to convey the ideal of Christian marriage and child-rearing practices to West African communities. The Basel missionaries argued that their own children contributed to the esteem and acceptance of the Basel Mission in Cameroon and on the Gold Coast, claiming that abundance of offspring was a major signal of social and cultural prestige in West Africa.[92]

Children and youth were equally important for the mission community at home. By singing in missionary choirs, collecting offerings for the *Kindermissionskollekte*—children's mission collection—and selling evangelical publications, they contributed significantly to the Basel Mission's success.[93] While boys created handicrafts in all-male youth missionary associations, girls participated in so-called *Jungfrauenvereine*—maiden associations—and sewed goods for fundraising events. The Basel leadership placed great importance on anchoring the mission among the young generation. Missionaries on home leave and itinerant preachers regularly attended Sunday schools to give lectures, show images and demonstrate objects originating from Africa, since Sunday schools were believed to provide a convenient setting to capture children's attention and curiosity.[94]

---

[91] Susanne Wille, Dienen, kämpfen, beten: Die ersten unverheirateten Schwestern im Dienst der Basler Mission an der Goldküste 1857–1917, Licentiate Thesis, University of Zurich, 2001, p. 18.

[92] The children born to Basel missionaries abroad were sent back to Switzerland once they had reached school age. Between 1853 and 1914, more than 1,200 mission children had to separate from their parents overseas and migrate to the mission's children's house in Basel. Dagmar Konrad, Schweizer Missionskinder des 19. Jahrhunderts, in: Schweizerische Gesellschaft für Wirtschafts- und Sozialgeschichte 29 (2015), p. 163–185, here p. 164; Konrad, Im Dienst des Herrn, p. 66.

[93] Zusammenfassung der Referate. Reisepredigerkonferenz in Freudenstadt 1910, BMA, QH-14.1.

[94] Patrick Harries, Dompter les sauvages domestiques. Le rôle de l'Afrique dans les Écoles du dimanche en Suisse romande, 1860–1920, in: Sandra Bott/Thomas David/Claude Lutzelschwab/Janick Marina Schaufelbuehl (eds.), Suisse—Afrique (18e–20e siècles): De la traite des Noirs à la fin du régime de l'apartheid/Schweiz—Afrika (18.–20. Jahrhundert): Vom Sklavenhandel zum Ende des Apartheid-Regimes, Münster 2005, p. 227–246.

2.2.4 Beyond the City

The Basel Mission emerged at the initiative of the Pietist *Deutsche Christentumsgesellschaft* during the nineteenth-century evangelical revival in Europe. Wealthy and influential patrician families from Basel favoured the establishment of a mission seminary in the city on the Rhine but the Basel Mission rapidly evolved into a grassroots movement. Thanks to the fervent support of associations and support groups, and a wide-ranging publication network, the Basel Mission was not only firmly anchored in urban society but also found numerous supporters in the Alemannic countryside. The Pietist movement retained particular strength in the villages and small towns of southern Germany.[95] While patrician men from the city of Basel dominated the Committee, more than half of the overseas staff, all the Inspectors and most of the theology lecturers in the Basel Mission seminary were recruited from the Wurttemberg area before 1914.[96]

Members of voluntary societies anchored the foreign mission within local contexts by organising bazaars, festivals and exhibitions dedicated to the evangelising cause abroad.[97] The young men who would go on to become Basel missionaries frequently attended these events. The first Basel Mission doctor Rudolf Fisch, for example, was initially introduced to the mission as a teenager when he attended a Basel Mission festival in the Swiss town of Suhr in October of 1873. He vividly recounted the event in his memoirs: "The thought of heathen mission bathed my future in a bright, hopeful light."[98] Upon completing his apprenticeship as a

---

[95] Eckhard Hagedorn, Nur eine "Schwabenkaserne"? Die Bedeutung der Basler Mission für den deutschen Südwesten, in: Uri Robert Kaufmann (ed.), Die Schweiz und der deutsche Südwesten. Wahrnehmung, Nähe und Distanz im 19. und 20. Jahrhundert, Ostfildern 2006, p. 97–108.

[96] Paul Jenkins, The Basel Mission in West Africa and the Idea of the Christian Village Community, in: Godwin Shiri (ed.), Wholeness in Christ. The Legacy of the Basel Mission in India, Mangalore 1985, p. 13–25, here p. 18.

[97] As Karolin Wetjen and Rebekka Habermas have shown for Central and Northern Germany, smaller towns and villages learnt about the colonies from missionaries and, in particular, from what contemporaries called "mission friends", who supported the numerous informal as well as officially recognised mission associations. Karolin Wetjen, Das Globale im Lokalen: Die Unterstützung der Äusseren Mission im ländlichen lutherischen Protestantismus um 1900, Göttingen 2013; Habermas, Colonies in the Countryside.

[98] Rudolf Fisch, Self-composed CV until 1911, p. 3, BMA, Personal File Rudolf Fisch BV 985.

saddler in the summer of 1874, Fisch attended another Basel Mission festival in Rothrist, where he witnessed the account of a missionary from the Gold Coast that deeply impressed him. The missionary talked about Paulo Mohenu, a "notorious fetish priest" who had converted to Christianity. Years later, Fisch would care for the old Paulo Mohenu in his final days in Aburi on the Gold Coast.[99]

Fisch applied to join the Basel Mission seminary as soon as he turned eighteen and started his missionary training in August of 1875, together with another twenty-two young men, most of whom were peasants and artisans originating from Wurttemberg.[100] The Committee favoured a homogenous group of pupils, believing that uniformity in beliefs, education and experience contributed to the predictability and efficiency of training.[101] Their education took a minimum of five years to complete, and included Latin, Greek, Hebrew, English, German, medicine, arithmetic, geometry, physics, geography, history, pedagogics, anthropology, Bible classes and catechism.[102] Considering the seminary's extensive curriculum and the position of missionaries as Europeans in colonial territories, the missionary profession certainly presented students with the prospect of climbing the social ladder.[103]

Representatives from the industrial working class of large urban areas were notably absent in the seminary. They were nonetheless part of the web of mission; either by donating to the halfpenny collection, or as objects of philanthropic activities. The Christian welfare network connected the bourgeois and academic elite, who were directing the Basel Mission, with both urban blue-collar workers and Pietist rural communities. The Basel Mission created horizontal as well as vertical entanglements between people and groups of different class, gender, denomination and location. Certainly, the highly diverse coalition that provided the moral and financial underpinning of the Basel Mission did not share identical

---

[99] Ibid., p. 3–4; Rudolf Fisch, Letter to Committee, 03.07.1886, BMA, D-1.45.6.

[100] Fisch, Self-composed CV until 1911, p. 4–5.

[101] Miller, Missionary Zeal, p. 45–54.

[102] Curricula of the evangelical missionary school, in: Seminar BM, Studienpläne und Reformvorschläge, BMA, QS-03.07.

[103] According to Christraud Geary, most Basel missionaries in Cameroon came from the peasantry or old *Mittelstand* and were "upwardly mobile and education-minded." Christraud M. Geary, Impressions of the African Past: Interpreting Ethnographic Photographs from Cameroon, in: Visual Anthropology 3 (1990) 3, p. 289–315, here p. 296.

interests or expectations with the decision-makers at the headquarters in Basel but the meshing of their worldviews was sufficient to keep them together for over a century of common effort.

In contrast to earlier missionary organisations, which depended on nobility and royal patronage, missionary societies emerging in the nineteenth century were voluntary organisations, funded by small donations from a large number of people. Both their outreach and their organisation depended on a new social geography and understanding of theology.[104] Purity was a key element of Pietist faith and practice, which allowed the Basel Mission to create and strengthen a sense of community in their circle of supporters. The leading figures of the Pietist movement justified their evangelising fervour by arguing that the Reformation had not been completed. According to them, too much emphasis had been placed upon purity of doctrine rather than upon purity of life, which led many people, who lived in conscious sin, to depend upon the merits of Christ for salvation.[105]

2.3   PURITY, HEALING AND DEATH

Purity is an eminently religious concept, which in almost all faiths is aimed at indicating the proximity or distance of humans from God, thus also marking moral and social differences between people.[106] Pietists asserted that what set them apart from the rest of society, which they dismissively called "the world," was their practical approach to purity.[107] Purity in

---

[104] Susan Thorne, Religion and Empire at Home, in: Catherine Hall/Sonya O. Rose (eds.), At Home with Empire. Metropolitan Culture and the Imperial World, Cambridge 2006, p. 143–165, here p. 148–149.

[105] David Crowner/Gerald Christianson, General Introduction, in: ibid. (eds.), The Spirituality of the German Awakening, Mahwah 2003, p. 5–41, here p. 10–14.; Gerhard Härle, Reinheit der Sprache, des Herzens und des Leibes. Zur Wirkungsgeschichte des rhetorischen Begriffs *puritas* in Deutschland von der Reformation bis zur Aufklärung, Tübingen 1996, p. 99–126.

[106] Mary Douglas, Purity and Danger. An Analysis of Concepts of Pollution and Taboo, London/New York 1966; Härle, Reinheit der Sprache, des Herzens und des Leibes; Peter Burschel/Christoph Marx (eds.), Reinheit. Veröffentlichungen des Instituts für Historische Anthropologie, Wien/Köln/Weimar, Böhlau 2011; Andrew Brower Latz/Arseny Ermakov (eds.), Purity: Essays in Bible and Theology, Eugene 2014; Valentin Groebner, Wer redet von der Reinheit? Eine kleine Begriffsgeschichte, Wien 2019.

[107] Hartmut Lehmann, Absonderung und neue Gemeinschaft, in: ibid (ed.), Geschichte des Pietismus, vol. 4: Glaubenswelt und Lebenswelten, Göttingen 2004, p. 488–497.

the Pietist sense of the word was a universal concept, not only encompassing theological tenets but also social norms and cultural practices that outranked church life or confessional purity. Pietism was characterised by an unusual measure of "worldly asceticism," as Max Weber noted over a century ago.[108] It offered a holistic ideology, strongly based on ideas of purity and sin, which manifested itself in a specific attitude towards the body, healing and death.

2.3.1   Pietist Purity

One of the few remaining textbooks in the Basel Mission archives is Friedrich Reiff's *Die christliche Glaubenslehre als Grundlage der christlichen Weltanschauung*.[109] Reiff was the Basel Mission's head theology teacher and member of the Committee from 1864 to 1875.[110] His 1873 publication in two volumes provides a systematic summary of the theological tenets conveyed in the Basel Mission seminary. The heart took centre stage in the Pietist narrative of sin and purity, as Reiff's manual illustrates. He defined sin as "the abandonment of God caused by selfishness and the orientation towards worldly affairs, which are glorified instead of Him."[111] The only effective way to counteract sinful behaviour, according to Reiff, was to recognise the inherent sinfulness of one's heart, since it constituted "truly the actual moral-religious organ."[112]

---

[108] Weber interpreted this as a precondition for the formation of a capitalistic spirit and the genesis of the modern world. See Max Weber, Die Protestantische Ethik und der "Geist" des Kapitalismus, in: Archiv für Sozialwissenschaft und Sozialpolitik 20 (1904), p. 1–54; Ibid., Die Protestantische Ethik und der "Geist" des Kapitalismus, in: Archiv für Sozialwissenschaft und Sozialpolitik 21 (1905), p. 1–110. For a similar argument, see Ernst Troeltsch, Die Soziallehren der christlichen Kirchen und Gruppen. Gesammelte Schriften, vol. 1, Tübingen 1912, p. 773–789; 827–835; 918–926. On Weber's interpretation of Pietism, see Hartmut Lehmann, Max Webers Pietismusinterpretation, in: ibid. (ed.), Max Webers "Protestantische Ethik". Beiträge aus der Sicht eines Historikers, Göttingen 1996, p. 50–65.

[109] Friedrich Reiff, Die christliche Glaubenslehre als Grundlage der christlichen Weltanschauung, 2 vol., Basel 1873.

[110] Julia Ulrike Mack, Menschenbilder. Anthropologische Konzepte und stereotype Vorstellungen vom Menschen in der Publizistik der Basler Mission 1816–1914, Zürich 2013, p. 91–92.

[111] Reiff, Die christliche Glaubenslehre, vol. 2, p. 79.

[112] Ibid., vol. 1, p. 438.

Pietists were noted for an intense emotional fervour that began with a personal conversion experience or "spiritual rebirth," as they called it.[113] All believers had to testify to this fundamental change, which after a deep recognition of sin had led them to repent by making a unique and final decision to submit to God. Pietists attached great importance to self-examination as the path to the divine. They believed that moral consciousness originated in the heart and thus emphasised the need to educate the heart through close reading of Scripture and individual piety. To be a born-again Christian meant living a life of ceaseless self-awareness, constantly striving for improvement and betterment in both the spiritual and material realms. Yet, as might be expected, Pietist conversions were in reality often more varied, complex and problematic than in theory.[114]

Pietist conversion not only entailed an internal spiritual rebirth but also went hand in hand with an external transformation encompassing all aspects of life, away from old worldly habits into a vigorous Christian life that expressed itself through asceticism, discipline and social deeds.[115] Pietists upheld the importance of "loyalty in small things" and rejected what they considered unchristian impulses and behaviour such as aggression, sexuality, passion, indulgence, insults and curses, pub visits, the consumption of spirits and gambling. These practices of renunciation were a means for Pietists to give visible, outward expression to their spiritual ideal of purity. By displaying a shared code of conduct, Pietists expressed community affiliation and distanced themselves from the perceived impurity in the world. Purity regulations kept things apart and marked them as incompatible.[116]

[113] As Hartmut Lehmann has expounded, the full meaning of specific Pietist words such as "spiritual rebirth" or "God's Kingdom" is difficult to evaluate. Hartmut Lehmann, Einführung, in: ibid. (ed.), Geschichte des Pietismus, vol. 4: Glaubenswelt und Lebenswelten, Göttingen 2004, p. 1–18, here p. 9.

[114] Jonathan Strom, German Pietism and the Problem of Conversion, University Park, Pennsylvania 2018; Judith Becker, Conversio im Wandel. Basler Missionare zwischen Europa und Südindien und die Ausbildung einer Kontaktreligiosität, 1834–1860, Göttingen 2015.

[115] Markus Matthias, Bekehrung und Wiedergeburt, in: Hartmut Lehmann (ed.), Geschichte des Pietismus, vol. 4: Glaubenswelt und Lebenswelten, Göttingen 2004, p. 49–79.

[116] Maria Lugones, Purity, Impurity, and Separation, in: Signs 19 (1994) 2, p. 458–479; Angelika Malinar/Martin Vöhler, Einleitung: Un/Reinheit. Konzepte und Praktiken

In everyday life, however, purity practices were constantly at risk of being ignored, diluted and compromised. To prevent this, the maintenance of Pietist purity crucially relied on rigid social ethics, discernible in the organisational structure of the Basel Mission, which reproduced the patriarchal hierarchy of Pietist families and communities.[117] The Committee members justified their right to occupy the centre and to prevail over the organisation's affairs on the grounds that they had been directly called by God to create and control the organisation.[118] They believed that the agrarian Pietist background of most mission candidates made them amenable to hierarchical discipline and thus served God's plan. The personal qualifications that governed admission and life in the Basel Mission seminary reveal the premium that was placed on the acceptance of authority as something religiously and organisationally indispensable.[119]

Pietist purity expressed itself, among other ways, in readiness to obey established authority. The decisive criterion for acceptance to the Basel Mission seminary was a candidate's convincing account of spiritual rebirth that signalled complete emotional surrender to the larger Pietist cause. In the Committee's eyes, a true Christian, and therefore suitable mission contender, was not merely a baptised person but a born-again individual, who recognised their inherent sinfulness and their dependency on God's grace. Applicants had to describe the exact moment of their own conversion and the authenticity of the account had to be confirmed by a witness, usually the candidate's own local minister, who was known to the Basel Mission.[120] Practices of self-examination were a vital component of Pietist

im Kulturvergleich, in: ibid. (eds.), Un/Reinheit. Konzepte und Praktiken im Kulturvergleich, Paderborn 2009, p. 9–18.

[117] Miller, Missionary Zeal, p. 54–60.

[118] Eiselen, "Zur Erziehung einer zuverlässigen, wohldisziplinierten Streiterschar", p. 49.

[119] Plan der neuen Gestaltung der Hausordnung des Missionshauses in Basel, Mai 1860, BMA, Q-9.31; Verordnungen über die persönliche Stellung der Missionare, Basel 1886, BMA, Q-9.21.7; Haus-Ordnung der evangelischen Missions-Anstalt zu Basel, Basel 1888, BMA, X.III.12; Hausordnung der evangelischen Missions-Anstalt zu Basel, Basel 1912, BMA, X.III.12a.

[120] Miller, Missionary Zeal, p. 94.

faith. Whether openly dialogical or solitary, introspection was by no means a private affair but always shared within the community.[121]

Pietists corresponded, sometimes over great distances, with spiritual friends and leaders, and kept diaries, which they shared during edification assemblies and devotional hours.[122] By publicly confessing an awareness of their own sins and exhibiting an earnest desire for sanctification, through diaries and correspondences, they affirmed their membership in the Pietist community. The autobiographies written by the young men who wished to join the Basel Mission seminary show that many of them were familiar with the use of devotional literature and practices of pious introspection.[123] They often contrasted their own spiritual rebirth with drunkenness, laziness, disobedience, personal vanity and petty theft in the world around them. Entering the seminary and becoming an active and committed Christian meant turning one's back on such temptations and living a life under the discipline and mutual criticism of Pietist fellowship.[124]

In the period from 1880 to 1914, between 30 and 80 men applied for a place at the Basel Mission seminary each year, of which between 14 and 25 were admitted as pupils.[125] The Committee cited a lack of "moral integrity" and "divine vocation" as the most common reasons for turning down applicants.[126] Those who did gain entry to the boarding school were subject to a detailed set of strict house rules, which stipulated order, abstinence and thrift. Purity, health and cleanliness were explicitly linked in these guidelines, with each pupil required "to wash his body diligently, in order to keep it pure and healthy."[127] The rigid regulations,

---

[121] On the Protestant tradition of introspection from the Reformation to Pietism, see Hölscher, Geschichte der protestantischen Frömmigkeit in Deutschland, p. 65, 68–72, 76.

[122] Gleixner, Pietismus und Bürgertum, p. 124–145.

[123] On the basic narrative patterns of Pietist autobiographic writing, see Magnus Schlette, Die Selbst(er)findung des Neuen Menschen. Zur Entstehung narrativer Identitätsmuster im Pietismus, Göttingen 2005.

[124] Jenkins, The Basel Mission in West Africa and the Idea of the Christian Village Community.

[125] Schlatter, Geschichte der Basler Mission, vol. 1, p. 346.

[126] Eiselen, "Zur Erziehung einer zuverlässigen, wohldisziplinierten Streiterschar", p. 57–58.

[127] Haus-Ordnung der evangelischen Missions-Anstalt zu Basel, Basel 1888, p. 8, BMA, X.III.12.

including a meticulous daily timetable, dress code and severe sanctions in case of lapses, posed a major challenge to the mission contenders. Only about a third of them completed their training.[128] Purity regulations were a means for the leaders of the Basel Mission to create a sense of belonging by drawing lines of inclusion and exclusion.

In her classic 1966 study *Purity and Danger*, Mary Douglas showed that concepts of purity were never merely expressions of experience but also instruments to systematise perceptions and synchronise them within a community. She applied Emile Durkheim's arguments about the distinctiveness of the sacred and the profane in order to explore the system of boundary maintenance that ensured the purity of social categories through the exclusion of objects and people that did not belong.[129] Purity is the utopian dream of precision in cognitive organisation. While the properties of purity remain elusive, the consequences of impurity are more concrete and elaborated in detail. Concepts of purity thus become particularly effective in contrast to impurity.[130]

2.3.2   Healing and Deliverance Theology

The meaning of purity for the Basel Mission gained another layer of complexity with the appropriation of scientific medicine and the training of medical missionaries in the 1880s. Although healing had been part of Pietism ever since the movement gained momentum, most adherents had reservations about the morality and efficacy of scientific medicine.[131] In the early nineteenth century, a strand of Pietism had emerged, led by Christian Blumhardt, which explained the existence of illness as well as antisocial or immoral behaviour with reference to Satan. Blumhardt focused on the liberation of the sick from the Devil and established the

---

[128] Eiselen, "Zur Erziehung einer zuverlässigen, wohldisziplinierten Streiterschar", p. 68–69. Also see Josef Haller, Das Leben im Basler Missionshaus, Basel 1897.

[129] Douglas, Purity and Danger.

[130] They are what Reinhart Koselleck called "asymmetrical antonyms"—binary terms with a universal claim—conceived to exclude mutual recognition. Reinhart Koselleck, Vergangene Zukunft. Zur Semantik geschichtlicher Zeiten, Frankfurt a. M. 1989.

[131] On the healing tradition in Wurttemberg Pietism, see Katharina Ernst, Krankheit und Heilung. Die medikale Kultur der württembergischen Pietisten im 18. Jahrhundert, Stuttgart 2013.

first systematic healing theology in Wurttemberg.[132] His healing and deliverance ministry was not an isolated phenomenon within Pietism but an example of a much wider practice throughout Germany and Switzerland in the nineteenth century.[133]

Even more significant than Christian Blumhardt to the development of Pietist healing concepts and practices was his nephew, Johann Blumhardt, who became the most important healing and deliverance practitioner in Wurttemberg in the mid-nineteenth century.[134] Thousands of believers visited him annually in healing pilgrimages, which flourished from the 1840s until his death. Blumhardt viewed healing as a purely supernatural process and strongly questioned the effectiveness of scientific means of restoration.[135] The tension between his healing ministry and the medical establishment was exacerbated when the medical community successfully lobbied church authorities to prevent Johann Blumhardt from performing Pietist healing rituals, such as laying on hands and praying for the afflicted, in his parish in 1846.[136]

Mission and healing were both significant aspects of Pietism. Bad Boll, where Johann Blumhardt relocated in 1852, became the centre of healing,

---

[132] These themes within Christian Blumhardt's theology of healing and deliverance can be traced back to the earlier works of Friedrich Christoph Oetinger and even earlier to writings of Johann Albrecht Bengel. But neither Oetinger nor Bengel put healing and deliverance at the centre of their theology as Christian Blumhardt did.

[133] Another major figure from Blumhardt's era whose name was closely associated with him was Dorothea Trudel. Between 1851 and 1856 Trudel opened two healing homes in Mannedorf in the canton of Zurich to care for the sick. See Johann Christoph Blumhardt, Die Heilung von Kranken durch Glaubensgebet. Mit Zeugnissen aus der Gegenwart, 2nd ed., Leipzig 1924, p. 71–76.

[134] Frank D. MacChia, Spirituality and Social Liberation. The Message of the Blumhardts in the Light of Wuerttemberg Pietism, Metuchen 1993; Dieter Ising, Johann Christoph Blumhardt. Leben und Werk, Göttingen 2002; Christoffer H. Grundmann, "Jesus ist Sieger!" Heilungen im Wirken des Pfarrers Johann Christoph Blumhardt (1805–1880), in: Irmtraut Sahmland/Hans-Jürgen Schrader (eds.), Medizin- und kulturgeschichtliche Konnexe des Pietismus. Heilkunst und Ethik, arkane Traditionen, Musik, Literatur und Sprache, Göttingen 2016, p. 235–251.

[135] Johann Christoph Blumhardt, Krankheit und Heilung an Leib und Seele. Auszüge aus Briefen, Tagebüchern und Schriften, ed. by Dieter Ising, Leipzig 2014.

[136] Daniel J. Koehler, Pilgrimage of Protestants. Miracles and Religious Community in J. C. Blumhardt's Württemberg, 1840–1880, in: Michael Geyer/Lucian Hölscher (eds.), Die Gegenwart Gottes in der modernen Gesellschaft. Transzendenz und religiöse Vergemeinschaftung in Deutschland, Göttingen 2006, p. 60–85, here p. 75.

whilst Basel developed as the hub of missionary activities.[137] Many figures in the Pietist movement, such as Johann and Christian Blumhardt, participated in both of these spheres. Christian Blumhardt was one of the founding members of the Basel Mission and the first Inspector from 1815 until his death in 1838. His nephew Johann Blumhardt worked at the mission seminary from 1830 to 1837, teaching Hebrew, mathematics, physics and chemistry. After leaving Basel to work as a healing and deliverance theologian, he remained closely attached to the Mission.[138]

Medical staff were part of the earliest Pietist evangelising projects overseas. The Tranquebar mission to India—a joint venture established in 1706 between Pietists from Halle, Danish reformed circles and the Anglican Society for Promoting Christian Knowledge—included medical practitioners. Likewise, the Pietist *Herrnhuter Brüdergemeine*—Moravian Church—dispatched orderlies to Western India, Ceylon and Astrakhan from 1735.[139] The Basel Mission first employed a medical man in 1822, who practised in the Caucasus region for nine years.[140] The first medical practitioner working for the Basel Mission in West Africa was Christian Friedrich Heinze. He arrived on the Gold Coast in 1831, after the loss of

[137] Richard Toellner, Medizin und Pharmazie, in: Hartmut Lehmann (ed.), Geschichte des Pietismus, vol. 4: Glaubenswelt und Lebenswelten, Göttingen 2004, p. 332–356, here p. 346.

[138] Blumhardt collected weekly offerings for the Basel Mission every Saturday evening at Bad Boll. He was a frequent speaker at mission festivals, informed various congregations of the work of the mission, wrote a handbook about its history and maintained close contact with missionaries throughout his life.

[139] Christoffer H. Grundmann, Pietism, Revivalism, and Medical Missions. The Concern for the Corporeality of Salvation in A. H. Francke, P. Parker, and G. Dowontt, in: Christian T. Collins Winn et al. (eds.), The Pietist Impulse in Christianity, Eugene 2011, p. 296–306; Ibid., Von der caritas in missionibus zur ärztlichen Mission—Ein Gang durch die Frühgeschichte missionsärztlicher Arbeit in Übersee unter besonderer Berücksichtigung Halles, in: Richard Toellner (ed.), Die Geburt einer sanften Medizin. Die Franckeschen Stiftungen zu Halle als Begegnungsstätte von Medizin und Pietismus im frühen 18. Jahrhundert, Halle 2004, p. 124–140; Toellner, Medizin und Pharmazie, p. 348.

[140] For Rudolf Friedrich Hohenacker's personal file, see BMA, BV 0019.

the entire initial batch of four missionaries there. Ironically, he succumbed to what was referred to as "the fever" within six weeks of his arrival.[141]

Medicine became an increasingly materialistic concept during the course of the nineteenth century, questioning the tenets of spiritual healing. While the link between Pietist healing, medical aid and missionary endeavours overseas had existed from the start, the use of scientific medicine—that is the conceptualisation and treatment of the body as a biological organism that could be scientifically understood—remained taboo for most of the nineteenth century. After the death of Heinze, the Committee refrained from employing medical staff since they feared that medical science would undermine their holistic approach to healing. They recognised, nevertheless, that medical knowledge was crucial to the survival of the missionaries in the field. They integrated basic medical notions and practices into missionary training, without at the same time giving up on their religious holism or subscribing to the scientific view of the body held by the medical community.[142]

From 1845, all mission contenders were given medical lectures that followed Pietist tenets of healing as part of their five-year course at the seminary in Basel.[143] Carl Streckeisen, the general practitioner of the institution, provided the lessons, which included "healing," "pastoral medicine" and "clinic," meaning the teaching of students at the bedside.[144] Streckeisen also arranged for portable pharmacies and medical boxes to be sent to the mission stations abroad. They contained technical literature, drugs and medical instruments such as "bloodletting fleams" and "cupping glasses."[145] The medical procedures, which the missionaries had acquired during their formation in Basel, however, proved generally

[141] Marion Baschin, "[...] und war ein Stück Grümpel mehr im Lande". Die gescheiterten Versuche einer homöopathischen Ausbildung für Missionare der Basler Mission, in: Robert Jütte (ed.), Medizin, Gesellschaft und Geschichte. Jahrbuch des Instituts für Geschichte der Medizin der Robert Bosch Stiftung, vol. 29, Stuttgart 2011, p. 229–274, here p. 242; Friedrich Hermann Fischer, Der Missionsarzt Rudolf Fisch und die Anfänge medizinischer Arbeit der Basler Mission an der Goldküste (Ghana), Herzogenrath 1991, p. 27; Schlatter, Geschichte der Basler Mission, vol. 3, p. 26.

[142] On the relationship between Christianity, healing and scientific medicine, see Amanda Porterfield, Healing in the History of Christianity, Oxford 2005.

[143] Fischer, Der Missionsarzt Rudolf Fisch, p. 110; Schlatter, Geschichte der Basler Mission, vol. 1, p. 29.

[144] Medizinischer Unterricht, in: Lehrfächer 1864–1907, BMA, QS-3.18.4.

[145] Schlatter, Geschichte der Basler Mission, vol. 1, p. 375.

ineffective and oftentimes even harmful when applied during their stays in West Africa. Moreover, there was never enough medicine to meet the needs of the missionaries and the people they sought to serve with these supplies.

2.3.3   Deadly Mission

"Tropical fevers," the Basel missionaries on the Gold Coast lamented in 1838, had cost them eight out of ten lives in the first decade of their enterprise. Throughout the eighteenth and nineteenth centuries, what the missionaries referred to as "tropical fevers" represented a large variety of diseases that Europeans dreaded when venturing into the tropics. Death was omnipresent and continued to threaten the existence of the Basel Mission in West Africa into the twentieth century.[146] Missionary Karl Stolz commented on the passing of his friend Ferdinand Ernst in Cameroon in 1910: "This is Africa! We are dying while greeting each other. Tonight, we bury one of us and tomorrow morning we are receiving another one."[147] The Basel missionaries' conviction in their divine mission and their Pietist faith resulted in an apparent outward resilience to grief and misfortunes.

While suffering and death certainly fed missionary narratives of martyrdom and sacrifice, the high mortality rate also meant that Africans were unlikely to view European missionaries and their medicine as inherently superior. In 1870, the Basel missionary Elias Schrenk, stationed in Christiansborg, addressed a request for a scientifically trained mission doctor to the Committee, stating: "We lack the charisma of biblical healing, we also lack scientific medicine, we cannot treat seriously ill people with good conscience, therefore we must solicit for a doctor."[148] Schrenk explicitly expressed what many Basel missionaries on the Gold Coast perceived as a frustrating period for the mission. Their letters and reports show that they regularly felt overwhelmed and helpless against the diseases they encountered, fearing not only for their own health but

---

[146] 141 missionaries and their wives died on the Gold Coast between 1828 and 1913, not counting children. See Jenkins, A Short History of the Basel Mission, p. 6.

[147] Karl Hauss, Der Pionier der Balimission. Aus dem Leben von Ferdinand Ernst, Basel 1910, p. 41.

[148] Elias Schrenk, Request for a mission doctor, Christiansborg, 24.11.1870, BMA, D-1.22a.50.

also deploring that it undermined their credibility in the eyes of potential converts.

The Committee received numerous requests for the dispatch of a mission doctor from missionaries on the Gold Coast, based on three main arguments. Firstly, the missionaries emphasised that a medical missionary would be able to provide vital medical care to the members of the missionary community in a centrally located sanatorium.[149] Hitherto, the Basel missionaries relied on the health services provided by the colonial government in Christiansborg and on the skills of African medical men. They were always acutely conscious of their lack of training for the medical work they found so necessary. The specialised books in the medical boxes, for instance, proved useless since they required prior medical training that the missionaries did not possess. Therefore, they solicited the employment of a mission doctor, who would be able to counteract the high mortality rate among them, which lay around fifty per cent in the mid-nineteenth century.[150]

Secondly, the letters highlighted the exploration of tropical diseases, especially the different types of fevers, as an important assignment. Interestingly, they also encouraged the study of certain West African remedies since they had experienced their efficacy first-hand.[151] The letters written by Basel missionaries on the Gold Coast, particularly before the 1880s, show that they had an open mind about African concepts and methods of healing. They often preferred African over European remedies, believing that they were more suitable for local diseases than the medicine available at colonial health facilities. People on the Gold Coast, in turn, took kindly to the Basel missionaries' healing practices, since they showed many similarities with their own. Laxatives made from Glauber salt, which the missionaries brought with them, for example, proved highly popular since bowel cleansing was an important bodily practice on the Gold Coast.[152]

---

[149] Johann Gottlieb Christaller, Letter to Committee, Akropong, 01.09.1866, BMA, D-1.18b.10.

[150] Christoph Wilhelm Locher, Letter to Committee, Christiansborg, March 1863, BMA, D-1.13b.84; Johann Georg Widmann, Letter to Committee, Akropong, 06.11.1843, BMA, D-1.2.11.

[151] Johann Adam Mader, Letter to Committee, Akropong, 27.06.1865, BMA, D-1.17.4.

[152] Johannes Christian Dieterle, Letter to Committee, Akropong, 21.05.1849, BMA, D-1.3.17; Charles Alexander Gordon, Some Observations on Medicine and Surgery as

Thirdly, the Basel missionaries in West Africa stressed the potential of mission medicine as a tool of conversion. They argued that by combining the effectiveness of scientific medicine with the narrative of biblical healing, people on the Gold Coast could be persuaded of the superiority of Christian medicine and faith. They noticed that members of their parishes often found themselves drawn back to what they called "witch doctors" when their remedies proved ineffective against their ills.[153] Mission medicine, in their eyes, offered a way of demonstrating the validity of Christian explanations and methods. Historians, however, have debated how effective medicine was as a tool of conversion because, for much of the nineteenth century, it was not obviously more effective than African systems of healing.[154]

The British government physician Francis J. G. Gunn, who was stationed on the Gold Coast from 1863 to 1865, lent substance to the Basel missionaries' appeals for a medical missionary. In a letter to the Committee in 1865, he regretted that missionaries were placed in medical charge "who really must be acting in total darkness and therefore destroying as often as saving life."[155] Gunn affronted the leadership in Basel by asking: "Who are the murderers in the sight of God: the staff members who have been deployed improperly or the society that has placed them in this uncomfortable situation?"[156] Confronted with these allegations, the Inspector of the Basel Mission at the time, Joseph Josenhans, pointed at the social make-up of the mission pupils, most of

Practised by the Natives of the Portion of the West Coast of Africa, in: Edinburgh Medical Journal 2 (1856/1857), p. 529–537, here p. 532; Hermann Vortisch, Statistik und Bericht über das erste Halbjahr 1904 der ärztlichen Mission auf der Goldküste, in: Archiv für Schiffs- und Tropenhygiene 9 (1905), p. 346–354, here p. 352; Rudolf Fisch, Über die Darmparasiten der Goldküstenneger, in: Archiv für Schiffs- und Tropenhygiene 12 (1908), p. 711–718, here p. 712.

[153] Elias Schrenk, Request for a mission doctor, Christiansborg 24.11.1870, BMA, D-1.22a.50.

[154] Vaughan, Curing Their Ills; Hunt, A Colonial Lexicon of Birth Ritual, Medicalization and Mobility in the Congo; White, Speaking with Vampires; Worboys, Colonial and Imperial Medicine; Livingston, Debility and the Modern Imagination in Botswana.

[155] Francis J. G. Gunn, Letter to Committee, Abokobi, 15.05.1865, BMA, D-1.17.11.

[156] Ibid.

whom did not have an academic formation. He expounded that integrating a training programme for scientific doctors into the seminary was
too formidable a challenge, both organisationally and financially.[157]

Why not then, as Gunn suggested, recruit a medical man connected
with the Basel Mission?[158] Indeed, an opportunity had arisen in 1845
when Streckeisen, the medical teacher in the seminary, asked to be sent to
the Gold Coast "to promote the gospel among the Negroes by means of
medical help."[159] The Committee acknowledged that he was "a serious,
favourable, altruistic man" but refused to send him overseas doubting
that he was "actually converted."[160] Streckeisen's request was treated
with suspicion as to his true motivations and ambitions. The leaders in
Basel feared that his medical work would outshine the overriding aim of
their work in West Africa, the salvation of souls. Since Streckeisen had not
officially testified to his spiritual rebirth or undergone the close scrutiny
of training and life in the seminary, they were not willing to take this risk.

More importantly, the employment of an academically qualified physician endangered the social hierarchy within the Basel Mission. According
to a Committee report dating from 1873, the decision-makers in Basel
feared that the "autonomous nature and decision-making ability of
academically trained doctors" would undermine their authority.[161] As
a result of this, mission contenders interested in medical work were
asked to choose between their missionary vocation and a medical career,
which generally resulted in their exclusion from the Basel Mission.[162]
Furthermore, incorporating university graduates, mostly people from the
urban middle and upper classes, into the missionary enterprise would
have undermined the Committee's recruitment strategy, which was based
on finding amenable candidates from a homogenous rural background,
skilled in crafts, agriculture and construction.

The African General Conference, consisting of Basel missionaries based
in West Africa, actively supported Gunn's demand, pointing inter alia

---

[157] Fischer, Der Missionsarzt Rudolf Fisch, p. 109–112.

[158] Frances J. G. Gunn, Letter to Committee, Abokobi 15.05.1865, BMA, D-1.17.11.

[159] Committee report, 12.11.1845, BMA, Komitee-Protokoll 1845, §531.

[160] Ibid., 18.11.1846, BMA, Komitee-Protokoll 1846, §572.

[161] Ibid., 15.01.1873, BMA, Komitee-Protokoll 1873, §27.

[162] Fischer, Der Missionsarzt Rudolf Fisch, p. 111; Schlatter, Die Geschichte der Basler
Mission, vol. 1, p. 233.

at the prohibitive prices of British colonial and military doctors. Their conference proceedings presented manifold arguments for the sending of a medical missionary, including his contribution to the sciences, his financial autonomy, the medical education and training of Africans, the fight against "quackery" and the "enhancement of European medicine with African medicinal herbs."[163] In his response to the African General Conference in 1865, Inspector Josenhans maintained, nonetheless, that healing was primarily a spiritual matter:

> Be patient, my dear brothers! Although it is true that a capable physician provides better care than an incapable one, the LORD alone is the right physician; those who are as close to Him as you missionaries should trust in His special help and certainly feel confident that, despite the lack of a capable physician at your side, you will not miss out on anything essential, now or in eternity.[164]

In West Africa, however, the primacy of saving souls over healing bodies seemed displaced. Clearly, the success of the Basel Mission crucially depended on the survival of the missionaries in the field. By the 1880s, Pietist healing had been considerably depreciated by the growing persuasiveness and effectiveness of scientific theories, practices and technologies, leaving the leaders of the Basel Mission no choice but to integrate the training and methods of scientific medicine into their evangelising project. Continuous missionary work was simply inconceivable without effective health care. The Basel missionaries' confrontation with the pervasive problem of illness and death in West Africa laid the foundation for the reformulation of Pietist concepts of healing and purity by exposing them to scientific theories of disease and hygiene.

---

[163] Schlatter, Die Geschichte der Basler Mission, vol. 3, p. 187.

[164] Jospeh Josenhans, Letter to Christoph Wilhelm Locher, 18.09.1865, BMA, D-2.5, p. 72.

REFERENCES

Hans Anstein, Das Jubiläum der Halbbatzenkollekte, in: Der Evangelische Heidenbote 78 (1905), p. 9.

Hans Anstein, Fünfzig Jahre Stadt-Mission in Basel. Rückblick auf die Tätigkeit der Evangelischen Gesellschaft für Stadt-Mission in Basel in den Jahren 1859 bis 1909, Basel 1909.

Marion Baschin, "[…] und war ein Stück Grümpel mehr im Lande". Die gescheiterten Versuche einer homöopathischen Ausbildung für Missionare der Basler Mission, in: Robert Jütte (ed.), Medizin, Gesellschaft und Geschichte. Jahrbuch des Instituts für Geschichte der Medizin der Robert Bosch Stiftung, vol. 29, Stuttgart 2011, p. 229–274.

Judith Becker, "Gehet hin in alle Welt…". Sendungsbewusstsein in der evangelischen Missionsbewegung der ersten Hälfte des 19. Jahrhunderts, in: Evangelische Theologie 72 (2012) 2, p. 134–154.

Judith Becker, Zukunftserwartungen und Missionsimpetus bei Missionsgesellschaften in der ersten Hälfte des 19. Jahrhunderts, in: Wolfgang Breul/ Jan Carsten Schnurr (eds.), Geschichtsbewusstsein und Zukunftserwartungen in Pietismus und Erweckungsbewegung, Göttingen 2013, p. 244–270.

Judith Becker, Conversio im Wandel. Basler Missionare zwischen Europa und Südindien und die Ausbildung einer Kontaktreligiosität, 1834–1860, Göttingen 2015.

Judith Becker, Frauen in der Mission und Mädchenschulen, in: Christine Christ-von Wedel/Thomas K. Kuhn (eds.), Basler Mission. Menschen, Geschichte, Perspektiven 1815–2015, Basel 2015, p. 57–62.

Gustav Adolf Benrath, Die Erweckung innerhalb der deutschen Landeskirchen, in: Ulrich Gäbler (ed.), Geschichte des Pietismus, vol. 3: Der Pietismus im neunzehnten und zwanzigsten Jahrhundert, Göttingen 2000, p. 150–271.

Johann Christoph Blumhardt, Die Heilung von Kranken durch Glaubensgebet. Mit Zeugnissen aus der Gegenwart, 2nd ed., Leipzig 1924.

Johann Christoph Blumhardt, Krankheit und Heilung an Leib und Seele. Auszüge aus Briefen, Tagebüchern und Schriften, ed. by Dieter Ising, Leipzig 2014.

Irina Bossart, "Wuchern mit dem anvertrauten Pfunde" oder Krisenbewältigung durch Evangelisierung. Die Basler Stadtmission in der zweiten Hälfte des 19. Jahrhunderts, Doctoral Thesis, University of Basel, 2009.

Irina Bossart, 150 Jahre Basler Stadtmission. "… hervorgerufen durch den Ernst der Zeit", in: Basler Stadtbuch 130 (2009), ed. by Christoph Merian Stiftung, p. 143–145.

Martin Brecht/Friedrich de Boor/Klaus Deppermann/Harmut Lehmann/ Andreas Lindt/Johannes Wallmann (eds.), Die Basler Christentumsgesellschaft, Göttingen 1982.

Martin Brecht/Klaus Deppermann/Ulrich Gäbler/Hartmut Lehmann (eds.), Geschichte des Pietismus, 4 vol., Göttingen 1993–2004.

Peter Burschel/Christoph Marx (eds.), Reinheit. Veröffentlichungen des Instituts für Historische Anthropologie, Wien/Köln/Weimar, Böhlau 2011.

Heinrich Christ, Mission und Geld. Die Missions-Handlungs-Gesellschaft, in: Christine Christ-von Wedel/Thomas K. Kuhn (eds.), Basler Mission. Menschen, Geschichte, Perspektiven 1815–2015, Basel 2015, p. 93–98.

Heinrich Christ, Zwischen Religion und Geschäft. Die Basler Missions-Handlungs-Gesellschaft und ihre Unternehmensethik, 1859–1917, Basel 2015.

Christopher Clark/Michael Ledger-Lomas, The Protestant International, in: Abigail Green/Vincent Viaene (eds.), Religious Internationals in the Modern World. Globalization and Faith Communities since 1750, Basingstoke 2012, p. 23–52.

John Comaroff/Jean Comaroff, Of Revelation and Revolution, vol. 1: Christianity, Colonialism and Consciousness in South Africa, Chicago 1991.

Jeffrey Cox, Global Christianity in the Contact Zone, in: Judith Becker (ed.), European Missions in Contact Zones: Transformation Through Interaction in a (Post-)Colonial World, Göttingen 2015, p. 27–44.

David Crowner/Gerald Christianson, General Introduction, in: ibid. (eds.), The Spirituality of the German Awakening, Mahwah 2003, p. 5–41.

Justin A. Davis, Pietism and the Foundations of the Modern World, Eugene 2019.

Mary Douglas, Purity and Danger. An Analysis of Concepts of Pollution and Taboo, London/New York 1966.

Christine Egger/Martina Gugglberger, Editorial, in: ibid. (eds.), Missionsräume, in: Österreichische Zeitschrift für Geschichtswissenschaft 24 (2013) 2, p. 5–18.

Tobias Eiselen, "Zur Erziehung einer zuverlässigen, wohldisziplinierten Streiterschar für den Missionskrieg". Basler Missionarsausbildung im 19. Jahrhundert, in: Werner Ustorf (ed.), Mission im Kontext. Beiträge zur Sozialgeschichte der Norddeutschen Missionsgesellschaft im 19. Jahrhundert, Bremen 1986, p. 47–120.

Katharina Ernst, Krankheit und Heilung. Die medikale Kultur der württembergischen Pietisten im 18. Jahrhundert, Stuttgart 2013.

Matthäus Feigk, Von Edinburgh nach Oegstgeest. Die transnationalen missionarischen Netzwerke Europas am Beispiel der Basler Mission 1910–1920, in: Linda Ratschiller/Karolin Wetjen (eds.), Verflochtene Mission. Perspektiven auf eine neue Missionsgeschichte, Köln/Weimar/Wien 2018, p. 45–64.

Rudolf Fisch, Über die Darmparasiten der Goldküstenneger, in: Archiv für Schiffs- und Tropenhygiene 12 (1908), p. 711–718.

Friedrich Hermann Fischer, Der Missionsarzt Rudolf Fisch und die Anfänge medizinischer Arbeit der Basler Mission an der Goldküste (Ghana), Herzogenrath 1991.

Andrea Franc, Wie die Schweiz zur Schokolade kam. Der Kakaohandel der Basler Handelsgesellschaft mit der Kolonie Goldküste (1893–1960), Basel 2008.

Ulrike Freitag/Achim von Oppen, Introduction: 'Translocality'. An Approach to Connection and Transfer in Area Studies, in: ibid. (eds.), Translocality. The Study of Globalising Processes from a Southern Perspective, Leiden 2010, p. 1–24.

Norbert Friedrich/Traugott Jähnichen, Geschichte der sozialen Ideen im deutschen Protestantismus, in: Helga Grebing (ed.), Geschichte der sozialen Ideen in Deutschland. Sozialismus—katholische Soziallehre—protestantische Sozialethik. Ein Handbuch, 2nd ed., Wiesbaden 2005, p. 867–1102.

Mary Fulbrook, Piety and Politics: Religion and the Rise of Absolutism in England, Württemberg and Prussia, Cambridge 1984.

Christraud M. Geary, Impressions of the African Past: Interpreting Ethnographic Photographs from Cameroon, in: Visual Anthropology 3 (1990) 3, p. 289–315.

Alexa Geisthövel/Ute Siebert/Sonja Finkbeiner, "Menschenfischer". Über die Parallelen von äusserer und innerer Mission um 1900, in: Rolf Lindner (ed.), "Wer in den Osten geht, geht in ein anderes Land". Die Settlementbewegung in Berlin zwischen Kaiserreich und Weimarer Republik, Berlin 1997, p. 27–50.

Gesellschaft für das Gute und Gemeinnützige (ed.), Über die Fabrikarbeiter-Verhältnisse der Baseler Industrie. Berichterstattung einer von der Baselerischen Abteilung der Schweizerischen Gemeinnützigen Gesellschaft aufgestellten Kommission, Basel 1843.

Andreas Gestrich, Pietismus und ländliche Frömmigkeit in Württemberg im 18. und frühen 19. Jahrhundert, in: Norbert Haag/Sabine Holtz/Wolfgang Zimmermann/Dieter R. Bauer (eds.), Ländliche Frömmigkeit. Konfessionskulturen und Lebenswelten, Stuttgart 2002, p. 343–357.

Michael Gladwin, Mission and Colonialism, in: Joel D. S. Rasmussen/Judith Wolfe/Johannes Zachhuber (eds.), The Oxford Handbook of Nineteenth-Century Christian Thought, Oxford 2017, p. 282–304.

Ulrike Gleixner, Pietismus und Bürgertum. Eine historische Anthropologie der Frömmigkeit, Göttingen 2005.

Charles Alexander Gordon, Some Observations on Medicine and Surgery as Practised by the Natives of the Portion of the West Coast of Africa, in: Edinburgh Medical Journal 2 (1856/1857), p. 529–537.

Lionel Gossman, Basel in the Age of Burckhardt: A Study in Unseasonable Ideas, Chicago 2000.

Arnd Götzelmann, Die Soziale Frage, in: Ulrich Gäbler (ed.), Geschichte des Pietismus, vol. 3: Der Pietismus im neunzehnten und zwanzigsten Jahrhundert, Göttingen 2000, p. 272–307.

Abigail Green/Vincent Viaene, Rethinking Religion and Globalization, in: ibid. (eds.), Religious Internationals in the Modern World. Globalization and Faith Communities since 1750, Basingstoke 2012, p. 1–19.

Valentin Groebner, Wer redet von der Reinheit? Eine kleine Begriffsgeschichte, Wien 2019.

Christoffer H. Grundmann, Von der caritas in missionibus zur ärztlichen Mission—Ein Gang durch die Frühgeschichte missionsärztlicher Arbeit in Übersee unter besonderer Berücksichtigung Halles, in: Richard Toellner (ed.), Die Geburt einer sanften Medizin. Die Franckeschen Stiftungen zu Halle als Begegnungsstätte von Medizin und Pietismus im frühen 18. Jahrhundert, Halle 2004, p. 124–140

Christoffer H. Grundmann, Pietism, Revivalism, and Medical Missions. The Concern for the Corporeality of Salvation in A. H. Francke, P. Parker, and G. Dowontt, in: Christian T. Collins Winn et al. (eds.), The Pietist Impulse in Christianity, Eugene 2011, p. 296–306.

Christoffer H. Grundmann, "Jesus ist Sieger!" Heilungen im Wirken des Pfarrers Johann Christoph Blumhardt (1805–1880), in: Irmtraut Sahmland/ Hans-Jürgen Schrader (eds.), Medizin- und kulturgeschichtliche Konnexe des Pietismus. Heilkunst und Ethik, arkane Traditionen, Musik, Literatur und Sprache, Göttingen 2016, p. 235–251.

Waltraud Haas, Erlitten und erstritten. Der Befreiungsweg von Frauen in der Basler Mission 1816–1966, Basel 1994.

Rebekka Habermas, Mission im 19. Jahrhundert. Globale Netze des Religiösen, in: Historische Zeitschrift 287 (2008) 3, p. 629–679.

Rebekka Habermas, Colonies in the Countryside: Doing Mission in Imperial Germany, in: Journal of Social History 50 (2017), p. 502–517.

Eckhard Hagedorn, Nur eine "Schwabenkaserne"? Die Bedeutung der Basler Mission für den deutschen Südwesten, in: Uri Robert Kaufmann (ed.), Die Schweiz und der deutsche Südwesten. Wahrnehmung, Nähe und Distanz im 19. und 20. Jahrhundert, Ostfildern 2006, p. 97–108.

Josef Haller, Das Leben im Basler Missionshaus, Basel 1897.

Gerhard Härle, Reinheit der Sprache, des Herzens und des Leibes. Zur Wirkungsgeschichte des rhetorischen Begriffs puritas in Deutschland von der Reformation bis zur Aufklärung, Tübingen 1996.

Patrick Harries, Dompter les sauvages domestiques. Le rôle de l'Afrique dans les Écoles du dimanche en Suisse romande, 1860–1920, in: Sandra Bott/ Thomas David/Claude Lutzelschwab/Janick Marina Schaufelbuehl (eds.), Suisse—Afrique (18e–20e siècles): De la traite des Noirs à la fin du régime de l'apartheid/Schweiz—Afrika (18.–20. Jahrhundert): Vom Sklavenhandel zum Ende des Apartheid-Regimes, Münster 2005, p. 227–246.

Ernst Hauri, Die Evangelische Gesellschaft für Stadtmission in Basel. Kurze Darstellung ihrer Entwicklung von 1859–1959, Basel 1959.

Julia Hauser, German Religious Women in Late Ottoman Beirut. Competing Missions, Leiden 2015.

Karl Hauss, Der Pionier der Balimission. Aus dem Leben von Ferdinand Ernst, Basel 1910.

Hans Hauzenberger, Basel und die Bibel. Die Bibel als Quelle ökumenischer, missionarischer, sozialer und pädagogischer Impulse in der ersten Hälfte des 19. Jahrhunderts, Basel 1996.

Erika Hebeisen, Leidenschaftlich fromm. Die pietistische Bewegung in Basel 1750–1830, Köln/Weimar/Wien 2005.

Urs Hofmann, "Nur das Evangelium vermag die soziale Frage zu lösen". Die reformierte Kirche und die Armenpolitik im 19. und frühen 20. Jahrhundert, in: Josef Mooser/Simon Wenger (eds.), Armut und Fürsorge in Basel. Armutspolitik vom 13. Jahrhundert bis heute, Basel 2011, p. 134–142.

Lucian Hölscher, Geschichte der protestantischen Frömmigkeit in Deutschland, München 2005.

Richard Hölzl, Imperiale Kommunikationsarbeit. Zur medialen Rahmung von Mission im 19. und 20. Jahrhundert, in: medien&zeit 31 (2016) 2, p. 3–17.

Nancy Rose Hunt, A Colonial Lexicon of Birth Ritual, Medicalization and Mobility in the Congo, Durham 1999.

Dieter Ising, Johann Christoph Blumhardt. Leben und Werk, Göttingen 2002.

Sara Janner, Korporative und private Wohltätigkeit. "Stadtgemeinde" und Stadtbürgertum als Träger der Armenpflege im 19. Jahrhundert, in: Josef Mooser/Simon Wenger (eds.), Armut und Fürsorge in Basel. Armutspolitik vom 13. Jahrhundert bis heute, Basel 2011, p. 101–109.

Sara Janner, Zwischen Machtanspruch und Autoritätsverlust. Zur Funktion von Religion und Kirchlichkeit in Politik und Selbstverständnis des konservativen alten Bürgertums im Basel des 19. Jahrhunderts, Basel 2012.

Sara Janner, GGG 1777–1914. Basler Stadtgeschichte im Spiegel der "Gesellschaft für das Gute und Gemeinnützige", Basel 2015.

Paul Jenkins, The Basel Mission in West Africa and the Idea of the Christian Village Community, in: Godwin Shiri (ed.), Wholeness in Christ. The Legacy of the Basel Mission in India, Mangalore 1985, p. 13–25.

Paul Jenkins, Short History of the Basel Mission, Basel 1989.

Paul Jenkins, Württemberg als Hauptsäule der historischen Basler Mission—transregionale Erwägungen über Entwicklungen bis 1914, in: Blätter für württembergische Kirchengeschichte 116 (2016), p. 29–54.

Christine Keim, Frauenmission und Frauenemanzipation. Eine Diskussion in der Basler Mission im Kontext der frühen ökumenischen Bewegung (1901–1928), Münster 2005.

Andrew Kloes, The German Awakening: Protestant Renewal after the Enlightenment, 1815–1848, Oxford 2020.

Daniel J. Koehler, Pilgrimage of Protestants. Miracles and Religious Community in J. C. Blumhardt's Württemberg, 1840–1880, in: Michael Geyer/Lucian Hölscher (eds.), Die Gegenwart Gottes in der modernen Gesellschaft. Transzendenz und religiöse Vergemeinschaftung in Deutschland, Göttingen 2006, p. 60–85.

Dagmar Konrad, Missionsbräute. Pietistinnen des 19. Jahrhunderts in der Basler Mission, Münster 2001.

Dagmar Konrad, Im Dienst des Herrn: Schweizer Missionarsfamilien des 19. Jahrhunderts in Übersee, in: Christine Christ-von Wedel/Thomas K. Kuhn (eds.), Basler Mission. Menschen, Geschichte, Perspektiven 1815–2015, Basel 2015, p. 63–68.

Dagmar Konrad, Schweizer Missionskinder des 19. Jahrhunderts, in: Schweizerische Gesellschaft für Wirtschafts- und Sozialgeschichte 29 (2015), p. 163–185.

Marcel Köppli, Protestantische Unternehmer in der Schweiz des 19. Jahrhunderts. Christlicher Patriarchalismus im Zeitalter der Industrialisierung, Zürich 2012.

Reinhart Koselleck, Vergangene Zukunft. Zur Semantik geschichtlicher Zeiten, Frankfurt a. M. 1989.

Thomas K. Kuhn, Religion und neuzeitliche Gesellschaft. Studien zum sozialen und diakonischen Handeln in Pietismus, Aufklärung und Erweckungsbewegung, Tübingen 2003.

Thomas K. Kuhn/Veronika Albrecht-Birkner (eds.), Zwischen Aufklärung und Moderne: Erweckungsbewegungen als historiographische Herausforderung, Berlin 2017.

Thomas K. Kuhn/Martin Sallmann (eds.), Das "fromme Basel". Religion in einer Stadt des 19. Jahrhunderts, Basel 2002.

Andrew Brower Latz/Arseny Ermakov (eds.), Purity: Essays in Bible and Theology, Eugene 2014.

Hartmut Lehmann, Pietismus und weltliche Ordnung in Württemberg vom 17. bis zum 20. Jahrhundert, Stuttgart 1969.

Hartmut Lehmann, Max Webers Pietismusinterpretation, in: ibid. (ed.), Max Webers "Protestantische Ethik". Beiträge aus der Sicht eines Historikers, Göttingen 1996, p. 50–65.

Hartmut Lehmann, Engerer, weiterer und erweiterter Pietismusbegriff, in: Pietismus und Neuzeit 29 (2003), p. 18–37.

Hartmut Lehmann, Einführung, in: ibid. (ed.), Geschichte des Pietismus, vol. 4: Glaubenswelt und Lebenswelten, Göttingen 2004, p. 1–18.

Hartmut Lehmann, Absonderung und neue Gemeinschaft, in: ibid (ed.), Geschichte des Pietismus, vol 4: Glaubenswelt und Lebenswelten, Göttingen 2004, p. 488–497.

Martin Lengwiler, Wissenschaft und Sozialpolitik. Der Einfluss von Gelehrtengesellschaften und Experten auf die Sozialpolitik im 19. Jarhundert, in: Josef Mooser/Simon Wenger (eds.), Armut und Fürsorge in Basel. Armutspolitik vom 13. Jahrhundert bis heute, Basel 2011, p. 111–122.

Julie Livingston, Debility and the Modern Imagination in Botswana, Bloomington 2005.

Maria Lugones, Purity, Impurity, and Separation, in: Signs 19 (1994) 2, p. 458–479.

Frank D. MacChia, Spirituality and Social Liberation. The Message of the Blumhardts in the Light of Wuerttemberg Pietism, Metuchen 1993.

Julia Ulrike Mack, Menschenbilder. Anthropologische Konzepte und stereotype Vorstellungen vom Menschen in der Publizistik der Basler Mission 1816–1914, Zürich 2013.

Angelika Malinar/Martin Vöhler, Einleitung: Un/Reinheit. Konzepte und Praktiken im Kulturvergleich, in: ibid (eds.), Un/Reinheit. Konzepte und Praktiken im Kulturvergleich, Paderborn 2009, p. 9–18.

Matthias Manz, Basel. Von der Helvetik bis zur Kantonstrennung (1798–1833), in: Historisches Lexikon der Schweiz, https://hls-dhs-dss.ch/de/articles/007387/2016-01-13/#HVonderHelvetikbiszurKantonstrennung281798-183329, version 13.01.2016 (last access: 22.07.2022).

Markus Matthias, Bekehrung und Wiedergeburt, in: Hartmut Lehmann (ed.), Geschichte des Pietismus, vol. 4: Glaubenswelt und Lebenswelten, Göttingen 2004, p. 49–79.

John Middleton, One Hundred and Fifty Years of Christianity in a Ghanaian Town, in: Africa 53 (1983) 3, p. 2–19.

Giorgio Miescher, Hermann Ludwig Rottmann. Zu den Anfängen der Basler Missions-Handels-Gesellschaft in Christiansborg (Ghana), in: Lilo Roost Vischer/Anne Mayor/Dag Henrichsen (eds.), Werkschau Afrikastudien, vol. 2: Brücken und Grenzen, Münster 1999, p. 345–362.

Jon Miller, Missionary Zeal and Institutional Control. Organizational Contradictions in the Basel Mission on the Gold Coast, 1828–1917, London/New York 2003.

Josef Mooser, Der "christliche Unternehmer" Karl Sarasin. Sozialer Protestantismus in der Schweiz und in Deutschland, 1860–1880, in: Thomas K. Kuhn/Martin Sallmann (eds.), Das "fromme Basel". Religion in einer Stadt des 19. Jahrhunderts, Basel 2002, p. 73–92

Josef Mooser, Armenpflege zwischen Freiwilligkeit und Verstaatlichung. Träger und Reformen der Armenpolitik im Umbruch zur Grossstadt um 1900, in: ibid./Simon Wenger (eds.), Armut und Fürsorge in Basel. Armutspolitik vom 13. Jahrhundert bis heute, Basel 2011, p. 177–204.

Karen Nolte, "Local Missionaries". Community Deaconesses in Early 19th Century Health Care, in: Martin Dinges/Robert Jütte (eds.), The Transmission of Health Practices (c. 1500 to 2000), Stuttgart 2011, p. 105–116.

Claudia Opitz, Von der Aufklärung zur Kantonstrennung, in: Georg Kreis/Beat von Wartburg (eds.), Basel. Geschichte einer städtischen Gesellschaft, Basel 2000, p. 150–185.

Albert Ostertag, Jahresbericht der Stadtmission vom 1. April 1868, Basel 1869.

Martin W. Pernet, Nietzsche und das "fromme" Basel, Basel 2014.

Andrew Porter, 'Cultural Imperialism' and Protestant Missionary Enterprise, 1780–1914, in: The Journal of Imperial and Commonwealth History 25 (1997) 3, 367–391.

Amanda Porterfield, Healing in the History of Christianity, Oxford 2005.

Line Nyhagen Predelli/Jon Miller, Piety and Patriarchy: Contested Gender Regimes in Nineteenth-Century Evangelical Missions, in: Mary Taylor Huber/Nancy C. Lutkehaus (eds.), Gendered Missions. Women and Men in Missionary Discourse and Practice, Ann Arbor 1999, p. 67–112.

Catherine M. Prelinger, The Nineteenth-Century Deaconessate in Germany. The Efficacy of a Family Model, in: Ruth Ellen B. Joeres/Mary Jo Manyes (eds.), Germany Women in the Eighteenth and Nineteenth Centuries, Bloomington 1986, p. 215–229.

Simone Prodolliet, Wider die Schamlosigkeit und das Elend der heidnischen Weiber. Die Basler Frauenmission und der Export des europäischen Frauenideals in die Kolonien, Zürich 1987.

Alexandra Przyrembel, Der Missionar Johann Hinrich Wichern, die Sünde und das unabänderliche Elend der städtischen Unterschichten um 1850, in: WerkstattGeschichte 57 (2011), p. 53–67.

Friedrich Reiff, Die christliche Glaubenslehre als Grundlage der christlichen Weltanschauung, vol. 2, Basel 1873.

Karl Rennstich, Mission—Geschichte der protestantischen Mission in Deutschland, in: Ulrich Gäbler (ed.), Geschichte des Pietismus, vol. 3: Der Pietismus im neunzehnten und zwanzigsten Jahrhundert, Göttingen 2000, p. 308–319.

Dana L. Robert, Christian Mission: How Christianity Became a World Religion, Chichester 2009.

Ernst Matthias Rüsch, "Conversation über das Eine, was not tut". Evangelisch-reformierte Italienerseelsorge im Kanton Zürich im 19. und 20. Jahrhundert, Zürich 2010.

Philipp Sarasin, Stadt der Bürger. Bürgerliche Macht und städtische Gesellschaft, Basel 1846–1914, Göttingen 1997.

Martin Schaffner, Die Basler Arbeiterbevölkerung im 19. Jahrhundert. Beiträge zur Geschichte ihrer Lebensformen, Basel/Stuttgart 1972.

Bernhard C. Schär, Tropenliebe. Schweizer Naturforscher und niederländischer Imperialismus in Südostasien um 1900, Frankfurt a. M./New York 2015.

Bernhard C. Schär, Philanthropie postkolonial. Macht und Mitleid zwischen der Schweiz und Indien, 1850–1900, in: Alix Heiniger/Sonja Matter/ Stéphanie Ginalski (eds.), Die Schweiz und die Philanthropie. Reform, soziale Vulnerabilität und Macht (1850–1930), Basel 2017, p. 127–140.

Martin Scharfe, Die Religion des Volkes. Kleine Kultur- und Sozialgeschichte des Pietismus, Gütersloh 1980.

Wilhelm Schlatter, Geschichte der Basler Mission 1815–1915, vol. 3, Basel 1916.

Magnus Schlette, Die Selbst(er)findung des Neuen Menschen. Zur Entstehung narrativer Identitätsmuster im Pietismus, Göttingen 2005.

Beatrice Schumacher, Braucht es uns? Selbstbilder, Arbeitsweisen und organisatorische Strukturen der Schweizerischen Gemeinnützigen Gesellschaft (1810–1970), in: ibid. (ed.), Freiwillig verpflichtet. Gemeinnütziges Denken und Handeln in der Schweiz seit 1800, Zürich 2010, p. 37–69.

Anke Schürer-Ries, Die Sammlerinnen und Sammler für die Balser Mission, in: Christine Christ-von Wedel/Thomas K. Kuhn (eds.), Basler Mission. Menschen, Geschichte, Perspektiven 1815–2015, Basel 2015, p. 99–100.

Mrinalini Sebastian, Reading Archives from a Postcolonial Feminist Perspective: "Native" Bible Women and the Missionary Ideal, in: Journal of Feminist Studies in Religion 19 (2003) 1, p. 5–25.

William O. Shanahan, Der deutsche Protestantismus vor der sozialen Frage 1815–1871, München 1962.

Douglas H. Shantz, An Introduction to German Pietism: Protestant Renewal at the Dawn of Modern Europe, Baltimore 2013.

Ulrike Sill, Encounters in Quest of Christian Womanhood: The Basel Mission in Pre- and Early Colonial Ghana, Leiden/Boston 2010.

Jonathan Strom, German Pietism and the Problem of Conversion, University Park, Pennsylvania 2018.

Karl Stückelberger, Die Armen- und Krankenfürsorge in Basel, Basel 1906.

Susan Thorne, "The Conversion of Englishmen and the Conversion of the World Inseparable". Missionary Imperialism and the Language of Class in Early Industrial Britain, in: Frederick Cooper/Ann Laura Stoler (eds.), Tensions of Empire. Colonial Cultures in a Bourgeois World, Berkeley et al. 1997, p. 238–262.

Susan Thorne, Congregational Missions and the Making of an Imperial Culture in Nineteenth-Century England, Stanford 1999.

Susan Thorne, Religion and Empire at Home, in: Catherine Hall/Sonya O. Rose (eds.), At Home with Empire. Metropolitan Culture and the Imperial World, Cambridge 2006, p. 143–165.

Richard Toellner, Medizin und Pharmazie, in: Hartmut Lehmann (ed.), Geschichte des Pietismus, vol. 4: Glaubenswelt und Lebenswelten, Göttingen 2004, p. 332–356.

Luca Trevisan, Das Wohnungselend der Basler Arbeiterbevölkerung in der zweiten Hälfte des 19. Jahrhunderts, Basel 1989.

Ernst Troeltsch, Die Soziallehren der christlichen Kirchen und Gruppen. Gesammelte Schriften, vol. 1, Tübingen 1912.

Beatrice Tschudi-Barbatti, Die Halbbatzen-Kollekte. Ein Kapitel aus der Finanzgeschichte der Basler Mission, Licentiate Thesis, University of Zurich, 1992.

Megan Vaughan, Curing Their Ills. Colonial Power and African Illness, Cambridge 1991.

Hermann Vortisch, Statistik und Bericht über das erste Halbjahr 1904 der ärztlichen Mission auf der Goldküste, in: Archiv für Schiffs- und Tropenhygiene 9 (1905), p. 346–354.

Gustav Wanner, Die Basler Handels-Gesellschaft A.G. 1859–1959, Basel 1959.

Max Weber, Die Protestantische Ethik und der "Geist" des Kapitalismus, in: Archiv für Sozialwissenschaft und Sozialpolitik 20 (1904), p. 1–54.

Max Weber, Die Protestantische Ethik und der "Geist" des Kapitalismus, in: Archiv für Sozialwissenschaft und Sozialpolitik 21 (1905), p. 1–110.

Regina Wecker, 1833 bis 1910. Die Entwicklung zur Grossstadt, in: Georg Kreis/Beat von Wartburg (eds.), Basel. Geschichte einer städtischen Gesellschaft, Basel 2000, p. 196–224.

Horst Weigelt, Die Diasporaarbeit der Herrnhuter Brüdergemeine und die Wirksamkeit der Deutschen Christentumsgesellschaft im 19. Jahrhundert, in: Ulrich Gäbler (ed.), Geschichte des Pietismus, vol. 3: Der Pietismus im neunzehnten und zwanzigsten Jahrhundert, Göttingen 2000, p. 113–148.

Karolin Wetjen, Das Globale im Lokalen: Die Unterstützung der Äusseren Mission im ländlichen lutherischen Protestantismus um 1900, Göttingen 2013.

Luise White, Speaking with Vampires. Rumor and History in Colonial Africa, Berkley 2000.

Susanne Wille, Dienen, kämpfen, beten: Die ersten unverheirateten Schwestern im Dienst der Basler Mission an der Goldküste 1857–1917, Licentiate Thesis, University of Zurich, 2001.

Christian T. Collins Winn et al. (eds.), The Pietist Impulse in Christianity, Eugene 2011.

Michael Worboys, Colonial and Imperial Medicine, in: Deborah Brunton (ed.), Medicine Transformed. Health, Disease and Society in Europe 1880–1930, Manchester/New York 2004, p. 211–238.

Andreas Würgler, Die Tagsatzung der Eidgenossen: Politik, Kommunikation und Symbolik einer repräsentativen Institution im europäischen Kontext, Epfendorf 2010.

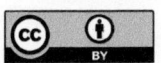

CHAPTER 3

The Scientific Space of Knowledge: Medical Missionaries, Tropical Medicine and the Age of Hygiene

3.1 Medicine, Missionaries and the Microscope

The Basel Mission doctors embodied the link between the evangelical missionary movement and the consolidation of scientific medicine in the late nineteenth century. Once they had completed their course at the mission seminary in Basel, they went on to study medicine at European universities. They thus participated in a scientific space of knowledge, in which hygiene came to dominate a wide range of research areas from sanitation, medical topographies and population studies to the emergence of tropical medicine around 1900. With the rise of germ theory and laboratory sciences, medicine gained considerable trust and authority from the 1870s. The microscope became the symbol of a new understanding of the human body as scientists began to focus on the bacteriological causes of disease. Significantly, the Basel Mission only started promoting scientific medicine as an inherent part of evangelicalism once medicine had gained a new status and sense of moral direction.

© The Author(s) 2023
L. M. Ratschiller Nasim, *Medical Missionaries and Colonial Knowledge in West Africa and Europe, 1885–1914*,
Cambridge Imperial and Post-Colonial Studies,
https://doi.org/10.1007/978-3-031-27128-1_3

3.1.1   Scientific Medicine and Pietism

The origins of both Pietism and scientific medicine can be traced back to the end of the seventeenth century.[1] Over the following centuries, however, Pietists became increasingly critical of scientific developments within the medical field, which appeared to contradict their approach to healing. From about 1800, medical scientists began to abandon the idea that ill health originated in an imbalance of fluids or energies—the so-called humoral theory, which had dominated medicine in Europe since classical times—and to think of disease as localised phenomena, based on organic changes in the solid organs and tissues of the body.[2] They now understood disease in terms of processes that occurred at the cellular level and focused on combatting disease agents with the help of a growing understanding of anatomy and biology. Infectious diseases resulted from the action of microscopic pathogens, while other complaints resulted from malfunctions within the complex physiological processes of the body.[3]

The scientification of the body and specialisation of medicine compromised the Pietist approach to healing, which emphasised the unity of body and soul and treated human beings in their entirety. Pietists opposed reducing living nature to the inorganic laws of physics or chemistry and stressed the importance of holistic medicine.[4] In general, they mostly disregarded scientific developments affecting society at large, unless these

---

[1] Robert K. Merton argued in his 1938 book *Science, Technology and Society in 17th-century England* for a positive correlation between the rise of Pietism and early experimental science, similar to Max Weber's famous claim on the link between Protestant ethic and the capitalist economy. The Merton thesis has resulted in continuous debates. See I. Bernard Cohen (ed.), Puritanism and the Rise of Modern Science: The Merton Thesis, New Brunswick/London 1990.

[2] L. S. Jacyna, Localization of Disease, in: Deborah Brunton (ed.), Medicine Transformed. Health, Disease and Society in Europe, 1800–1930, Manchester/New York 2004, p. 1–30; Roy Porter, What is Disease? in: ibid (ed.), The Cambridge History of Medicine, Cambridge 2006, p. 71–102.

[3] Philipp Sarasin/Jakob Tanner (eds.), Physiologie und industrielle Gesellschaft. Studien zur Verwissenschaftlichung des Körpers im 19. und 20. Jahrhundert, Frankfurt a. M. 1998; Michael Worboys, Spreading Germs: Disease Theories and Medical Practice in Britain, 1865–1900, Cambridge 2000.

[4] Jürgen Helm, "Dass auch zugleich die Gottseligkeit dadurch gebauet wird". Pietismus und Medizin in der ersten Hälfte des achtzehnten Jahrhunderts, in: Berichte zur Wissenschaftsgeschichte 26 (2003) 3, p. 199–211; Johanna Geyer-Kordesch, Pietismus, Medizin und Aufklärung im 18. Jahrhundert. Das Leben und Werk Georg Ernst Stahls, Tübingen 2000.

developments openly contradicted biblical stories, in which case they fought and rejected them. Technology, on the other hand, especially its artisanal and industrial use, was incorporated in the Pietist way of life, regardless of its scientific origins. Pietists tapped into ideas, practices and technologies considered inevitable or useful in an increasingly technical and industrial society while emphasising that healing was to remain a largely spiritual affair.[5]

One site in which the confrontations between Pietist healing and scientific medicine became particularly obvious was in hospitals, which began to grow in both size and number from the mid-nineteenth century. Two historical processes led to a wave of hospital creations in Germany and Switzerland. Firstly, Pietists began to work towards the creation of nursing orders similar to those in Catholic countries, where hospital nursing had long been provided by religious orders as part of the Christian service ideal. In contrast to the longstanding and extensive hospital care provided by Catholic nursing orders, this philanthropic tradition was largely lacking in Protestant churches until the nineteenth century, when Protestant charities started to dedicate themselves to medical care.[6]

The second process concerned the increasingly important role of the hospital for scientific research. The application of scientific thinking and experiments for the production of medical knowledge, which originated in early modern scholarship, became part of clinical medicine. Knowledge of disease no longer relied on subjective judgements made by doctors' unaided senses and clinical skills. Instead, the study of the body's processes was the subject of laboratory research, whereby physiological phenomena were explored through experiments and objectively measured. Experimentally ascertained knowledge became more and more constitutive for the medical image of the human body and the conception of health and illness.[7]

---

[5] On medical and cultural developments within Pietism, see Irmtraut Sahmland/ Hans-Jürgen Schrader (eds.), Medizin- und kulturgeschichtliche Konnexe des Pietismus. Heilkunst und Ethik, arkane Traditionen, Musik, Literatur und Sprache, Göttingen 2016.

[6] The creation of Protestant nursing orders was chiefly the work of pastor Theodor Fliedner and his wife, Friederike, who created the Deaconesses' Institute in Kaiserswerth, Prussia, in 1836. Gary B. Ferngren, Medicine and Religion. A Historical Introduction, Baltimore 2014, p. 166; Roy Porter, Hospitals and Surgery, in: ibid. (ed.), The Cambridge History of Medicine, Cambridge 2006, p. 176–210, here p. 195.

[7] Roy Porter, Medical Science, in: ibid. (ed.), The Cambridge History of Medicine, Cambridge 2006, p. 136–175; Deborah Brunton, The Rise of Laboratory Medicine, in:

By 1900, the hospital had transformed from being on the margins of medical care, offering shelter to the poorest, into a respected bourgeois institution of medical science and an indispensable site of health care.[8] In Basel, the *Bürgerspital*—the citizens' hospital—founded in 1842, became the main institution for medical care and research. It was closely connected to the medical curricula at the University of Basel, which was founded in the fifteenth century. The hospital's management lay with the *Bürgergemeinde*, which was dominated by Basel's pious elite. The multi-faceted role of the hospital as a place of research, teaching and nursing led to conflicts between the proponents of Christian health care, who defined the spirit of the hospital as a site of healing and sanctification, and doctors, who increasingly understood the hospital as an instrument for scientific research and practice, and consequently aspired to take over management.[9]

The history of the hospital suggests a relationship of complex inter-action rather than of mutual ignorance between Pietist and scientific approaches to medicine.[10] The hospital and the medical mission were two significant fields in which Pietism and scientific medicine interacted over time. The breakthrough of scientific medicine in the late nineteenth century did not simply devalue or replace religion. The so-called scientific revolution and the progressive medicalisation of society were embedded in a historical context that also gave birth to the evangelical revival and the missionary movement. The shaping influence of Enlightenment modes of thought, which ushered in a new confidence about the validity of experiments, fuelled Christian mission and activism.[11] Pietism was a

---

ibid. (ed.), Medicine Transformed. Health, Disease and Society in Europe, 1800–1930, Manchester/New York 2004, p. 92–118.

[8] Hilary Marland, The Changing Role of the Hospital, 1800–1900, in: Deborah Brunton, (ed.), Medicine Transformed. Health, Disease and Society in Europe, 1800–1930, Manchester/New York 2004, p. 31–60.

[9] Toellner, Medizin und Pharmazie.

[10] The influential anthropologists Jean and John Comaroff have argued that medicine began to replace the church as the guardian of public and private health in the course of the nineteenth century. See Comaroff/Comaroff, Of Revelation and Revolution, vol. 2, p. 325. Yet the importance of Christian medical work at that time both abroad and at home suggests that it is too simple to think about science and religion in antagonistic terms.

[11] Brian Stanley, Christian Missions and the Enlightenment, Grand Rapids 2001. On the important influence of Enlightenment thinking on the German Protestant awakening and

driver of social change and conceived of as experimental faith, a maxim subsequently applied to the "experiment" of foreign mission during the evangelical awakening.[12]

3.1.2   The Question of a Medical Mission

In a seminal speech at the International Conference of the Evangelical Alliance on the 5th of September 1879 in Basel, the eminent professor for practical theology in Bonn, Theodor Christlieb, asked: "Why do we, in the German missions, not have any mission doctors or a medical mission society yet like the English and the American missions do?"[13] The creation of the Edinburgh Medical Missionary Society almost forty years earlier in 1841 had initiated a wave of society foundations dedicated to evangelical medical mission in both North America and Great Britain.[14] To Christlieb, who had worked as a pastor in London for seven years and gained important insights into the work of British mission societies, part of the reason lay in the lack of support for the missionary movement at German universities.[15] He deplored that "the thought of mission" was subject "to deadly mockery" in the country's medical faculties. Professors and students of medicine, he observed, "believe in a

---

particularly its social vision, see Martin Greschat, Die Vorgeschichte der Inneren Mission, in: ibid. (ed.), Die christliche Mitgift Europas—Traditionen und Zukunft, Stuttgart 2000, p. 87–105.

[12] Inductive methods emanating from seventeenth century natural sciences further enabled evangelicals to move from the particulars of experience to establishing general laws. See Gladwin, Mission and Colonialism, p. 285; Mark Hutchinson/John Wolffe, A Short History of Global Evangelicalism, Cambridge 2012, p. 1–23; Davis, Pietism and the Foundations of the Modern World.

[13] Theodor Christlieb, Der gegenwärtige Stand der evangelischen Heidenmission, in: Allgemeine Missionszeitschrift 6 (1879), p. 481–582, here p. 512.

[14] Given their dedication to medical philanthropy through nursing orders, it is not surprising that Catholics pioneered medical missions. As early as the sixteenth century, the Jesuits had established more than 150 hospitals in Mexico alone. Ferngren, Medicine and Religion, p. 169; David Hardiman, Introduction, in: ibid. (ed.), Healing Bodies, Saving Souls. Medical Missions in Asia and Africa, Amsterdam/New York 2006, p. 5–57, here p. 12–13.

[15] Thomas Schirrmacher, Theodor Christlieb und seine Missionstheologie, Wuppertal 1985, p. 113.

naturalistic superstition, in which Christianity has ceased to be a 'scientific' standpoint."[16]

In 1889, the British magazine *Medical Missions at Home and Abroad* commented on the situation of medical missions on the European continent: "It may be difficult for us to realise, but there is no room to question the fact that the missionary idea has yet to find its way into the medical circles of university life on the Continent."[17] In contrast to the United Kingdom, doctors in Europe were generally regarded as critical of evangelism and medicine often seemed to be at the forefront of secularisation, as its assumptions became more materialistic.[18] Christlieb used the comparison with Britain to accuse German academics of their lack of support: "They follow Darwin in all matters, except in his sympathy for the mission, which recently brought him to donate 100 Marks to the London South American Mission Society."[19] Frustrated by the refusal of medical faculties to contribute to the success of the missionary movement, Christlieb concluded his speech by asking: "So, what can we hope for?"[20]

Christlieb's speech was based on an extensive study comparing Protestant missions around the world. It was printed in numerous languages and came to constitute a key text for the missionary movement at the end of the nineteenth century. The first English versions appeared in London in 1880 and in Calcutta and Edinburgh in 1882.[21] His writings were used extensively for educational purposes in the seminary in Basel. Based on his own Pietist background, he established the necessity for a medical mission in line with Pietist beliefs. He emphasised that spiritual salvation and physical healing were inseparable, and that missionary work had to pay attention to both.[22] His arguments lent theological substance to the

---

[16] Christlieb, Der gegenwärtige Stand der evangelischen Heidenmission, p. 513.

[17] Medical Missionary Association (ed.), Medical Missions at Home and Abroad, London 1889, p. 3.

[18] Hardiman, The Mission Hospital 1880–1960, p. 200.

[19] Christlieb, Der gegenwärtige Stand der evangelischen Heidenmission, p. 513.

[20] Ibid.

[21] Theodor Christlieb, Protestant Foreign Missions. Their Present State, A Universal Survey, London 1880; Ibid., Protestant Missions to the Heathen. A General Survey of their Recent Progress and Present State Throughout the World, Calcutta/Edinburgh 1882.

[22] Wolfgang U. Eckart, "Reichgottesarbeit" nicht Reichsarbeit—Theodor Christlieb und die Idee einer deutschen ärztlichen Mission in der Wilhelminischen Epoche, in: Richard

longstanding demands by the Basel missionaries in West Africa, who had been calling for the dispatch of a mission doctor for decades.

Christlieb's appeal reflected a conceptual shift in the Pietist approach to healing, away from Blumhardt's deliverance theology to the integration of medical sciences into the evangelical worldview. The head theology teacher in the Basel Mission seminary, Reiff, noted in 1873 that "scientific education" was not a "necessary evil" but a precious asset "provided that above all the heart is in the right place."[23] The growing significance of scientific medicine from the 1870s prompted a change of attitude towards scientific methods and academic training. Pietists now started to appropriate scientific medicine, where it seemed to serve God's plan. Towards the end of his life, Johann Blumhardt believed that doctors served as instruments through whom God provided healing.[24] He became disillusioned with the effectiveness of healing through prayer and was convinced that medicine played a significant role in healing, even to the point of recommending that most of the sick that came to Bad Boll should consult physicians. By the time of his death in 1880, Pietist healing and deliverance practices had begun to wane.[25]

In Basel, the election of a new Inspector, Otto Schott, in 1879 facilitated the conception and implementation of a medical mission with scientifically trained physicians.[26] Schott believed in a close connection between saving souls and healing bodies, assuring the many critical members of the Committee that "medical aid is a good means to dispel the heathens' doubts about the gospel and to demonstrate Christian charity and love."[27] The dispatch abroad of scientific medical personnel was seen by some Pietists as an expression of religious weakness, arguing that health risks should be borne with true faith in God. Schott retorted that God had also given man his faculties for dealing with avoidable

Toellner (ed.), Die Geburt einer sanften Medizin. Die Franckeschen Stiftungen zu Halle als Begegnungsstätte von Medizin und Pietismus im frühen 18. Jahrhundert, Halle 2004, p. 151–158.

[23] Reiff, Die christliche Glaubenslehre, vol. 1, Basel 1873, p. vi.

[24] Koehler, Pilgrimage of Protestants.

[25] Adam Mohr, Missionary Medicine and Akan Therapeutics: Illness, Health and Healing in Southern Ghana's Basel Mission, 1828–1918, in: Journal of Religion in Africa 39 (2009) 4, p. 429–461, here p. 449.

[26] Schlatter, Geschichte der Basler Mission, vol. 1, p. 303–315.

[27] Committee report, 28.04.1880, BMA, Komitee-Protokoll 1880, §158.

dangers, and that it would amount to irresponsible behaviour not to use these faculties. He depicted medical advancement as providential, God's purpose being that scientific medicine would become "a mighty instrument to open up the way and keep open the way for the message of Christ."[28]

Inspired by English and American mission societies, Christlieb and Schott provided theological arguments for the benefit of medical missions. They conceived of medical missionaries as evangelising forces, who had the power to both heal and preach. In doing so, they paved the way for the integration of academically qualified mission doctors into the evangelising agenda. The training and methods of scientific medicine were gradually incorporated into the syllabus of the Basel Mission seminary. While earlier medical classes were based on Pietist principles of healing, the curriculum from the late 1880s included scientifically based approaches to medicine. Starting in 1887, students in senior class had to take a "first aid course," and from 1897 all students were expected to attend weekly lectures on hygiene and "surgical classes with practical exercises."[29] Scientific medicine was now considered vital to the advancement of the missionary cause and the Basel Mission started recruiting candidates for a medical mission in 1880.

Rudolf Fisch, a pupil who had joined the mission seminary in 1875, attracted the Committee's attention. He started his medical studies at the University of Basel, once he had completed his five-year missionary training in the autumn of 1880.[30] That same year, a theology student from Tubingen, Alfred Eckhardt, applied to become a medical missionary with the Basel Mission. Upon receiving a favourable response from the Basel leadership, Eckhardt began his medical studies at the University of Tubingen.[31] Despite the pressing circumstances in West Africa demanding urgent action, the lengthy duration of medical studies meant that the launch of a medical mission abroad would have to wait until 1885.

---

[28] Ibid.

[29] Medizinischer Unterricht, BMA, Lehrfächer 1864–1907, QS-3.18.4; Schlatter, Geschichte der Basler Mission, vol. 1, p. 376.

[30] Committee report, 13.10.1880, BMA, Komitee-Protokoll 1880, §449.

[31] Personal File Alfred Eckhardt, BMA, BV 1139.

3.1.3   The Medical Research Expedition of 1882–1883

In the summer of 1881, four Basel missionaries on the Gold Coast passed away in the space of four weeks; among them the pharmacist Alphons Schmidt, who, by virtue of his medical knowledge, had helped many missionaries dealing with illness.[32] *Der Evangelische Heidenbote* reported on the fatalities in West Africa in detail and appeared particularly concerned about the passing of the senior missionary of the *Norddeutsche Missionsgesellschaft* in Togo, who had attended the seminary in Basel.[33] Urged into action by this wave of fatalities, Karl Sarasin—the founder of the *Halbbazten-Kollekte*—donated 10,000 Swiss francs to the Basel Mission for a "medical expert report" of the area.[34] The Committee used Sarasin's contribution to commission the 26-year-old general practitioner and zealous Pietist Ernst Mähly to assess the specific health challenges on the Gold Coast.[35]

Sarasin, who embodied the entanglements between liberal capitalism, conservative politics and evangelical fervour, recognised the value of a medical mission overseas. In a letter to Mähly, he explained that he hoped that his donation would help to achieve in West Africa what he had failed to do in Basel, "to contribute to a progressive transformation of hygienic conditions based on the fundamental principles of Max von Pettenkofer."[36] Pettenkofer, a chemist, pharmacist and physician, had become the first German professor for hygiene in 1865 at the Ludwig-Maximilian-University in Munich and the director of the first Hygiene Institute founded there in 1879. Considered to be a pioneer of hygiene and public health, he analysed the cholera epidemics in Munich (1836–1837; 1853–1854) and convinced Ludwig II of Bavaria that soil quality could be improved significantly by centralising the sewage system and drinking water supply.[37]

---

[32] Fischer, Der Missionsarzt Rudolf Fisch, p. 127.

[33] Anonymous, Die afrikanischen Todesfälle, in: Der Evangelische Heidenbote 54 (1881), p. 69–71, 74–78.

[34] Committee report, 06.07.1881, BMA, Komitee-Protokoll 1881, §305.

[35] For a short biography of Ernst Mähly, see Hans Werner Debrunner, Schweizer im kolonialen Afrika, Basel 1991, p. 175–178.

[36] Karl Sarasin, Letter to Ernst Mähly, 20.08.1883, BMA, D-1.39.K.

[37] Locher, Max von Pettenkofer; Weyer-von Schoultz, Max von Pettenkofer.

Sarasin, who initiated and supervised numerous public health measures in his hometown, was convinced that hygiene held the key to prosperity. He had striven for the establishment of a new sewer system in the old town of Basel during his time as head of the health department but was eventually defeated by political rivals. He subsequently retired from all his political offices, focussing instead more vigorously on Christian philanthropy.[38] His charitable commitment both abroad and at home was clearly driven by his Pietist faith and wish for social harmony, which—hardly coincidentally—also increased economic productivity and benefitted his global silk empire.

Mähly thoroughly prepared his medical research expedition for over a year by studying the relevant literature, examining death reports in the mission archives and compiling statistics. By doing so, he hoped to calculate the most opportune time for home leaves and marriages as well as the most convenient locations for mission stations.[39] In the summer of 1882, he spent four months at Pettenkofer's Hygiene Institute in Munich and then travelled to Edinburgh to study English publications and meet British doctors who had practised in the tropics.[40] Mähly's preparations also consisted of gathering and studying information from the Gold Coast. He asked the Basel missionary Karl Schönfeld, who was due to return from Christiansborg to Basel in May of 1882, to bring him some African remedies.[41]

There is no indication in the records as to whether Schönfeld fulfilled Mähly's request. What we do know, however, is that Schönfeld assisted Mähly by providing him with a medical brochure about the most prevalent diseases in West Africa and advice on how to prevent and treat them. For this, he had asked the British colonial doctor Charles Scovell Grant to sum up his experiences on the Gold Coast in a booklet. Grant's brochure offered practical advice on hygiene, which Schönfeld reproduced and sent to every Basel Mission station in West Africa. Grant edited his work into

---

[38] Shanahan, Der deutsche Protestantismus, p. 76, 378–388.

[39] Ernst Mähly, Letter to Inspector Schott, 05.11.1881, BMA, D-1.39.K.

[40] Ernst Mähly, Letter to Committee, Munich, 15.05.1882, BMA, D-1.39.J.8.

[41] Karl Schönfeld, Letter to Ernst Mähly, Christiansborg, 09.03.1882, BMA, D-1.39.J.5.

a published manual, which found wide recognition, appearing in three English and two French editions.[42]

In March of 1882, Mähly submitted to the Committee a proposed research programme for his medical expedition. The proposal was very much along the lines of a classic hygiene survey, popularised by Pettenkofer, his former teacher.[43] A characteristic feature of this type of survey, distinguishing them from earlier approaches and observation techniques, was the systematic statistical evaluation of life records, reflecting the contemporary preoccupation with medical topographies based on ethnographic, demographic and sometimes epidemiological data.[44] Once in West Africa, Mähly planned to complement his preliminary results by studying the living conditions of the Basel missionaries on the ground, including their clothing, diet, means of travel, dwellings, schools and latrines.[45] He also intended to visit every mission station, in order to assess their respective "geographical position" and "meteorological character" in relation to the surrounding vegetation and the quality of soil, air and water.[46]

In November 1882, Mähly arrived in Christiansborg together with Hermann Prätorius, the Basel Mission's newly appointed Inspector for Africa, and the merchant Wilhelm Preiswerk.[47] The main objective of their inspection visit was to assess the potential for increasing autonomy of the parishes on the Gold Coast by conducting community visits and conferences with African pastors and community elders. The news of the arrival of a European doctor spread quickly, gaining Mähly the moniker *tschofåtscha*—father of roots—among the Basel Mission communities on the Gold Coast. *Der Evangelische Heidenbote* reported in 1883: "His reputation draws sick people from all quarters and it looks like he is about

---

[42] Charles Scovell Grant, West African Hygiene. Or, Hints on the Preservation of Health, and the Treatment of Disease on the West Coast of Africa, London 1882, 1884, 1887; Ibid., Petit guide d'hygiène pratique dans l'Ouest Africain, Paris 1882, 1893.

[43] Ernst Mähly, Programme for the Medical Inspection, March 1882, BMA, D-1.39.K.

[44] Mark Harrison, Climates and Constitutions: Health, Race, Environment and British Imperialism in India, 1600–1850, Delhi 1999, p. 92–93.

[45] Ernst Mähly, Programme for the Medical Inspection, March 1882, D-1.39.K.

[46] Ibid.; Committee report, 14.09.1881, BMA, Komitee-Protokoll 1881, §409.

[47] The Committee created the position of an Inspector for Africa because of the growing importance of the missionary activities on this continent. Schlatter, Geschichte der Basler Mission, vol. 3, p. 156–160.

to become the most popular person on the Gold Coast. He is literally besieged by people seeking help wherever he goes."[48]

While the significance of a mission doctor for the status of the Basel Mission on the Gold Coast became increasingly clear, illness and death continued to menace the lives of European personnel. Mähly, Prätorius and Preiswerk witnessed the passing of five young mission members in the first three months after their arrival, three of which they attributed to bilious fever.[49] They also regularly reported on how diseases such as dysentery and various fevers personally affected them. The tragic irony of their inspection visit, which lasted nearly two years, was that the Africa Inspector Prätorius succumbed shortly before their departure from the Gold Coast in April 1883. In his autopsy, Mähly found four liver abscesses, indicating that the cause of death had been amoebic dysentery.[50] Mähly's medical research expedition marked the first scientifically-based attempt within the Basel Mission to characterise and prevent so-called tropical diseases, laying the foundation for a systematic medical mission in West Africa.

Upon his return to Basel, Mähly shared his insights with the mission doctor assigned for the Gold Coast, Rudolf Fisch, who completed his medical studies in the summer of 1884.[51] In November, Mähly drew up a plan for equipment regulation, including guidelines for clothing and household items, which the Basel Mission implemented swiftly.[52] During the following months, he compiled a 61-page long report on "The hygienic conditions of the African mission area."[53] The Committee used Mähly's insights to prepare the launch of the medical mission on the Gold Coast. His advice on tropical hygiene and his theories about the

---

[48] Hermann Prätorius, Mittheilungen aus der afrikanischen Visitationsreise, in: Der Evangelische Heidenbote 56 (1883), p. 9–11, 17–19, 25–28, 33–35, 41–43, here p. 18–19.

[49] Ibid., p. 33–35.

[50] Wilhelm Preiswerk, Letter to Committee, Christiansborg, 08.04.1883, BMA, D-1.39.F.15; Ernst Mähly, Letter to Committee, Abetifi, 28.05.1883, BMA, D-1.39.K.

[51] Committee report, 11.06.1884, BMA, Komitee-Protokoll 1884, §210.

[52] Ernst Mähly, Propositions for the equipment of African missionaries, BMA, D-1.39.k; Committee report, 19.11.1884, BMA, Komitee-Protokoll 1884, §435a.

[53] Ernst Mähly, The hygienic conditions of the African mission area, BMA, D-1.39.K. Partially printed in Mähly, Die Gesundheitsverhältnisse auf der Goldküste. Also see Fischer, Der Missionsarzt Rudolf Fisch, p. 136–142.

aetiologies of tropical diseases provided a valuable base on which to carry out further research.[54]

3.1.4   The Institutionalisation of Mission Medicine

The Basel Mission broke fresh ground in the German-speaking evangelical missionary movement when they started deploying academically trained mission doctors in the 1880s. The implementation of a systematic scientific medical mission proved immensely challenging, as the Committee expounded in the specialised publications *An die Freunde des Ärztlichen Zweiges der Basler Mission* (1891–1894) and *Unsere ärztliche Mission* (1895–1898). Medical mission continued to draw scant interest in German-speaking Europe, while demanding considerable medical expertise and funds. Therefore, the Basel Mission appealed for the establishment of an aid organisation that would guarantee an independent, financially sustainable medical mission. Supporters gathered to form a Society for Medical Mission in Stuttgart in 1898, devoted exclusively to the ideological, practical and financial assistance of the Basel medical mission.[55]

The society in Stuttgart was chaired by the industrialist Paul Lechler and managed by Eugen Liebendörfer, the first Basel medical missionary sent to India in 1886.[56] According to the statutes, the first of the four main activities of the organisation was the provision of financial aid to medical missionary students. Second, the society was to use its funds to purchase books, instruments, drugs and bandaging material. Third, it had to ensure the continuing education of medical missionaries in the fields of medicine, surgery and tropical hygiene. Last but not least, the medical aid organisation aimed to facilitate the foundation of new medical stations and hospitals in the mission fields.[57]

---

[54] Schlatter, Geschichte der Basler Mission, vol. 1, p. 376–377.

[55] Eckart, Medizin und Kolonialimperialismus, p. 97–112.

[56] Maya Trapp, Die Bedeutung der Basler Ärztlichen Mission in ihren südindischen Missionsgebieten in der Zeit von 1886–1914, in: Richard Toellner (ed.), Die Geburt einer sanften Medizin. Die Franckeschen Stiftungen zu Halle als Begegnungsstätte von Medizin und Pietismus im frühen 18. Jahrhundert, Halle 2004, p. 141–150.

[57] Verein für ärztliche Mission (ed.), Bericht über das 1. Geschäftsjahr, Stuttgart 1899, p. 23.

The formation of the Society for Medical Mission in Stuttgart, the first of its kind in German-speaking Europe, initiated the founding of several aid organisations devoted to medical missions throughout Switzerland and Germany.[58] They joined forces in 1909 by creating an umbrella association, the *Verband der deutschen Vereine für ärztliche Mission*, to advocate for common concerns. By the eve of the First World War, a total of 14 benevolent societies for medical mission counted 8000 active members and generated yearly donations of some 75,000 Marks.[59] The progressive institutionalisation of mission medicine culminated in the founding of the German Institute for Medical Mission in 1906 in Tubingen, still operating today.

The Tubingen Institute offered accommodation to medical students thought to be suited for missionary service and ran courses for non-medical missionaries covering surgery, birth assistance, internal medicine and tropical medicine over two semesters.[60] It also established a tropical clinic for the recovery of missionaries, where 372 patients were treated between 1906 and 1914. The Tubingen Institute housed a vast body of medical expertise about the tropics, bringing together funds, personnel and knowledge on a transnational level. By 1914, a total of 74 missionaries from 14 mission societies had graduated as doctors and 43 missionary sisters had qualified in nursing and midwifery in Tubingen.[61] The growing significance attached to tropical diseases and hygiene was also reflected in the founding of the *Institut für Schiffs- und Tropenkrankheiten* in Hamburg in 1901, which became a close ally of the Tubingen Institute.[62]

The German Institute for Medical Mission was valued as a serious partner in the field of tropical medicine and an important resource in the

---

[58] Verband der deutschen Vereine für ärztliche Mission (ed.), Jahrbuch der Ärztlichen Mission 1914, Gütersloh 1914, p. 137.

[59] Eckart, Medizin und Kolonialimperialismus, p. 97.

[60] The formation of the German Institute for Medical Mission, BMA, G.II.17a; Gottlieb Olpp, Über die Ausbildungsstätten des missionsärztlichen Personals in der europäischen Heimat einst und jetzt, in: Verband der deutschen Vereine für ärztliche Mission (ed.), Jahrbuch der Ärztlichen Mission, Gütersloh 1914, p. 14–26, BMA, G.II.13.

[61] Schlatter, Geschichte der Basler Mission, vol. 1, p. 381.

[62] Wolfgang U. Eckart, Die Anfänge der deutschen Tropenmedizin. Die Gründung des Hamburger Instituts für Schiffs- und Tropenkrankheiten, in: Heinz Schott (ed.), Meilensteine der Medizin, Dortmund 1996, p. 411–418; Ibid., Medizin und Kolonialimperialismus, p. 73–90.

context of colonial policies. On the occasion of its official inauguration in 1909, the German State Secretary for Colonial Affairs, Bernhard Dernburg, expressed his "great satisfaction," stating that the progress that had been made at the Tubingen Institute marked "a significant new step for the cultural development of the German colonies."[63] Paul Lechler, the founder of the German Institute for Medical Mission, asserted that his institution wished to support the "adequate working ability of natives" by exploring the health conditions in the colonies. Over the course of a lively telegram exchange between Tubingen and Berlin, the Kaiser replied to one of Lechler's telegrams: "His majesty the Kaiser and King takes keen interest in the German Institute for Medical Mission established there and wishes rich success to this significant education facility for the benefit of both the German colonies and the entire fatherland."[64]

3.2   THE FORMATION OF TROPICAL MEDICINE AND HYGIENE

Tropical medicine emerged as a medical specialisation at the end of the nineteenth century and was, at first, instituted primarily and largely for the benefit of European administrators and the military rather than for the welfare of the colonised. The distinctive characteristic of tropical medicine, which was based on the idea that certain diseases were caused by pathogens that were endemic or peculiar to the tropics, is that it developed as a result of the convergence of two different fields of knowledge. On the one hand, it drew on the medical, environmental and cultural experiences and acumen that Europeans had gathered in warm climates over the last centuries. Climate, particularly tropical climate, had been an important preoccupation of missionaries, explorers and traders ever since the earliest colonial endeavours. On the other hand, it incorporated newly emergent germ theory and parasitology, which shifted medical attention from climate and environment to bacteria and parasites.[65]

[63] Bernhard Dernburg, Letter to Paul Lechler, 06.07.1909, BMA, QH-3.1.

[64] Rudolf von Valentini, Telegram to Paul Lechler, 22.10.1909, BMA, QH-3.1.

[65] Pratik Chakrabarti, Medicine and Empire, 1600–1960, Basingstoke 2014, p. 141–163.

3.2.1   The Question of Acclimatisation

"Knowledge of Africa began with the know-how needed to survive the climate," as Johannes Fabian phrased it.[66] The question of acclimatisation, that is the concern for the survival and capability of white personnel in the tropics, lay at the origin of the field of tropical medicine.[67] It can be traced back to the early modern period, when naval surgeons tried to conserve the health of Europeans during expeditions. In the early nineteenth century, it was mainly British and French physicians in India and Africa who contributed to the question of maintaining white health in tropical climates.[68] By 1900, more than fifty acclimatisation societies had formed around the globe. Their findings went hand in hand with land appropriation, economic exploitation and the formalisation of colonial administration.[69]

Geographically, the tropics were broadly defined as the regions within the lines known as the Tropic of Cancer and the Tropic of Capricorn. However, beyond mere regions on the map, the tropics were widely discussed as medical and cultural concepts in European literature. The tropics consequently did not only cover a specific geographical location but also a conceptual space, which was seen as both environmentally and culturally alien from temperate zones.[70] Travelogues and expedition reports conjured up contrasting ideas about the tropics, a space at once exotic and repulsive, alluring and threatening. The sun, heat and

[66] Johannes Fabian, Out of Our Minds. Reason and Madness in the Exploration of Central Africa, Berkley et al. 2000, p. 59.

[67] Bruchhausen, Die "hygienische Eroberung" der Tropen, p. 207–208.

[68] Warwick Anderson, Climates of Opinion. Acclimatization in Nineteenth-Century France and England, in: Victorian Studies 35 (1992) 2, p. 135–157; Michael A. Osborne, Nature, the Exotic and the Science of French Colonialism, Bloomington 1994.

[69] Christopher Lever, They Dined on Eland: The Story of Acclimatization Societies, London 1992; Michael A. Osborne, Acclimatizing the World: A History of Paradigmatic Colonial Science, in: Osiris 15 (2000), p. 135–151.

[70] David Arnold, Inventing Tropicality, in: ibid. (ed.), The Problem of Nature. Environment, Culture, and European Expansion, London 1996, p. 141–168; Ibid., The Tropics and the Traveling Gaze: India, Landscape, and Science, 1800–1856, Seattle 2006; Nancy Leys Stepan, Picturing Tropical Nature, Ithaca 2001; Georgina H. Endfield/David J. Nash, Missionaries and Morals: Climatic Discourse in Nineteenth-Century Central Southern Africa, in: Annals of the Association of American Geographers 92 (2002) 4, p. 727–742; Felix Driver/Luciana Martins (eds.), Tropical Visions in an Age of Empire, Chicago/London 2005.

humidity of the tropics accounted for their apparent luxuriance, verdure and productivity and yet were simultaneously thought to be a leading cause of the deterioration of Europeans' health. In the Basel missionaries' testimonies about West Africa, life in the tropics seemed not so much a decadent luxury than a sore trial and often even a death sentence, reflected in the contemporary moniker given to the Guinea Coast: the "white man's grave."[71]

Rudolf Virchow held a disillusioning lecture on acclimatisation at the 58th Assembly of German Natural Scientists and Physicians in 1885. An influential physician, anthropologist and liberal politician of his time, Virchow was considered the accepted medical authority of the German Reich.[72] In his view, Germany had "substantially missed the time in world history" to pursue colonial politics. Nevertheless, now that the German government had "decided to acquire colonies," he emphasised that "one cannot adopt a passive attitude" since "the sciences" had to provide the basis on which "the order of the new polity abroad" would be built. Despite his scepticism, Virchow promoted further scientific investigation into the "medicine of exotic diseases."[73]

Virchow's appeal marked the beginning of intensified research efforts into tropical medicine but, contrary to his intentions, it was not the universities that first took his call to heart but mainly colonial interest groups.[74] The German Colonial Society initiated and financed an international questionnaire-based survey related to the issue of acclimatisation in 1886. Doctors, who were members of the *Deutsche Kolonialverein* and stayed in tropical regions, were asked to assess hygienic conditions and to report on the possibility of acclimatisation. The Colonial Society hoped that the survey, conducted by the physician and writer Ernst Below, would provide evidence for the ability of Europeans to settle in the tropics. In Below's view, the purpose of research into tropical medicine and hygiene was to produce biological validation and scientific legitimacy for the

---

[71] Philip D. Curtin, "The White Man's Grave": Image and Reality, 1780–1850, in: The Journal of British Studies 1 (1961), p. 94–110.

[72] Constantin Goschler, Rudolf Virchow. Mediziner—Anthropologe—Politiker, Köln/Weimar/Wien 2009.

[73] Rudolf Virchow, Über Acclimatisation, in: Tageblatt der 58. Versammlung deutscher Naturforscher und Ärzte, Strassburg 1885, p. 540–554, here p. 540.

[74] Eckart, Medizin und Kolonialimperialismus, p. 74–75.

expansion of the "white race" in the "tropical belt," so that in the future, it would no longer belong to "yellow and black people alone."[75]

Virchow, who, in contrast to most of his colleagues, was not a member of the German Colonial Society, assisted Below nonetheless, helping to prepare a second study in 1889 and a third one in 1891.[76] The results of the first survey on acclimatisation were published in a special issue of the *Deutsche Kolonialzeitung* in 1886. Ernst Mähly, who had conducted his own evaluation a few years earlier, contributed to this issue, arguing that the notion of "climate fever" should be replaced by the term "malarial fever," since it was not caused by any specific environmental conditions, such as altitude, soil, humidity or vegetation, but occurred all over the Gold Coast, affecting Europeans as much as Africans: "We have to recognise that the germ causing fever is a specific, independent and ubiquitous thing, which can be favoured or impaired by external geographical conditions but, most likely and sadly, not produced or destroyed."[77] Mähly formulated a fever theory that drew practical conclusions from laboratory findings and recent clinical research.

The germ theory of disease, emerging in French and German scientific circles in the 1870s, suggested that microbes rather than climatic factors were the enemies of European acclimatisation in the tropics. Mähly, whose advice on tropical hygiene was widely published in medical, colonial and missionary journals, argued that all efforts had to be concentrated on limiting the number of malarial agents entering one's body, while simultaneously strengthening one's physical condition to overcome the inevitable fevers.[78] The Basel Mission doctors were up to speed with the

---

[75] Ernst Below, Die praktischen Ziele der Tropenhygiene, in: Verhandlungen der Gesellschaft deutscher Naturforscher und Ärzte, 68. Versammlung, Frankfurt a. M., 21.–26. September 1896, ed. by Albert Wangerin/Otto Taschenberg, part 1, Leipzig 1896, p. 91–120, here p. 96.

[76] Otto Schellong, Die Klimatologie der Tropen nach den Ergebnissen des Fragebogenmaterials im Auftrage der Deutschen Kolonialgesellschaft, Berlin 1891, p. 3, BArch R 8023/1005; Ernst Below, Die Ergebnisse der tropenhygienischen Fragebogen. Besonders vom Gesichtspunkte des internationalen Seuchenschutzes aus betrachtet, Leipzig 1892, p. 5, BArch R8023/1006.

[77] Mähly, Akklimatisation und Klimafieber, in: Deutsche Kolonialzeitung 3 (1886), p. 72–83, here p. 78; Mähly, Die Gesundheitsverhältnisse auf der Goldküste, p. 408.

[78] Mähly, Die Gesundheitsverhältnisse auf der Goldküste; Ibid., Über das sogenannte "Gallenfieber" an der Goldküste, in: Correspondenz-Blatt für Schweizer Ärzte 15 (1885), p. 73–79, 108–116; Ibid., Akklimatisation und Klimafieber, in: Deutsche Kolonialzeitung

fast-changing scientific landscape of their time. They trained at renowned institutions, studied state-of-the-art medicine and had access to transnational scientific networks. Alfred Eckhardt, who became the second Basel Mission doctor to practise on the Gold Coast, completed his studies in Berlin, where he assisted with Robert Koch's first lecture on hygiene, took a class in bacteriology and passed his final exams with Rudolf Virchow in 1887.[79]

3.2.2   Scientific Networks

The author of the first German monograph on tropical diseases was the mission doctor Rudolf Fisch, who worked for the Basel Mission on the Gold Coast for 26 years. His *Tropische Krankheiten* first appeared in 1891 and subsequently went through four editions, remaining a best-seller in the field of tropical medicine and hygiene for over 20 years.[80] A review, written by Otto Schellong, a renowned physician, anthropologist and linguist, in the *Deutsche Kolonialzeitung*, praised the "hitherto unequalled, clear approach to the matter" and explained that the manual reflected "Fisch's serenity gained from many years of experience as a physician in the tropics."[81] The importance attached to first-hand experience of distant places was crucial to medical missionaries' acquisition of scientific credibility in the field of tropical medicine. What David Arnold has called the "power of localism" was an important feature in the formative era of tropical medicine and explains why the Basel Mission doctors were successful in establishing themselves as experts in the field.[82]

3 (1886), p. 72–83; Ibid., Gesundheitszustand bzw. Sterblichkeit auf der Goldküste; Ibid., Akklimatisation und Klimafieber, in: Evangelisches Missionsmagazin 30 (1886), p. 129–147.

[79] Alfred Eckhardt, Letters to Committee, 05.04.1886, 04.02.1887, 22.03.1887, Personal File Alfred Eckhardt, BMA, BV 1139.

[80] Rudolf Fisch, Tropische Krankheiten. Anleitung zu ihrer Verhütung und Behandlung speziell für die Westküste von Afrika, für Missionare, Kaufleute, Pflanzer und Beamte, 1st ed., Basel 1891; 2nd ed., Basel 1894; 3rd ed., Basel 1903; 4th ed., Basel 1912.

[81] Otto Schellong, Besprechung der Bücher von R. Fisch und P. Kohlstock, in: Deutsche Kolonialzeitung 4 (1891), p. 182–184, here p. 183.

[82] David Arnold, Introduction. Tropical Medicine before Manson, in: ibid. (ed.), Warm Climates and Western Medicine. The Emergence of Tropical Medicine 1500–1900, Amsterdam/Atlanta 1996, p. 1–19, here p. 6.

Fisch's medical manual, dedicated to "missionaries, traders, planters and officials," provided practical assistance to Europeans in West Africa. The book was structured around the cause, progression, prevention and treatment of "the four most common African diseases," which included malaria, dysentery and diseases of the liver and spleen. The prevention of malaria was discussed in its own chapter entitled "tropical hygiene" and the appendix offered pharmaceutical advice on the use of specific drugs. Despite qualifying diseases as "tropical" or "African," most of these conditions were not confined to these regions. In fact, all the diseases mentioned in Fisch's book were prevalent in Europe at that time.[83]

The claim that tropical diseases represented a distinct area of medical practice was first made by the British physician Patrick Manson in 1897, then practising at the Seaman's Hospital in Greenwich and medical adviser to the Colonial Office.[84] Manson's manual on *Tropical Diseases*, which contained the first cogent discussion of what came to be known as tropical medicine in the English-speaking world, was published in 1898. Yet in 1907, Manson reflected that "tropical disease" was not a scientific category but one that was "useful and practical."[85] Tropical medicine was an ambiguous category in terms of research methodology and lineage, based more on its specific social, historical and political context rather than epistemological distinctions. The question of European acclimatisation and the later concern for the health of colonial subjects in tropical colonies gave rise to a problem-oriented network, which brought together experts from different nations, located in both metropolitan societies in Europe and colonial settings in the tropics.

The foundation of the Liverpool School of Tropical Medicine in 1898, the London School of Tropical Medicine in 1899 and the *Institut für Schiffs- und Tropenkrankheiten* in Hamburg in 1901 required a constant flow of knowledge across the globe. The growing significance of international congresses, academic exchanges and medical publishing facilitated

---

[83] For studies on malaria in Europe, for instance, see Bauche, Medizin und Herrschaft; James L.A. Webb, Humanity's Burden: A Global History of Malaria, Cambridge/New York 2009.

[84] Haynes, Imperial Medicine, p. 85–124.

[85] Michael Worboys, Germs, Malaria and the Invention of Mansonian Tropical Medicine. From "Diseases in the Tropics" to "Tropical Diseases", in: David Arnold, (ed.) Warm Climates and Western Medicine. The Emergence of Tropical Medicine 1500–1900, Amsterdam/Atlanta 1996, p. 181–207, here p. 196.

the circulation of people, ideas and practices.[86] The *Archiv für Schiffs-und Tropenhygiene*, the most important publication for tropical medicine in the German-speaking world, illustrates that the preoccupation with tropical diseases and their prevention crossed professional, institutional, linguistic, national and imperial boundaries. The journal, founded in 1897 and supported by the German Colonial Society, attracted an international and interdisciplinary field of contributors who published not only in German but also in English, French, Italian, Spanish, Portuguese and Dutch.[87]

The Basel Mission doctors regularly contributed to the *Archiv für Schiffs- und Tropenhygiene*.[88] In contrast to most colonial doctors and metropolitan scientists, they witnessed and explored tropical diseases on the ground in West Africa over an extended period of time. They produced data, surveys and theories on the health conditions in their mission areas and circulated them in transimperial networks. Both the global scope and local entrenchment of their mission represented a valuable resource for the formation of a medical speciality devoted to the health conditions in tropical colonies. Simultaneously, their role as scientific brokers between distant colonial sites and metropolitan institutions provided their mission with a new spirit and purpose, linking them with powerful centres of knowledge at home. By contributing to scientific journals, metropolitan institutions and international conferences, the Basel Mission doctors shaped ideas and practices in the field of tropical medicine and hygiene.

The longstanding exclusion of religious actors from the historiography of nineteenth-century science, however, has concealed the significance of missionaries for the formation of tropical medicine. Highlighting the problem is Norman Etherington's assumption that because "the theory and practice of mission medicine diverged so sharply from mainstream scientific models, it tends to be neglected by general histories of

---

[86] Neill, *Networks in Tropical Medicine*, p. 12–43.

[87] Including the most prominent experts in tropical medicine such as Patrick Manson and Alphonse Laveran.

[88] Between 1897 and 1914, Rudolf Fisch published 9 articles and was mentioned in at least 9 articles by other authors, Hermann Vortisch authored 8 articles and was referred to at least 5 times, Friedrich Hey was quoted in 6 articles.

medicine and even in books devoted specifically to imperial medicine."[89] Michael Jennings has addressed this supposed divergence for British Tanganyika and shown that colonial authorities deliberately portrayed mission medicine as curative for evangelising purposes, while their own medical services were framed as preventive. Yet as Jennings has suggested, no such clear demarcation existed.[90] While basic first aid and curative care were indeed part and parcel of mission medicine, medical missionaries also formed an important network through which ideas and practices of tropical medicine were generated and circulated.[91]

3.2.3   Miasma, Germs and Tropical Hygiene

Rudolf Fisch's four editions of *Tropische Krankheiten*, appearing between 1891 and 1912, demonstrate the radical change that medical knowledge about tropical diseases underwent in these two decades. In his foreword to the 1891 edition, his colleague Alfred Eckhardt wrote: "We would not advise anyone to use this book in fifteen years' time. We live in a grand time; just now the study of Koch's great discoveries goes out into the world."[92] Eckhardt, who was not on the Gold Coast but on home leave in Berlin when he wrote these lines, witnessed the initial enthusiasm surrounding Robert Koch's new tuberculosis remedy in 1890–1891 up close, which made him confident that remedies for other pathogens identified under the microscope would follow.[93] Koch and the French

[89] Norman Etherington, Education and Medicine, in: ibid. (ed.) Missions and Empire, Oxford 2005, p. 261–284, here p. 277.

[90] Michael Jennings, "Healing of Bodies, Salvation of Souls". Missionary Medicine in Colonial Tanganyika, 1870s–1939, in: Journal of Religion in Africa 38 (2008), p. 27–56; Ibid., Cooperation and Competition: Missions, the Colonial State and Constructing a Health System in Colonial Tanganyika, in: Anna Greenwood (ed.), Beyond the State. The Colonial Medical Service in British Africa, Manchester 2016, p. 153–173.

[91] Ryan Johnson, Colonial Mission and Imperial Tropical Medicine. Livingstone College, London, 1893–1914, in: Social History of Medicine 23 (2010) 3, p. 549–556.

[92] Alfred Eckhardt, Vorwort, in: Fisch, Tropische Krankheiten, 1st ed., p. xi.

[93] Christoph Gradmann, Krankheit im Labor. Robert Koch und die medizinische Bakteriologie, Göttingen 2005; Ibid., Laboratory Disease. Robert Koch's Medical Bacteriology, Baltimore 2009.

microbiologist Louis Pasteur became the figureheads of a new understanding of disease, which held that specific microbes caused many of the illnesses afflicting human beings and animals.[94]

In contrast to longstanding miasma theories of disease, where disease-causing airs emanated from swamps and rotting vegetable matter, germ theory suggested that diseases were not specifically linked to climate and could, therefore, be overcome by medical science. They could be identified under the microscope and eradicated with the application of bacteriology, which put laboratories at the heart of scientific research and public health policies both at home and abroad. Koch and his assistant, Paul Kohlstock, deepened their investigation into what they called "bacteriological hygiene" at the Imperial Health Office and at the Berlin Institute for Infectious Diseases in the late 1890s. Their research activities focussed on cholera, pest and malaria and included expeditions to South Africa, Egypt, India and German East Africa.[95] Some doctors and scientists, however, held on to the importance of soil, water and air against the bacteriological claims to absoluteness.[96]

The infamous controversy between Koch and Pettenkofer illustrates that research in tropical medicine was long divided between proponents of bacteriology and advocates of environmental causes. Pettenkofer insisted on incorporating environmental and climatic factors into the germ theory of disease, arguing that microbes had to transform or ferment

[94] Koch's bacteriology and Pasteur's microbiology gained wide persuasiveness and had profound effects because the germ theory synthesised natural and social determinants, which previously ran next to each other or mutually excluded each other. This synthesis cannot be understood detached from the cultural framework in which it happened. Therefore, history of science is always history of knowledge. See Bruno Latour, Les microbes. Guerre et Paix, suivi de Irréductions, Paris 1984; Ibid., Science in Action; Ibid., The Pasteurization of France, Cambridge 1988.

[95] Christoph Gradmann, Das reisende Labor: Robert Koch erforscht die Cholera 1883/84, in: Medizinhistorisches Journal 38 (2003) 1, p. 35–56; Wolfgang U. Eckart, Die Medizin und das "Grössere Deutschland". Kolonialpolitik und Tropenmedizin in Deutschland, 1884–1914, in: Berichte zur Wissenschaftsgeschichte 13 (1990), p. 129–139, here p. 129–132.

[96] Michael Worboys, Was There a Bacteriological Revolution in Late Nineteenth-Century Medicine? in: Studies in History and Philosophy of Biological and Biomedical Sciences 38 (2007) 1, p. 20–42; Christoph Gradmann, "Krieg den Bacterien!" Wunsch und Wirklichkeit der medizinischen Bakteriologie und der Labormedizin am Ende des 19. Jahrhunderts, in: "Sei Sauber ...!" Eine Geschichte der Hygiene und der öffentlichen Gesundheitsvorsorge in Europa, ed. by Musée d'Histoire de la Ville de Luxembourg, Köln 2004, p. 228–237.

under favourable conditions before they could become contagious and cause an epidemic. When Koch identified the cholera bacterium in 1882, Pettenkofer asserted that in order for the germ to cause disease it required an ideal composition of the soil, interaction with groundwater and an individual's susceptibility. To demonstrate his claim, Pettenkofer drank water containing cultures of the cholera bacillus in 1892. Though he felt a bit ill, he did not develop a full-blown case of cholera. His self-experiment led him to the conclusion that cholera was linked to the peculiar environment of India, where it was believed to originate, and could therefore not be contagious or endemic in Europe.[97]

Pettenkofer's theory was particularly significant for the conception of diseases in the tropics, since it combined longstanding theories of tropical climate as a cause for disease with more recent bacteriological findings. Medical officers in the colonies, who received Pettenkofer's work with great enthusiasm, now argued that the environmental conditions in tropical colonies favoured the growth of germs and parasites.[98] Paradoxically then, while Koch and Pasteur suggested that microbes could survive and be active anywhere, stressing the universality of their findings, tropical colonies increasingly came to be seen as reservoirs of germs and parasites.[99] Rather than devaluing all existing cosmologies about tropical diseases in one blow, therefore, the germ theory of disease led to a gradual transition, in which aetiologies identified by distinct pathogens under the microscope slowly came to replace symptomatic disease descriptions based on miasma theories.[100]

---

[97] On the history of the controversy, see Paul Steinbrück/Achim Thom (eds.), Robert Koch (1843–1910), Bakteriologe, Tuberkuloseforscher, Hygieniker. Ausgewählte Texte, Leipzig 1982, p. 20–21, 214–215; Ellen Jahn, Die Cholera in Medizin und Pharmazie im Zeitalter des Hygienikers Max von Pettenkofer, Stuttgart 1994.

[98] Most British medical men in nineteenth century India viewed cholera as a disease of locality. See Mark Harrison, A Question of Locality: The Identification of Cholera in British India, 1860–1890, in: David Arnold (ed.) Warm Climates and Western Medicine. The Emergence of Tropical Medicine 1500–1900, Amsterdam/Atlanta 1996, p. 133–159.

[99] Julyan G. Peard, Race, Place, and Medicine. The Idea of the Tropics in Nineteenth-Century Brazilian Medicine, Durham/London 1999; Anderson, Colonial Pathologies.

[100] The University of Basel hosted an Institute for Hygiene from 1892, which stood in Pettenkofer's tradition of statistical and geographical research rather than Koch's bacteriological hygiene. Silvia Berger, "Sie hätten in ein grosses Institut hineingehört". Robert Doerr und der Boom der Basler Hygiene, in: Susanna Burghartz/Georg Kreis (eds.), Geschichte der Universität Basel 1460–2010, January 2010, https://unigeschichte.unibas.ch/fileadmin/user_upload/pdf/Berger_DoerrBaslerHygiene.pdf (last access: 22.07.2022).

In 1890, Rudolf Fisch gave a lecture on "tropical malaria and its prophylaxis" at the 64th Assembly of German Natural Scientists and Physicians in Bremen.[101] Fisch opened his speech by stating that the Gold Coast, and West Africa more generally, were one of the most malaria-affected areas on earth. He claimed that the high air humidity favoured the occurrence of malarial plasmodia, which he argued were the cause for malarial diseases "beyond any doubt," emphasising "we ourselves have repeatedly detected the entities in the blood of malaria patients."[102] Fisch's assertion shows that he supported and adopted the new scientific theories emerging at the time. The French physician Charles Louis Alphonse Laveran had observed in 1880, while working in the military hospital in Constantine, Algeria, that people suffering from malaria presented parasites in their red blood cells. He therefore proposed that a protozoan organism, which he called "Oscillaria malariae," caused malaria.[103]

Simultaneously, Fisch assumed that these malarial plasmodia spread through poison and ferment, developed from decaying matter in the soil, occurring when rain evaporated, or arose from soil disturbed by agricultural and urban development.[104] While he established that malaria was endemic everywhere in West Africa, he recorded differences according to geographical locations, seasons, different types of soil, house building styles, wind directions and inundation areas around rivers, lagoons and creeks.[105] When Fisch gave his speech in Bremen in 1890, the transmission paths of malaria were still unknown, which is why most researchers relied on previous ideas about malaria as an environmental disease. In the formative period of tropical medicine, bacteriological findings went hand in hand with older views on the importance of climatic influences.

---

[101] His speech was printed in: Rudolf Fisch, Die Malaria der Tropen und ihre Prophylaxe, in: Verhandlungen der Gesellschaft Deutscher Naturforscher und Ärzte. 63. Versammlung zu Bremen 15.–20. September 1890, Leipzig 1891, p. 415–429.

[102] Fisch, Die Malaria der Tropen und ihre Prophylaxe, p. 415.

[103] Anne Marie Moulin, Tropical Without the Tropics. The Turning-Point of Pastorian Medicine in North Africa, in: David Arnold (ed.) Warm Climates and Western Medicine. The Emergence of Tropical Medicine 1500–1900, Amsterdam/Atlanta 1996, p. 160–180.

[104] Fisch, Tropische Krankheiten, 1st ed., p. 9–14.

[105] Ibid., Die Malaria der Tropen und ihre Prophylaxe, p. 416–417.

The significance attributed to tropical climate for the health of Europeans meant that the development of preventive measures was key to the question of acclimatisation.[106]

Medical recommendations discussed in the field of tropical hygiene advised Europeans travelling or settling in the colonies to adhere to an intense regime of measures and precautions to stay in good health in the tropics. Fisch highlighted the importance of these prophylactic methods by warning the readers of his *Tropische Krankheiten* of the adversarial tropical climate: "One must never forget that our body is in enemy territory in the tropics and that every weakening of its powers is used by the enemy to conquer it."[107] The ever growing body of knowledge on tropical hygiene around 1900 highlights that medical discourse and practice continued to be informed by the physical and conceptual peculiarities of the tropics.[108]

The Basel Mission doctors moved in transnational academic circles and participated in scientific debates of the time, dealing for instance with what many scientists of the period saw as the all-important problem of European acclimatisation. They became recognised health experts, most notably in the field of tropical hygiene, as notions and practices of hygiene prevailed in wider society in both Europe and Africa. In contrast to present-day usage, hygiene comprised all actions aimed at preserving and enhancing health. "Hygiene is the name of the science that is concerned with the maintenance and promotion of health for society as a whole as well as for the individual," as the Basel Mission doctor Friedrich Hey defined it. Its purpose therefore was "to examine the conditions of healthiness by considering the needs of human nature, the influence of the external world as well as the forces affecting our organism" and "provide means and ways that maintain and promote health."[109]

The Basel Mission doctors not only contributed to knowledge on tropical medicine and hygiene but also published a range of articles and books

---

[106] Anderson, Colonial Pathologies; Worboys, Colonial and Imperial Medicine; Peard, Race, Place, and Medicine.

[107] Fisch, Tropische Krankheiten, 1st ed., p. 28.

[108] James Beattie, Empire and Environmental Anxiety: Health, Science, Art and Conservation in South Asia and Australasia, 1800–1920, New York 2011, p. 39–71.

[109] Friedrich Hey, Der Tropenarzt. Ausführlicher Ratgeber für Europäer in den Tropen, sowie für Besitzer von Plantagen und Handelshäusern, Kolonialbehörden und Missionsverwaltungen, 1st ed., Offenbach 1906, p. 87.

that went beyond tropical specifics and dealt with more general medical questions, such as maternal health, natural healing and mental health.[110] Their scientific networks were not confined to the space of the tropics and their field of research was a sub-discipline of a growing interdisciplinary field dealing with hygiene, including studies on demography, nutrition and sexuality. The increasing importance attached to hygiene across all levels of European societies allowed the Basel Mission doctors to address a growing audience. Friedrich Hey's publication *Gesundheitsquell*, for example, went through eight editions and sold 58,000 copies from 1906 to 1933.[111] Hygiene broadened the interests of the Basel Mission doctors, allowing them to link themselves with the contemporary zeitgeist and to free themselves from accusations of puritan narrowness.

3.3 THE AGE OF HYGIENE

Hygiene—a term derived from the Greek Goddess of health Hygieia—took root as an essential tenet of bourgeois identity during the course of the eighteenth century.[112] It initially expressed concern for the self and was conceived as a practice of responsible and emancipated subjects.[113] By 1900, hygiene had become a fundamental dimension of people's lives across all levels of European societies. Although the concern for heath, the desire for cleanliness and the aspiration for purity are as old as humanity, the age of hygiene engendered a revolutionary programme that put the body at the heart of private as well as public worries and attention. The

---

[110] Friedrich Hey, Willst Du gesund werden? Dann nimm und lies: freies Wort eines Denkenden an Denkende, oder, Medizin und Naturheilkunde, Netstal 1904; Ibid., Wegweiser für den Christen über Leiden, Krankheiten, Heilung, Offenbach 1905; Ibid., Dr. med. Hey's "Frauenwohl". Ein aus Pflanzen bereitetes Präparat zur Verhinderung der Beschwerden der Schwangerschaft und zur Erleichterung der Geburt etc., Berlin 1907; Ibid., Meine Heilmethoden nebst Begründung, Bückeburg 1910; Hermann Vortisch, Mutter und Kind. Ein ärztlicher Ratgeber für junge Frauen, Hamburg 1920; Ibid., Die Nervosität als Störung zwischen Seele und Geist und ihre Überwindung, Hamburg 1921; Ibid., Die Relativitätstheorie und ihre Beziehung zur christlichen Weltanschauung, Hamburg 1921, to name but a few.

[111] Friedrich Hey, Dr. med. Hey's Gesundheitsquell, 8 ed., Leipzig 1906–1933.

[112] The term "hygiène" was introduced into public discourse during the Enlightenment with the publication of the last volumes of Diderot's and d'Alembert's *Encyclopédie* in 1765. See Sarasin, Reizbare Maschinen, p. 19.

[113] Frey, Der reinliche Bürger; Thomas Macho, Keimfrei, Zürich 2013, p. 41–43.

rise of preventive medicine was one of the most significant developments since 1800, forever altering health care, social policies and societies as a whole.[114] Hygiene found wide recognition in a "popular culture of knowledge" after 1840, as Philipp Sarasin has shown,and became a central feature of middle-class identity, propelled by a heterogenous group of stakeholders.[115]

3.3.1   The Hygiene Movement in Basel and Beyond

During the course of the nineteenth century, major epidemic outbreaks of typhus and cholera transformed hygiene from a personal matter into a public affair.[116] Basel's ruling class, who counted on private philanthropy to address social issues and had been reluctant to introduce public health measures, had no choice but to increase municipal interventions in the face of a cholera epidemic in 1855 that cost more than two hundred lives in the city. The municipal government appointed a committee for the combat of cholera, which was chaired by Karl Sarasin. The cholera committee introduced a range of immediate measures, including the erection of a cholera hospital and the disinfection of apartments and public institutions. They also initiated long-term interventions such as riverbed corrections, the construction of a sewage system and permanent street cleaning and waste collection by municipal staff.[117]

---

[114] Martin Lengwiler/Jeanette Madarász (eds.), Das präventive Selbst: Eine Kulturgeschichte moderner Gesundheitspolitik, Bielefeld 2010; Matthias Leanza, Die Zeit der Prävention: Eine Genealogie, Weilerswist 2017; Nicolai Hannig/Malte Thiessen (eds.), Vorsorgen in der Moderne. Akteure, Räume und Praktiken, Berlin/Boston 2017; Philipp Sarasin, Die Geschichte der Gesundheitsvorsorge. Das Verhältnis von Selbstsorge und staatlicher Intervention im 19. und 20. Jahrhundert, in: Cardiovascular Medicine 14 (2011) 2, p. 41–45; Martin Lengwiler/Stefan Beck, Historizität, Materialität und Hybridität von Wissenspraxen. Europäische Präventionsregime im 20. Jahrhundert, in: Geschichte und Gesellschaft 34 (2008), p. 489–523.

[115] Sarasin, Reizbare Maschinen, p. 95–172.

[116] Richard J. Evans' classic study on the 1892 cholera outbreak in Hamburg established the importance of the epidemic in the restructuring of Hamburg patrician politics. Richard D. Evans, Death in Hamburg. Society and Politics in the Cholera Years 1830–1910, Oxford 1987. For Zurich, see Flurin Condrau, Demokratische Bewegung, Choleraepidemie und die Reform des öffentlichen Gesundheitswesens im Kanton Zürich (1867), in: Sudhoffs Archiv 80 (1996) 2, p. 205–219.

[117] Lengwiler, Wissenschaft und Sozialpolitik, p. 118.

For many people, the experience of modernisation took the shape of a hygiene revolution. Their everyday habits radically changed, profoundly transforming the perception of their own body and environment. Hygiene became popular knowledge not so much because of breakthroughs by certain scientists or a paradigm shift within the sciences but rather because of the charitable commitment of a large and heterogenous group of social reformers and evangelical activists that resulted in a broad change in mindset. Experience showed that it was healthier to live in cities with fresh water, canalisation, waste disposal and clean streets long before pathogens could be identified under the microscope.[118]

Increasing industrialisation and urbanisation resulted in major economic and demographic transformations in most European societies. The hygiene movement bourgeoning across nineteenth-century Europe identified disease as an important cause for social destabilisation and political unrest.[119] The emergence, professionalisation and institutionalisation of social hygiene, eugenics and racial hygiene have been widely covered.[120] The beginnings of social hygiene were closely linked to political ideas developed during the attempted revolution of 1848–1849. In German-speaking Europe, physicians such as Salomon Neumann and Rudolf Virchow emphasised the social nature of medicine and advocated that it had to address the general working and living conditions of the entire population. Their voices carried considerable weight since diseased bodies were increasingly associated with political and social disorder.[121]

---

[118] Jürgen Osterhammel, Die Verwandlung der Welt. Eine Geschichte des 19. Jahrhunderts, München 2009, p. 291–292.

[119] Ute Frevert, Krankheit als politisches Problem 1770–1880. Soziale Unterschichten in Preussen zwischen medizinischer Polizei und staatlicher Sozialversicherung, Göttingen 1984, p. 334.

[120] For an overview, see Paul Weindling, Health, Race and German Politics between National Unification and Nazism, 1870–1945, Cambridge 1989; Wolfgang U. Eckart, Die Vision vom "gesunden Volkskörper". Seuchenprophylaxe, Sozial- und Rassenhygiene in Deutschland zwischen Kaiserreich und Nationalsozialismus, in: Susanne Roessiger/ Heidrun Merk (eds.), in: Hauptsache gesund! Gesundheitsaufklärung zwischen Disziplinierung und Emanzipation, Marburg 1998, p. 34–47; Jakob Tanner, Eugenik und Rassenhygiene in Wissenschaft und Politik seit dem ausgehenden 19. Jahrhundert. Ein historischer Überblick, in: Michael Zimmermann (ed.), Zwischen Erziehung und Vernichtung. Zigeunerpolitik und Zigeunerforschung im Europa des 20. Jahrhunderts, Stuttgart 2007, p. 109–121.

[121] Bryan S. Turner, The Body in Western Society: Social Theory and its Perspectives, in: Sarah Coakley (ed.), Religion and The Body, Cambridge 1997, p. 15–41, here p. 18.

The hygiene movement proved particularly successful in Switzerland, where it reached rural communities as well as urban populations. Beatrix Mesmer has argued that it took new hygiene norms merely two generations to prevail in Swiss society in the second half of the nineteenth century.[122] Textbooks on home economics, medical brochures and popular magazines, including *Die Familie* and *Der Hausfreund*, laid down detailed hygiene guidelines and served as a mouthpiece to the growing hygiene movement in Switzerland.[123] Physicians and scientists such as Jakob Laurenz Sonderegger, Louis Guillaume and Adolf Vogt, presented themselves as experts on the topic and popularised scientific explanations and justifications of hygiene. The increasing relevance of hygiene over the nineteenth century, which established health and cleanliness as new shared fundamental values, cemented the social status and moral authority of doctors and scientists.[124]

The increasing concern for preventive medicine and public health promotion in Switzerland was reflected in the creation of numerous associations. The *Gesellschaft für öffentliche Gesundheitspflege*—Society for Public Health Care—was formed in 1868 and the *Schweizerischer Centralverein für Naturheilkunde*—Swiss Central Association for Naturopathy—one year later. The Fourth International Hygiene Congress, held in Geneva in 1882, triggered the foundation of many local societies for hygiene across Switzerland, all connected with each other on national and transnational levels. Well-established organisations such as the *Naturforschende Gesellschaft* or the *Gemeinnützige Gesellschaft* included hygiene in their agendas; the latter introduced a standing committee on hygiene in 1891.[125]

Hygiene gained unprecedented social and political relevance in the nineteenth century because healthy workers and citizens constituted

---

[122] Mesmer, Reinheit und Reinlichkeit, p. 490.

[123] Beatrix Mesmer (ed.), Die Verwissenschaftlichung des Alltags. Anweisungen zum richtigen Umgang mit dem Körper in der schweizerischen Populärpresse 1850–1900, Zürich 1997.

[124] Labisch, Homo Hygienicus; Georges Vigarello, Concepts of Cleanliness: Changing Attitudes in France Since the Middle Ages, Cambridge 1988; Ute Frevert, Professional Medicine and the Working Classes in Imperial Germany, in: Journal of Contemporary History 20 (1985) 4, p. 637–658.

[125] Mesmer, Reinheit und Reinlichkeit, p. 474; Geneviève Heller, Hygiene. 19. und 20. Jahrhundert, in: Historisches Lexikon der Schweiz, http://www.hls-dhs-dss.ch/textes/d/D16310.php, version 17.12.2014 (last access: 22.07.2022).

the pillars of a successful industrial economy and society. Social statistics, which offered data on age-specific morbidity and mortality rates for example, allowed for remarkable cost–benefit calculations. From a macroeconomic perspective, child and adolescent mortality, for instance, appeared as a loss of future labour force and a waste of outlaid upbringing costs. Hygiene, therefore, was not only praised as an end in itself but as a means of achieving higher political and economic goals.[126]

The coupling of medical theories and political agendas turned hygiene and health into a public affair of the utmost concern. The Swiss Confederation passed factory and epidemic laws from the late 1870s, appointed an Advisory Hygiene Commission in 1891, enacted a federal monopoly on spirits gained from fruits and potatoes, created a Federal Health Department in 1894 and introduced health and accident insurance in the early twentieth century.[127] The hygiene movement, however, proved particularly effective on the cantonal and communal level. Swiss cantons and municipalities implemented the sanitation of drinking water, sewage, waste and burials, and conducted construction and food inspections. They also established and supervised their own *Sanitätspolizei*—health officers—to enforce new social norms of health and cleanliness. Schools, which were controlled by cantonal authorities, became crucial sites to anchor hygiene guidelines. School hygiene formed its own scientific discipline in Switzerland, organised as a society from 1899.[128]

Enthusiasm surrounding the germ theory of disease further encouraged governments to intensify their involvement in public health.[129]

---

[126] Alfons Labisch, Doctors, Workers and the Scientific Cosmology of the Industrial World: The Social Construction of 'Health' and the 'Homo Hygienicus', in: Journal of Contemporary History 20 (1985) 4, p. 599–615.

[127] Brigitte Ruckstuhl/Elisabeth Ryter, Von der Seuchenpolizei zu Public Health. Öffentliche Gesundheit in der Schweiz seit 1750, Zürich 2017.

[128] On school hygiene in Switzerland, see Monika Imboden, Die Schule macht gesund. Die Anfänge des schulärztlichen Dienstes der Stadt Zürich und die Macht hygienischer Wissensdispositive in der Volksschule 1860–1900, Zürich 2003; Michèle Hofmann, Gesundheitswissen in der Schule. Schulhygiene in der deutschsprachigen Schweiz im 19. und 20. Jahrhundert, Bielefeld 2016. For Germany, see Jürgen Bennack, Gesundheit und Schule. Zur Geschichte der Hygiene im preussischen Volksschulwesen, Köln 1990; Hideharu Umehara, Gesunde Schule und gesunde Kinder. Schulhygiene in Düsseldorf 1880–1933, Essen 2013.

[129] Paul Weindling, From Germ Theory to Social Medicine: Public Health, 1880–1930, in: Deborah Brunton (ed.), Medicine Transformed. Health, Disease and Society in Europe, 1800–1930, Manchester/New York 2004, p. 239–265.

Whereas sporadic action was taken against only a handful of diseases in the early nineteenth century, European states constantly monitored disease patterns by 1914. They made use of educational programmes and sanitary reforms as well as isolation and immunisation measures to reduce the lethality of a number of infectious diseases, such as typhus and cholera. Health became a seemingly depoliticised foundation of industrial, communal and national social policy because it rested on medical knowledge and was therefore supposedly value-free. State-sponsored measures, however, were not only implemented to protect individual citizens and promote public health but also used as tools for extending the state's influence and authority.[130]

3.3.2   Topographies of Dirt and Disease

In 1893, the English medical journalist Ernest Abraham Hart described cholera as a "filth disease carried by dirty people to dirty places."[131] Following the cholera epidemic of 1832, the governments in France, Prussia and England had conducted large-scale surveys to examine the living conditions that had led to this catastrophe. Various Swiss cities followed fifty years later, spearheaded by Basel in 1889.[132] The surveys examined which flats were hotbeds for germs by recording risk factors such as a lack of light, insufficiently aerated rooms and kitchens, latrines without drains, wash basins without water supply lines, inadequate sewer systems and soils soaked by waste water. Both filth and germs were seen as contributing to disease and the moral values associated with dirt came to dominate the image of people and places considered unhealthy. Municipal health services were put in place to inspect suspect flats and educate the parts of the population identified as threats to a healthy and civilised society.[133]

Hygiene reformers associated social disorder with disease, the latter being not merely an issue of dirt but also of the improper distribution

---

[130] Göckenjan, Kurieren und Staat machen; Axel C. Hüntelmann, Hygiene im Namen des Staates. Das Reichsgesdunheitsamt 1876–1933, Göttingen 2008.

[131] Ernest A. Hart, Cholera: Where It Comes From and How It Is Propagated, in: The British Medical Journal 2 (1 July 1893) 1696, p. 1–4, here p. 1.

[132] Lausanne followed in 1894, Berne in 1896, Winterthur and St. Gall in 1897.

[133] Koller, "Gesundes Wohnen"; Othmar Birkner, Hygiene im Schatten der Cholera, in: Kunst + Architektur in der Schweiz 55 (2004), p. 68–73.

of bodies in space. Their aim, therefore, was to regulate the circulation of matter or people that they deemed to be dangerous because of their contact with unknown people in unknown places.[134] The absence of clearly demarcated and visibly distinct persons, families and habitations was often deemed unhygienic and therefore unhealthy. Practically, this meant that both social policy at home and the civilising mission abroad had to transform people's domestic lives by creating the conditions and attitude required for cleanliness, thereby achieving a world in which all matter, beings and bodies were in their proper place.[135]

In order to venture into the private sphere, hygiene reformers needed to gain the support of middle-class women, who had to a large extent been ruled out of the labour market. They were identified as the most important allies in the quest for personal hygiene and domestic cleanliness and were targeted through weekly family newspapers, women's magazines and housekeeping manuals.[136] Hygiene, much like evangelicalism, was a field where women became publicly involved through membership and participation in societies such as the *Schweizer Gemeinnützige Frauen-verband*—Swiss Charitable Women's Association—founded in 1888. This organisation attracted political attention by pushing for the implementation of compulsory housekeeping instruction for girls in primary and secondary schools in all cantons.[137] The campaign rested on the

---

[134] Felix Driver, Moral Geographies: Social Science and the Urban Environment in Mid-Nineteenth Century England, in: Transactions of the Institute of British Geographers 13 (1988) 3, p. 275–287; David Armstrong, Public Health Spaces and the Fabrication of Identity, in: Sociology 27 (1993) 3, p. 393–410; William A. Cohen/Ryan Johnson (eds.), Filth: Dirt, Disgust, and Modern Life, Minneapolis 2005; Ben Campkin/Rosie Cox (eds.), Dirt: New Geographies of Cleanliness and Contamination, New York 2007; Friedrich Lenger, Stadthygiene: Gesundheit und städtischer Raum in Europa während der zweiten Hälfte des 19. Jahrhunderts, in: Heinz-Peter Schmiedebach, Medizin und öffentliche Gesundheit. Konzepte, Akteure, Perspektiven, Berlin/Boston 2018, p. 85–94.

[135] John Comaroff/Jean Comaroff, Ethnography and the Historical Imagination, Boulder 1992, p. 280–290.

[136] Alison Bashford has analysed how the nineteenth century hygiene movement was shaped by a gendered politics of health. See Alison Bashford, Purity and Pollution. Gender, Embodiment and Victorian Medicine, Basingstoke 2000. See further Nancy Tomes, The Gospel of Germs: Men, Women, and the Microbe in American Life, Cambridge 1999.

[137] Anne-Marie Stalder, Die Erziehung zur Häuslichkeit: Über den Beitrag des hauswirtschaftlichen Unterrichts zur Disziplinierung der Unterschichten im 19. Jahrhundert in der Schweiz, in: Schweizerische Zeitschrift für Geschichte 34 (1984), p. 370–384; Mesmer, Reinheit und Reinlichkeit, p. 489–490.

widespread view that the lack of housekeeping skills of working-class women led to domestic misery and alcoholism.[138] Housekeeping classes were introduced in public schools in the late nineteenth century and the First International Congress on Home Economics was held in Fribourg in 1908.[139]

Hygiene was used as a spatial system of ordering with inward and outward boundaries, which located filth in specific physical and cognitive spaces. Whilst what it meant to be clean and healthy was indicated by a variety of visible signs, the meaning of hygiene also relied on medical diagrams and topographies. They visualised hygiene in relation to gender, race, class and religion, and naturalised it as a state of being that corresponded to an imagined norm. Advocates of hygiene identified the female, non-white, poor and non-Christian parts of the world population as a threat to the civilised virtues of cleanliness, health and order.[140] These multi-relational markers of difference justified the stigmatisation of whole sections of the population on the grounds that they were dirty, unhealthy and therefore dangerous for public health and a functional polity.[141]

At the same time, hygiene allowed individuals and groups to unify their experiences, contributing to the formation of shared identities.[142] Ulrich im Hof argued in the early 1990s that hygiene significantly shaped how Swiss people have perceived themselves and others since the late

[138] Ute Frevert, "Fürsorgliche Belagerung": Hygienebewegung und Arbeiterfrauen im 19. und frühen 20. Jahrhundert, in: Geschichte und Gesellschaft 11 (1985) 4, p. 420–446.

[139] Anonymous, Erster internationaler Kongress für Haushaltungsunterricht. Vom Kongress in Freiburg angenommene Beschlüsse, in: Die Mädchenfortbildungsschule. Beilage zur Schweizerischen Lehrerinnen-Zeitung 13 (1908–1909), p. 7–8, 11–12, 14–15.

[140] For Switzerland and Basel in particular, see Véronique Mottier, Narratives of National Identity: Sexuality, Race and the Swiss Dream of Order, in: Swiss Journal of Sociology 26 (2000) 3, p. 533–556; Regina Wecker, "Erbkrankheit Armut". Eheverbote und eugenische Konzepte im Umgang mit Armen im 19. und 20. Jahrhundert, in: Josef Mooser/Simon Wenger (eds.), Armut und Fürsorge in Basel. Armutspolitik vom 13. Jahrhundert bis heute, Basel 2011, p. 205–215.

[141] Dana Berthold, Tidy Whiteness: A Genealogy of Race, Purity and Hygiene, in: Ethics & The Environment 15 (2010) 1, p. 1–26; Joanna de Groot, "Sex" and "Race": The Construction of Language and Image in the Nineteenth Century, in: Catherine Hall (ed.), Cultures of Empire. A Reader: Colonizers in Britain and the Empire in the Nineteenth and Twentieth Centuries, New York 2000, p. 37–60.

[142] Wolfgang Kaschuba, Nachwort: "Deutsche Sauberkeit"—Zivilisierung der Körper und der Köpfe, in: Georges Vigarello, Wasser und Seife, Puder und Parfüm. Geschichte der Körperhygiene seit dem Mittelalter, Frankfurt a. M./New York 1992, p. 292–326.

nineteenth century. According to him, work ethic, a legacy of the Reformation, merged with a new ethic of hygiene, which declared values such as health and cleanliness to be virtues of the hard-working and modest Swiss people. Although hygiene became a symbol of progress and modernity in all industrial nations, im Hof identified a "particular Swiss meaning" of hygiene on the grounds that it was elevated to a moral value.[143] This Swiss myth of hygiene has served as an effective political, cultural and social tool for the exclusion of minorities and the assertion of a national identity. Patricia Purtschert has recently shown how the figure of the Swiss housewife, originating in nineteenth-century colonial discourse, became a fixture of bourgeois national identity in the 1930s and continues to inform ideas of cleanliness, gender and race in Switzerland to this day.[144]

Proponents of the hygiene movement used fear of disease and social exclusion as a lever to instil a sense of responsibility in people, both for their own bodies and the health of the whole nation. However, their attempts at persuasion were not simply based on scientific arguments and rational explanations. On the contrary, they deliberately utilised emotions such as fear and disgust to leverage their political agenda, social norms and cultural values. Feelings of insecurity originating in demographic and social shifts helped to develop ever more specific hygiene rituals concerning the body, housing and nutrition. The constant exhortation by missionaries that boundaries were not to be transgressed constituted an important feature of the hygiene movement, as Alexandra Przyrembel has argued in her book on the taboo.[145] Theorists and agitators of hygiene adopted the missionary gospel of moral improvement, making hygiene the new signal of personal integrity and civic responsibility.

3.3.3   The New Godliness of Hygiene

Knowledge of hygiene was negotiated in social and geographic outposts between activists seeking to establish new—or rather change existing—bodily practices and the people they tried to transform. Missionaries

---

[143] Ulrich im Hof, Mythos Schweiz. Nation—Identität—Geschichte 1291–1991, Zürich 1991, p. 192–193.

[144] Purtschert, Kolonialität und Geschlecht im 20. Jahrhundert, p. 71–184.

[145] Alexandra Przyrembel, Verbote und Geheimnisse. Das Tabu und die Genese der europäischen Moderne, Frankfurt a. M. 2011.

promoted themselves as moral entrepreneurs and social reformers, who set out to locate, portray and tackle filth both at home and abroad. While city missionaries in Europe reported on the filth they encountered in depraved urban neighbourhoods, thereby emphasising the need to re-Christianise the lower social strata, missionaries in West Africa reported on the filth they perceived among the African population and thus underlined the necessity of their evangelising efforts abroad. These narratives of dirt made hygiene a universal imperative and allowed evangelicals to recode religious purity with social, political and scientific meanings.

The scale and density of the Basel Mission's networks and media sustained social causes such as the hygiene crusade, which evangelicals did not initiate but certainly appropriated. The cover image of a tractate published by the Basel Mission at least twice in 1879 and in 1887, entitled *Heidenmission in London*, shows a city missionary cleaning a street child under a water pump (Fig. 3.1).[146] Small and easy to carry around, tractates were an important informational resource and advertising tool through which the Basel Mission conveyed knowledge on a specific issue in a systematic, concise and clear manner.[147] The illustration highlights that the Basel Mission not only identified a lack of cleanliness, health and civilisation in Africa but also in European cities. They popularised a generalised image of the pitiful and needy proletariat that corresponded with the prevalent image of the poor heathens in the colonies. In their eyes, both needed to be saved from the filth and decay of their environment by evangelical initiatives.

The Basel Mission not only reported on the success of the London Medical Mission Society in "heathen lands" but also "in the poor quarters of England's big cities."[148] Organisations dedicated to propagating the gospel in their immediate vicinity in Basel, Hamburg, Paris or London, established shelters for children, city and railway missions and started visiting depraved neighbourhoods. In introducing visitation as a systematic practice of social control, Protestant philanthropists in Basel, and on

---

[146] Heidenmission in London, 2nd ed., Basel 1887, BMA, V.2b.47.

[147] Julia Mack, Publikationen und Unterrichtsmaterialien, in: Christine Christ-von Wedel/Thomas K. Kuhn (ed.), Basler Mission. Menschen, Geschichte, Perspektiven 1815–2015, Basel 2015, p. 119–124, here p. 121–122; Mack, Menschenbiler, p. 92–94.

[148] August Hermann Heinrich Wittenberg, Einiges aus der missionsärztlichen Arbeit in London, in: An die Freunde des Ärztlichen Zweiges der Basler Mission, Basel 1893, p. 30–31, here p. 30.

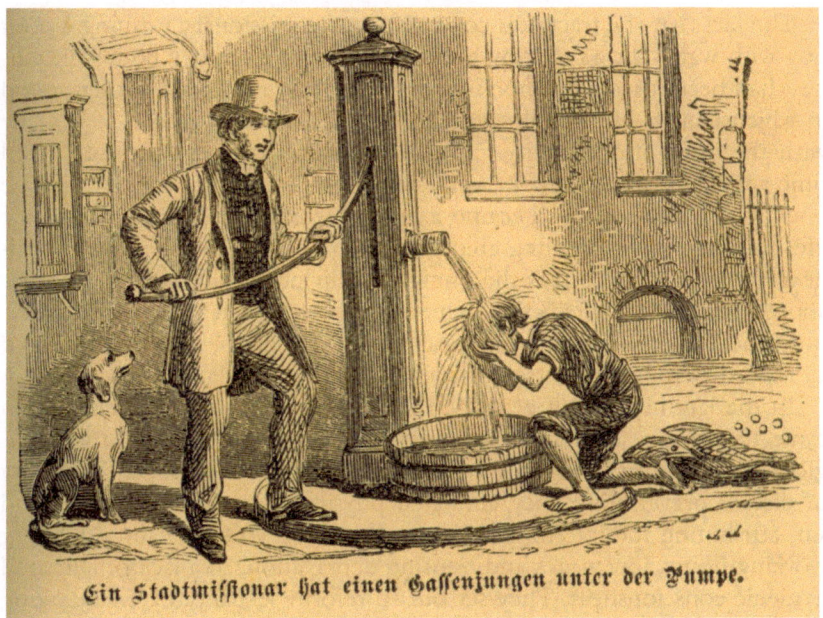

Fig. 3.1   Heidenmission in London, 2nd ed., Basel 1887, BMA, V.2b.47

the continent more generally, drew on models derived from Britain and Scotland, where this had been practised since the second half of the eighteenth century.[149] City missionaries, pastors and deaconesses active in the home mission movement chronicled their day-to-day community service in letters, pamphlets and work reports, which produced knowledge on the dirt and misery of the lower classes and established social topographies of poverty.[150]

---

[149] Bernd Weisbrod, "Visiting" and "Social Control". Statistische Gesellschaften und Stadtmissionen im Viktorianischen England, in: Christoph Sachsse/Florian Tennstedt (eds.), Sozial Sicherheit und soziale Disziplinierung. Beiträge zu einer historischen Theorie der Sozialpolitik, Frankfurt a. M. 1986, p. 181–208; Friedrich/Jähnichen, Geschichte der sozialen Ideen im deutschen Protestantismus, p. 890–892.

[150] Thorne, "The Conversion of Englishmen and the Conversion of the World Inseparable"; Comaroff/Comaroff, Home-Made Hegemony; Ibid., Of Revelation and Revolution, vol. 1; Przyrembel, Verbote und Geheimnisse.

The fact that the tractate's cover depicted a missionary washing a poor boy with water shows that by the late nineteenth century bodily cleanliness had been fused with moral purity. This fusion followed a long period in which Pietists had genuinely despised the close associations of hygiene with the body and sexuality.[151] Pietist purity had to be reprogrammed time and again, and equipped with suitable meanings in order to become operative. Since hygiene became a key dimension of private and public life, the Basel Mission integrated the material body and ideas of cleanliness into their concepts of the immaterial divine world and purity. Their appropriation of hygiene was helped by the fact that purity had always been more than a mere theological tenet for Pietists, governing instead all aspects of life from personal asceticism to social relationships.

In the late nineteenth century, those involved with the Basel Mission came to embrace hygiene as a Christian principle by merging their religious ideal of purity with medical and political arguments for the necessity of disease prevention. They conflated physical dirt with immorality and sin, attributing the inferior health conditions of workers, caused by long working hours, low wages and housing depravation, to a lack of faith and hygienic consciousness. They set out to reform sexuality by encouraging legal, Christian marriage and the creation of nuclear households, thus ostensibly putting an end to drunken indulgence in procreation. They also promoted the ideal of private property, beginning with the family home, and tried to reform gender relations and the social division of labour. Due to the comprehensive documentation of missionaries at home and abroad, purity—and more conspicuously impurity—were now visible on the streets and individual bodies. Cleanliness was, after all, next to godliness.[152]

The fact that missionaries succeeded in positioning themselves as important protagonists of the nineteenth-century hygiene movement reveals that the seemingly scientific arguments by medical experts, social reformers and political authorities worked in much the same way as older

---

[151] Smith, Clean, ch. 7, p. 185–223.

[152] Shin K. Kim, An Antiseptic Religion: Discovering a Hybridity on the Flux of Hygiene and Christianity, in: Journal of Religion and Health 47 (2008) 2, p. 253–262; Katharina Stornig, Cultural Conceptions of Purity and Pollution. Childbirth and Midwifery in a New Guinean Catholic Mission, 1896–c. 1930, in: Judith Becker (ed.), European Missions in Contact Zones: Transformation Through Interaction in a (Post-) Colonial World, Göttingen 2015, p. 107–123.

religious purity regulations. A quote from an article in the *Swiss Women's Magazine* in 1888 illustrates how religious convictions of sin and purity shaped nineteenth-century knowledge of hygiene: "Cleanliness develops a sense of shame as soon as any impurity occurs. [...] Anyone who views their body as temple of God that may not to be stained, will not tolerate the stains on their soul."[153] The body as a temple of God was a popular metaphor used by a wide range of people advocating new behaviours of hygiene. While it is unquestionable that hygiene gained wide societal relevance because of the growing significance of scientific medicine and the increasing scope of state interventions, the social assumptions and moral implications of hygiene were clearly rooted in longstanding religious beliefs of purity.

In this sense, hygiene was the nineteenth-century expression of religious purity, which used medical justifications to create a new social order and sense of belonging. Health guidelines, popularised by the hygiene movement, were tied to customs in the religious calendar: Saturday became the day for a purifying bath, Sunday was for fresh air and the revitalising of the bodily organs. Sunday walks and Saturday baths became rituals of a healthy lifestyle and anyone who did not observe them committed a greater sin than staying away from church, as a pastor from Basel warned in a sermon in 1903: "We want to be Christians but consider the first precepts of cleanliness as if they do not apply to us. First, we must keep ourselves and our children in order and clean, and only then can we speak of Christianity."[154] This citation underlines that old Pietist taboos surrounding the body as a sinful and unchaste matter had given way to a new ethic of hygiene that combined spiritual purity with physical cleanliness.

The systematisation of knowledge through encyclopaedias and handbooks allowed for the constitution of seemingly secular sciences by emancipating and demarcating them from theology and metaphysical beliefs.[155] Bruno Latour has described these methods of differentiation

---

[153] Anonymous, Reinheit und Reinlichkeit, in: Schweizer Frauen-Zeitung, 25.11.1888, p. 189.

[154] Georg Müller, Die Erziehung der Jugend zur körperlichen Gesundheit, in: Das Alpenhorn, 20.06.1903, p. 93.

[155] Philipp Sarasin suggested that "maybe sciences consist in nothing else than inventing terms and classifications and then successfully pretending that they reveal the innocent truth of things." Sarasin, Reizbare Maschinen, p. 99.

and secularisation as "practices of purification."[156] According to him, the cognitive division between religious, scientific and political domains of society is an expression of a modern pursuit for purity. In this sense, the manifestation of hygiene in the nineteenth century originated from the efforts of scientists who tried to purify society from religious ideas of purity by replacing them with secular arguments. Yet to this day, hygiene sits uneasily between ideal and reality, between the private and the public, and between the scientific and the moral, or religious, domains of society. The making of hygiene in the nineteenth century entailed a reformulation of Pietist notions of the body and purity, which in turn transformed the understanding of hygiene itself.

REFERENCES

Warwick Anderson, Climates of Opinion. Acclimatization in Nineteenth-Century France and England, in: Victorian Studies 35 (1992) 2, p. 135–157.

Warwick Anderson, Colonial Pathologies. American Tropical Medicine, Race, and Hygiene in the Philippines, Durham/London 2006.

Anonymous, Die afrikanischen Todesfälle, in: Der Evangelische Heidenbote 54 (1881), p. 69–71, 74–78.

Anonymous, Reinheit und Reinlichkeit, in: Schweizer Frauen-Zeitung, 25.11.1888, p. 189.

Anonymous, Erster internationaler Kongress für Haushaltungsunterricht. Vom Kongress in Freiburg angenommene Beschlüsse, in: Die Mädchenfortbildungsschule. Beilage zur Schweizerischen Lehrerinnen-Zeitung 13 (1908–1909), p. 7–8, 11–12, 14–15.

David Armstrong, Public Health Spaces and the Fabrication of Identity, in: Sociology 27 (1993) 3, p. 393–410.

David Arnold, Introduction. Tropical Medicine before Manson, in: ibid. (ed.), Warm Climates and Western Medicine. The Emergence of Tropical Medicine 1500–1900, Amsterdam/Atlanta 1996, p. 1–19.

David Arnold, Inventing Tropicality, in: ibid. (ed.), The Problem of Nature. Environment, Culture, and European Expansion, London 1996, p. 141–168.

David Arnold, The Tropics and the Traveling Gaze: India, Landscape, and Science, 1800–1856, Seattle 2006.

Alison Bashford, Purity and Pollution. Gender, Embodiment and Victorian Medicine, Basingstoke 2000.

---

[156] Latour, We Have Never Been Modern.

Manuela Bauche, Medizin und Herrschaft. Malariabekämpfung in Kamerun, Ostafrika und Ostfriesland 1890–1919, Frankfurt a. M. 2017.

James Beattie, Empire and Environmental Anxiety: Health, Science, Art and Conservation in South Asia and Australasia, 1800–1920, New York 2011.

Ernst Below, Die praktischen Ziele der Tropenhygiene, in: Verhandlungen der Gesellschaft deutscher Naturforscher und Ärzte, 68. Versammlung, Frankfurt a. M., 21.–26. September 1896, ed. by Albert Wangerin/Otto Taschenberg, part 1, Leipzig 1896, p. 91–120.

Jürgen Bennack, Gesundheit und Schule. Zur Geschichte der Hygiene im preussischen Volksschulwesen, Köln 1990.

Silvia Berger, "Sie hätten in ein grosses Institut hineingehört". Robert Doerr und der Boom der Basler Hygiene, in: Susanna Burghartz/ Georg Kreis (eds.), Geschichte der Universität Basel 1460–2010, January 2010, https://unigeschichte.unibas.ch/fileadmin/user_upload/pdf/Berger_ DoerrBaslerHygiene.pdf (last access: 22.07.2022).

Dana Berthold, Tidy Whiteness: A Genealogy of Race, Purity and Hygiene, in: Ethics & The Environment 15 (2010) 1, p. 1–26.

Othmar Birkner, Hygiene im Schatten der Cholera, in: Kunst + Architektur in der Schweiz 55 (2004), p. 68–73.

Walter Bruchhausen, Die "hygienische Eroberung" der Tropen. Gesundheitsschutz als europäischer Export in kolonialer und nachkolonialer Zeit, in: "Sei Sauber...!" Eine Geschichte der Hygiene und der öffentlichen Gesundheitsvorsorge in Europa, ed. by Musée d'Histoire de la Ville de Luxembourg, Köln 2004, p. 204–217.

Deborah Brunton, The Rise of Laboratory Medicine, in: ibid. (ed.), Medicine Transformed. Health, Disease and Society in Europe, 1800–1930, Manchester/New York 2004, p. 92–118.

Ben Campkin/Rosie Cox (eds.), Dirt: New Geographies of Cleanliness and Contamination, New York 2007.

Pratik Chakrabarti, Medicine and Empire, 1600–1960, Basingstoke 2014.

Theodor Christlieb, Der gegenwärtige Stand der evangelischen Heidenmission, in: Allgemeine Missionszeitschrift 6 (1879), p. 481–582.

Theodor Christlieb, Protestant Foreign Missions. Their Present State, A Universal Survey, London 1880.

Theodor Christlieb, Protestant Missions to the Heathen. A General Survey of their Recent Progress and Present State Throughout the World, Calcutta/ Edinburgh 1882.

Bernard Cohen (ed.), Puritanism and the Rise of Modern Science: The Merton Thesis, New Brunswick/London 1990.

William A. Cohen/Ryan Johnson (eds.), Filth: Dirt, Disgust, and Modern Life, Minneapolis 2005.

John Comaroff/Jean Comaroff, Of Revelation and Revolution, vol. 1: Christianity, Colonialism and Consciousness in South Africa, Chicago 1991.

John Comaroff/Jean Comaroff, Ethnography and the Historical Imagination, Boulder 1992.

John Comaroff/Jean Comaroff, Home-Made Hegemony: Modernity, Domesticity, and Colonialism in South Africa, in: Karen Tranberg Hansen (ed.), African Encounters with Domesticity, New Brunswick 1992, p. 37–74.

Flurin Condrau, Demokratische Bewegung, Choleraepidemie und die Reform des öffentlichen Gesundheitswesens im Kanton Zürich (1867), in: Sudhoffs Archiv 80 (1996) 2, p. 205–219.

Philip D. Curtin, "The White Man's Grave": Image and Reality, 1780–1850, in: The Journal of British Studies 1 (1961), p. 94–110.

Justin A. Davis, Pietism and the Foundations of the Modern World, Eugene 2019.

Hans Werner Debrunner, Schweizer im kolonialen Afrika, Basel 1991.

Felix Driver, Moral Geographies: Social Science and the Urban Environment in Mid-Nineteenth Century England, in: Transactions of the Institute of British Geographers 13 (1988) 3, p. 275–287.

Felix Driver/Luciana Martins (eds.), Tropical Visions in an Age of Empire, Chicago/London 2005.

Wolfgang U. Eckart, Die Medizin und das "Grössere Deutschland". Kolonialpolitik und Tropenmedizin in Deutschland, 1884–1914, in: Berichte zur Wissenschaftsgeschichte 13 (1990), p. 129–139.

Wolfgang U. Eckart, Die Anfänge der deutschen Tropenmedizin. Die Gründung des Hamburger Instituts für Schiffs- und Tropenkrankheiten, in: Heinz Schott (ed.), Meilensteine der Medizin, Dortmund 1996, p. 411–418

Wolfgang U. Eckart, Medizin und Kolonialimperialismus. Deutschland 1884–1945, Paderborn 1997.

Wolfgang U. Eckart, Die Vision vom "gesunden Volkskörper". Seuchenprophylaxe, Sozial- und Rassenhygiene in Deutschland zwischen Kaiserreich und Nationalsozialismus, in: Susanne Roessiger/Heidrun Merk (eds.), in: Hauptsache gesund! Gesundheitsaufklärung zwischen Disziplinierung und Emanzipation, Marburg 1998, p. 34–47.

Wolfgang U. Eckart, "Reichgottesarbeit" nicht Reichsarbeit—Theodor Christlieb und die Idee einer deutschen ärztlichen Mission in der Wilhelminischen Epoche, in: Richard Toellner (ed.), Die Geburt einer sanften Medizin. Die Franckeschen Stiftungen zu Halle als Begegnungsstätte von Medizin und Pietismus im frühen 18. Jahrhundert, Halle 2004, p. 151–158.

Georgina H. Endfield/David J. Nash, Missionaries and Morals: Climatic Discourse in Nineteenth-Century Central Southern Africa, in: Annals of the Association of American Geographers 92 (2002) 4, p. 727–742.

Norman Etherington, Education and Medicine, in: ibid. (ed.) Missions and Empire, Oxford 2005, p. 261–284.

Richard D. Evans, Death in Hamburg. Society and Politics in the Cholera Years 1830–1910, Oxford 1987.

Johannes Fabian, Out of Our Minds. Reason and Madness in the Exploration of Central Africa, Berkley et al. 2000.

Gary B. Ferngren, Medicine and Religion. A Historical Introduction, Baltimore 2014.

Rudolf Fisch, Die Malaria der Tropen und ihre Prophylaxe, in: Verhandlungen der Gesellschaft Deutscher Naturforscher und Ärzte. 63. Versammlung zu Bremen 15.–20. September 1890, Leipzig 1891, p. 415–429.

Rudolf Fisch, Tropische Krankheiten. Anleitung zu ihrer Verhütung und Behandlung speziell für die Westküste von Afrika, für Missionare, Kaufleute, Pflanzer und Beamte, 1st ed., Basel 1891; 2nd ed., Basel 1894; 3rd ed., Basel 1903; 4th ed., Basel 1912.

Friedrich Hermann Fischer, Der Missionsarzt Rudolf Fisch und die Anfänge medizinischer Arbeit der Basler Mission an der Goldküste (Ghana), Herzogenrath 1991.

Ute Frevert, Krankheit als politisches Problem 1770–1880. Soziale Unterschichten in Preussen zwischen medizinischer Polizei und staatlicher Sozialversicherung, Göttingen 1984.

Ute Frevert, "Fürsorgliche Belagerung": Hygienebewegung und Arbeiterfrauen im 19. und frühen 20. Jahrhundert, in: Geschichte und Gesellschaft 11 (1985) 4, p. 420–446.

Ute Frevert, Professional Medicine and the Working Classes in Imperial Germany, in: Journal of Contemporary History 20 (1985) 4, p. 637–658.

Manuel Frey, Der reinliche Bürger. Entstehung und Verbreitung bürgerlicher Tugenden in Deutschland, 1760–1860, Göttingen 1997.

Norbert Friedrich/Traugott Jähnichen, Geschichte der sozialen Ideen im deutschen Protestantismus, in: Helga Grebing (ed.), Geschichte der sozialen Ideen in Deutschland. Sozialismus—katholische Soziallehre—protestantische Sozialethik. Ein Handbuch, 2nd ed., Wiesbaden 2005, p. 867–1102.

Johanna Geyer-Kordesch, Pietismus, Medizin und Aufklärung im 18. Jahrhundert. Das Leben und Werk Georg Ernst Stahls, Tübingen 2000.

Michael Gladwin, Mission and Colonialism, in: Joel D. S. Rasmussen/Judith Wolfe/Johannes Zachhuber (eds.), The Oxford Handbook of Nineteenth-Century Christian Thought, Oxford 2017, p. 282–304.

Gerd Göckenjan, Kurieren und Staat machen. Gesundheit und Medizin in der bürgerlichen Welt, Frankfurt a. M. 1985.

Constantin Goschler, Rudolf Virchow. Mediziner—Anthropologe—Politiker, Köln/Weimar/Wien 2009.

Christoph Gradmann, Das reisende Labor: Robert Koch erforscht die Cholera 1883/84, in: Medizinhistorisches Journal 38 (2003) 1, p. 35–56.

Christoph Gradmann, "Krieg den Bacterien!" Wunsch und Wirklichkeit der medizinischen Bakteriologie und der Labormedizin am Ende des 19. Jahrhunderts, in: "Sei Sauber...!" Eine Geschichte der Hygiene und der öffentlichen Gesundheitsvorsorge in Europa, ed. by Musée d'Histoire de la Ville de Luxembourg, Köln 2004, p. 228–237.

Christoph Gradmann, Krankheit im Labor. Robert Koch und die medizinische Bakteriologie, Göttingen 2005.

Christoph Gradmann, Laboratory Disease. Robert Koch's Medical Bacteriology, Baltimore 2009.

Charles Scovell Grant, West African Hygiene. Or, Hints on the Preservation of Health, and the Treatment of Disease on the West Coast of Africa, London 1882, 1884, 1887.

Charles Scovell Grant, Petit guide d'hygiène pratique dans l'Ouest Africain, Paris 1882, 1893.

Martin Greschat, Die Vorgeschichte der Inneren Mission, in: ibid. (ed.), Die christliche Mitgift Europas—Traditionen und Zukunft, Stuttgart 2000, p. 87–105.

Joanna de Groot, "Sex" and "Race": The Construction of Language and Image in the Nineteenth Century, in: Catherine Hall (ed.), Cultures of Empire. A Reader: Colonizers in Britain and the Empire in the Nineteenth and Twentieth Centuries, New York 2000, p. 37–60.

Nicolai Hannig/Malte Thiessen (eds.), Vorsorgen in der Moderne. Akteure, Räume und Praktiken, Berlin/Boston 2017.

David Hardiman, Introduction, in: ibid. (ed.), Healing Bodies, Saving Souls. Medical Missions in Asia and Africa, Amsterdam/New York 2006, p. 5–57.

David Hardiman, The Mission Hospital 1880–1960, in: Mark Harrison/Margaret Jones/Helen Sweet (eds.), From Western Medicine to Global Medicine. The Hospital Beyond the West, Hyderabad 2009, p. 198–220.

Mark Harrison, A Question of Locality: The Identification of Cholera in British India, 1860–1890, in: David Arnold (ed.) Warm Climates and Western Medicine. The Emergence of Tropical Medicine 1500–1900, Amsterdam/Atlanta 1996, p. 133–159.

Mark Harrison, Climates and Constitutions: Health, Race, Environment and British Imperialism in India, 1600–1850, Delhi 1999.

Ernest A. Hart, Cholera: Where It Comes From and How It Is Propagated, in: The British Medical Journal 2 (1 July 1893) 1696, p. 1–4.

Douglas Melvin Haynes, Imperial Medicine. Patrick Manson and the Conquest of Tropical Disease, Philadelphia 2001.

Geneviève Heller, Hygiene. 19. und 20. Jahrhundert, in: Historisches Lexikon der Schweiz, http://www.hls-dhs-dss.ch/textes/d/D16310.php, version 17.12.2014 (last access: 22.07.2022).

Jürgen Helm, "Dass auch zugleich die Gottseligkeit dadurch gebauet wird". Pietismus und Medizin in der ersten Hälfte des achtzehnten Jahrhunderts, in: Berichte zur Wissenschaftsgeschichte 26 (2003) 3, p. 199–211.

Friedrich Hey, Willst Du gesund werden? Dann nimm und lies: freies Wort eines Denkenden an Denkende, oder, Medizin und Naturheilkunde, Netstal 1904.

Friedrich Hey, Wegweiser für den Christen über Leiden, Krankheiten, Heilung, Offenbach 1905.

Friedrich Hey, Der Tropenarzt. Ausführlicher Ratgeber für Europäer in den Tropen, sowie für Besitzer von Plantagen und Handelshäusern, Kolonialbehörden und Missionsverwaltungen, 1st ed., Offenbach 1906.

Friedrich Hey, Dr. med. Hey's "Frauenwohl". Ein aus Pflanzen bereitetes Präparat zur Verhinderung der Beschwerden der Schwangerschaft und zur Erleichterung der Geburt etc., Berlin 1907.

Friedrich Hey, Meine Heilmethoden nebst Begründung, Bückeburg 1910.

Friedrich Hey, Dr. med. Hey's Gesundheitsquell, 8 ed., Leipzig 1906–1933.

Ulrich im Hof, Mythos Schweiz. Nation—Identität—Geschichte 1291-1991, Zürich 1991.

Michèle Hofmann, Gesundheitswissen in der Schule. Schulhygiene in der deutschsprachigen Schweiz im 19. und 20. Jahrhundert, Bielefeld 2016.

Axel C. Hüntelmann, Hygiene im Namen des Staates. Das Reichsgesdunheitsamt 1876-1933, Göttingen 2008.

Mark Hutchinson/John Wolffe, A Short History of Global Evangelicalism, Cambridge 2012.

Monika Imboden, Die Schule macht gesund. Die Anfänge des schulärztlichen Dienstes der Stadt Zürich und die Macht hygienischer Wissensdispositive in der Volksschule 1860-1900, Zürich 2003.

L. S. Jacyna, Localization of Disease, in: Deborah Brunton (ed.), Medicine Transformed. Health, Disease and Society in Europe, 1800–1930, Manchester/New York 2004, p. 1–30.

Ellen Jahn, Die Cholera in Medizin und Pharmazie im Zeitalter des Hygienikers Max von Pettenkofer, Stuttgart 1994.

Michael Jennings, "Healing of Bodies, Salvation of Souls". Missionary Medicine in Colonial Tanganyika, 1870s–1939, in: Journal of Religion in Africa 38 (2008), p. 27–56.

Michael Jennings, Cooperation and Competition: Missions, the Colonial State and Constructing a Health System in Colonial Tanganyika, in: Anna Greenwood (ed.), Beyond the State. The Colonial Medical Service in British Africa, Manchester 2016, p. 153–173.

Ryan Johnson, Colonial Mission and Imperial Tropical Medicine. Livingstone College, London, 1893–1914, in: Social History of Medicine 23 (2010) 3, p. 549–556.

Wolfgang Kaschuba, Nachwort: "Deutsche Sauberkeit"—Zivilisierung der Körper und der Köpfe, in: Georges Vigarello, Wasser und Seife, Puder und Parfüm. Geschichte der Körperhygiene seit dem Mittelalter, Frankfurt a. M./New York 1992, p. 292–326.

Shin K. Kim, An Antiseptic Religion: Discovering a Hybridity on the Flux of Hygiene and Christianity, in: Journal of Religion and Health 47 (2008) 2, p. 253–262.

Daniel J. Koehler, Pilgrimage of Protestants. Miracles and Religious Community in J. C. Blumhardt's Württemberg, 1840–1880, in: Michael Geyer/Lucian Hölscher (eds.), Die Gegenwart Gottes in der modernen Gesellschaft. Transzendenz und religiöse Vergemeinschaftung in Deutschland, Göttingen 2006, p. 60–85.

Barbara Koller, Gesundes Wohnen. Ein Konstrukt zur Vermittlung bürgerlicher Werte und Verhaltensnormen und seine praktische Umsetzung in der Deutschschweiz 1880–1940, Zürich 1995.

Alfons Labisch, Doctors, Workers and the Scientific Cosmology of the Industrial World: The Social Construction of 'Health' and the 'Homo Hygienicus', in: Journal of Contemporary History 20 (1985) 4, p. 599–615.

Alfons Labisch, Homo Hygienicus. Gesundheit und Medizin in der Neuzeit, Frankfurt a. M. 1992.

Bruno Latour, Les microbes. Guerre et Paix, suivi de Irréductions, Paris 1984

Bruno Latour, Science in Action: How to Follow Scientists and Engineers Through Society, Milton Keynes 1987.

Bruno Latour, The Pasteurization of France, Cambridge 1988.

Bruno Latour, We Have Never Been Modern, Cambridge MA 1993.

Matthias Leanza, Die Zeit der Prävention: Eine Genealogie, Weilerswist 2017.

Friedrich Lenger, Stadthygiene: Gesundheit und städtischer Raum in Europa während der zweiten Hälfte des 19. Jahrhunderts, in: Heinz-Peter Schmiedebach, Medizin und öffentliche Gesundheit. Konzepte, Akteure, Perspektiven, Berlin/Boston 2018, p. 85–94.

Martin Lengwiler, Wissenschaft und Sozialpolitik. Der Einfluss von Gelehrtengesellschaften und Experten auf die Sozialpolitik im 19. Jarhundert, in: Josef Mooser/Simon Wenger (eds.), Armut und Fürsorge in Basel. Armutspolitik vom 13. Jahrhundert bis heute, Basel 2011, p. 111–122.

Martin Lengwiler/Stefan Beck, Historizität, Materialität und Hybridität von Wissenspraxen. Europäische Präventionsregime im 20. Jahrhundert, in: Geschichte und Gesellschaft 34 (2008), p. 489–523.

Martin Lengwiler/Jeanette Madarász (eds.), Das präventive Selbst: Eine Kulturgeschichte moderner Gesundheitspolitik, Bielefeld 2010.

Christopher Lever, They Dined on Eland: The Story of Acclimatization Societies, London 1992.

Wolfgang G. Locher, Max von Pettenkofer: Pionier der wissenschaftlichen Hygiene, Regensburg 2018.

Thomas Macho, Keimfrei, Zürich 2013.

Julia Ulrike Mack, Menschenbilder. Anthropologische Konzepte und stereotype Vorstellungen vom Menschen in der Publizistik der Basler Mission 1816–1914, Zürich 2013.

Julia Mack, Publikationen und Unterrichtsmaterialien, in: Christine Christ-von Wedel/Thomas K. Kuhn (ed.), Basler Mission. Menschen, Geschichte, Perspektiven 1815–2015, Basel 2015, p. 119–124.

Ernst Mähly, Die Gesundheitsverhältnisse auf der Goldküste, in: Evangelisches Missionsmagazin 29 (1885) p. 396–417, 445–461.

Ernst Mähly, Über das sogenannte "Gallenfieber" an der Goldküste, in: Correspondenz-Blatt für Schweizer Ärzte 15 (1885), p. 73–79, 108–116.

Ernst Mähly, Akklimatisation und Klimafieber, in: Deutsche Kolonialzeitung 3 (1886), p. 72–83.

Ernst Mähly, Akklimatisation und Klimafieber, in: Evangelisches Missionsmagazin 30 (1886), p. 129–147.

Ernst Mähly, Gesundheitszustand bzw. Sterblichkeit auf der Goldküste und in Westafrika überhaupt, in: Deutsche Kolonialzeitung 3 (1886), p. 555–559.

Hilary Marland, The Changing Role of the Hospital, 1800–1900, in: Deborah Brunton, (ed.), Medicine Transformed. Health, Disease and Society in Europe, 1800–1930, Manchester/New York 2004, p. 31–60.

Medical Missionary Association (ed.), Medical Missions at Home and Abroad, London 1889.

Beatrix Mesmer, Reinheit und Reinlichkeit. Bemerkungen zur Durchsetzung der häuslichen Hygiene in der Schweiz, in: Nicolai Bernard/Quirinus Reichen (eds.), Gesellschaft und Gesellschaften. Festschrift zum 65. Geburtstag von Professor Dr. Ulrich Im Hof, Bern 1982, p. 470–494.

Beatrix Mesmer (ed.), Die Verwissenschaftlichung des Alltags. Anweisungen zum richtigen Umgang mit dem Körper in der schweizerischen Populärpresse 1850–1900, Zürich 1997.

Adam Mohr, Missionary Medicine and Akan Therapeutics: Illness, Health and Healing in Southern Ghana's Basel Mission, 1828–1918, in: Journal of Religion in Africa 39 (2009) 4, p. 429–461.

Véronique Mottier, Narratives of National Identity: Sexuality, Race and the Swiss Dream of Order, in: Swiss Journal of Sociology 26 (2000) 3, p. 533–556.

Anne Marie Moulin, Tropical Without the Tropics. The Turning-Point of Pastorian Medicine in North Africa, in: David Arnold (ed.) Warm Climates and Western Medicine. The Emergence of Tropical Medicine 1500–1900, Amsterdam/Atlanta 1996, p. 160–180.

Georg Müller, Die Erziehung der Jugend zur körperlichen Gesundheit, in: Das Alpenhorn, 20.06.1903, p. 93.

Deborah J. Neill, Networks in Tropical Medicine. Internationalism, Colonialism, and the Rise of a Medical Specialty, 1890–1930, Stanford 2012.

Michael A. Osborne, Nature, the Exotic and the Science of French Colonialism, Bloomington 1994.

Michael A. Osborne, Acclimatizing the World: A History of Paradigmatic Colonial Science, in: Osiris 15 (2000), p. 135–151.

Jürgen Osterhammel, Die Verwandlung der Welt. Eine Geschichte des 19. Jahrhunderts, München 2009.

Julyan G. Peard, Race, Place, and Medicine. The Idea of the Tropics in Nineteenth-Century Brazilian Medicine, Durham/London 1999.

Roy Porter, What is Disease? in: ibid (ed.), The Cambridge History of Medicine, Cambridge 2006, p. 71–102.

Roy Porter, Medical Science, in: ibid (ed.), The Cambridge History of Medicine, Cambridge 2006, p. 136–175.

Roy Porter, Hospitals and Surgery, in: ibid (ed.), The Cambridge History of Medicine, Cambridge 2006, p. 176–210.

Hermann Prätorius, Mittheilungen aus der afrikanischen Visitationsreise, in: Der Evangelische Heidenbote 56 (1883), p. 9–11, 17–19, 25–28, 33–35, 41–43.

Alexandra Przyrembel, Verbote und Geheimnisse. Das Tabu und die Genese der europäischen Moderne, Frankfurt a. M. 2011.

Patricia Purtschert, Kolonialität und Geschlecht im 20. Jahrhundert. Eine Geschichte der weissen Schweiz, Bielefeld 2019.

Friedrich Reiff, Die christliche Glaubenslehre als Grundlage der christlichen Weltanschauung, 2 vol., Basel 1873.

Brigitte Ruckstuhl/Elisabeth Ryter, Von der Seuchenpolizei zu Public Health. Öffentliche Gesundheit in der Schweiz seit 1750, Zürich 2017.

Irmtraut Sahmland/Hans-Jürgen Schrader (eds.), Medizin- und kulturgeschichtliche Konnexe des Pietismus. Heilkunst und Ethik, arkane Traditionen, Musik, Literatur und Sprache, Göttingen 2016.

Philipp Sarasin, Reizbare Maschinen. Eine Geschichte des Körpers, 1765–1914, Frankfurt a. M. 2003.

Philipp Sarasin, Die Geschichte der Gesundheitsvorsorge. Das Verhältnis von Selbstsorge und staatlicher Intervention im 19. und 20. Jahrhundert, in: Cardiovascular Medicine 14 (2011) 2, p. 41–45.

Philipp Sarasin/Jakob Tanner (eds.), Physiologie und industrielle Gesellschaft. Studien zur Verwissenschaftlichung des Körpers im 19. und 20. Jahrhundert, Frankfurt a. M. 1998.

Otto Schellong, Besprechung der Bücher von R. Fisch und P. Kohlstock, in: Deutsche Kolonialzeitung 4 (1891), p. 182–184.

Thomas Schirrmacher, Theodor Christlieb und seine Missionstheologie, Wuppertal 1985.

Wilhelm Schlatter, Geschichte der Basler Mission 1815–1915, 3 vol., Basel 1916.

William O. Shanahan, Der deutsche Protestantismus vor der sozialen Frage 1815–1871, München 1962.
Virginia Smith, Clean. A History of Personal Hygiene and Purity, Oxford 2007.
Anne-Marie Stalder, Die Erziehung zur Häuslichkeit: Über den Beitrag des hauswirtschaftlichen Unterrichts zur Disziplinierung der Unterschichten im 19. Jahrhundert in der Schweiz, in: Schweizerische Zeitschrift für Geschichte 34 (1984), p. 370–384
Brian Stanley, Christian Missions and the Enlightenment, Grand Rapids 2001.
Paul Steinbrück/Achim Thom (eds.), Robert Koch (1843–1910). Bakteriologe, Tuberkuloseforscher, Hygieniker. Ausgewählte Texte, Leipzig 1982.
Nancy Leys Stepan, Picturing Tropical Nature, Ithaca 2001.
Katharina Stornig, Cultural Conceptions of Purity and Pollution. Childbirth and Midwifery in a New Guinean Catholic Mission, 1896–c. 1930, in: Judith Becker (ed.), European Missions in Contact Zones: Transformation Through Interaction in a (Post-)Colonial World, Göttingen 2015, p. 107–123.
Jakob Tanner, Eugenik und Rassenhygiene in Wissenschaft und Politik seit dem ausgehenden 19. Jahrhundert. Ein historischer Überblick, in: Michael Zimmermann (ed.), Zwischen Erziehung und Vernichtung. Zigeunerpolitik und Zigeunerforschung im Europa des 20. Jahrhunderts, Stuttgart 2007, p. 109–121.
Susan Thorne, "The Conversion of Englishmen and the Conversion of the World Inseparable". Missionary Imperialism and the Language of Class in Early Industrial Britain, in: Frederick Cooper/Ann Laura Stoler (eds.), Tensions of Empire. Colonial Cultures in a Bourgeois World, Berkeley et al. 1997, p. 238–262.
Richard Toellner, Medizin und Pharmazie, in: Hartmut Lehmann (ed.), Geschichte des Pietismus, vol. 4: Glaubenswelt und Lebenswelten, Göttingen 2004, p. 332–356.
Nancy Tomes, The Gospel of Germs: Men, Women, and the Microbe in American Life, Cambridge 1999.
Maya Trapp, Die Bedeutung der Basler Ärztlichen Mission in ihren südindischen Missionsgebieten in der Zeit von 1886–1914, in: Richard Toellner (ed.), Die Geburt einer sanften Medizin. Die Franckeschen Stiftungen zu Halle als Begegnungsstätte von Medizin und Pietismus im frühen 18. Jahrhundert, Halle 2004, p. 141–150.
Bryan S. Turner, The Body in Western Society: Social Theory and its Perspectives, in: Sarah Coakley (ed.), Religion and The Body, Cambridge 1997, p. 15–41.
Hideharu Umehara, Gesunde Schule und gesunde Kinder. Schulhygiene in Düsseldorf 1880–1933, Essen 2013.
Verein für ärztliche Mission (ed.), Bericht über das 1. Geschäftsjahr, Stuttgart 1899.

Verband der deutschen Vereine für ärztliche Mission (ed.), Jahrbuch der Ärztlichen Mission 1914, Gütersloh 1914.

Georges Vigarello, Concepts of Cleanliness: Changing Attitudes in France Since the Middle Ages, Cambridge 1988.

Rudolf Virchow, Über Acclimatisation, in: Tageblatt der 58. Versammlung deutscher Naturforscher und Ärzte, Strassburg 1885, p. 540–554.

Hermann Vortisch, Mutter und Kind. Ein ärztlicher Ratgeber für junge Frauen, Hamburg 1920.

Hermann Vortisch, Die Nervosität als Störung zwischen Seele und Geist und ihre Überwindung, Hamburg 1921.

Hermann Vortisch, Die Relativitätstheorie und ihre Beziehung zur christlichen Weltanschauung, Hamburg 1921.

James L.A. Webb, Humanity's Burden: A Global History of Malaria, Cambridge/New York 2009.

Regina Wecker, "Erbkrankheit Armut". Eheverbote und eugenische Konzepte im Umgang mit Armen im 19. und 20. Jahrhundert, in: Josef Mooser/ Simon Wenger (eds.), Armut und Fürsorge in Basel. Armutspolitik vom 13. Jahrhundert bis heute, Basel 2011, p. 205–215.

Paul Weindling, Health, Race and German Politics between National Unification and Nazism, 1870–1945, Cambridge 1989.

Paul Weindling, From Germ Theory to Social Medicine: Public Health, 1880–1930, in: Deborah Brunton (ed.), Medicine Transformed. Health, Disease and Society in Europe, 1800–1930, Manchester/New York 2004, p. 239–265.

Bernd Weisbrod, "Visiting" and "Social Control". Statistische Gesellschaften und Stadtmissionen im Viktorianischen England, in: Christoph Sachsse/Florian Tennstedt (eds.), Sozial Sicherheit und soziale Disziplinierung. Beiträge zu einer historischen Theorie der Sozialpolitik, Frankfurt a. M. 1986, p. 181–208.

Martin Weyer-von Schoultz, Max von Pettenkofer, 1818–1901. Die Entstehung der modernen Hygiene aus den empirischen Studien menschlicher Lebensgrundlagen, Frankfurt a. M. 2006.

August Hermann Heinrich Wittenberg, Einiges aus der missionsärztlichen Arbeit in London, in: An die Freunde des Ärztlichen Zweiges der Basler Mission, Basel 1893, p. 30–31.

Michael Worboys, Germs, Malaria and the Invention of Mansonian Tropical Medicine. From "Diseases in the Tropics" to "Tropical Diseases", in: David Arnold (ed.), Warm Climates and Western Medicine. The Emergence of Tropical Medicine 1500–1900, Amsterdam/Atlanta 1996, p. 181–207.

Michael Worboys, Spreading Germs: Disease Theories and Medical Practice in Britain, 1865–1900, Cambridge 2000.

Michael Worboys, Colonial and Imperial Medicine, in: Deborah Brunton (ed.), Medicine Transformed. Health, Disease and Society in Europe 1880–1930, Manchester/New York 2004, p. 211–238.

Michael Worboys, Was There a Bacteriological Revolution in Late Nineteenth-Century Medicine? in: Studies in History and Philosophy of Biological and Biomedical Sciences 38 (2007) 1, p. 20–42.

CHAPTER 4

The Colonial Space of Knowledge: The Medical Mission in West Africa, Imperial Entanglements and Colonial Cleanliness

4.1 Missionaries and Knowledge in a Colonial World

The Basel Mission doctors came of age in a period in which questions of hygiene dominated private lives and political agendas in European societies. At the same time, the increasing expansion and intensity of European imperialism overseas produced new knowledge on purity, health and cleanliness, which affected the development of hygiene. Christian missionaries stood at the forefront of the production of knowledge about lands and peoples previously unknown to Europeans. On the one hand, their expertise opened up new possibilities for colonial powers to access, widen and consolidate their spheres of influence. On the other, missionaries disseminated knowledge about the colonial world to a general public at home that became increasingly interested in people and places abroad. European societies developed narratives about the rest of the world based on texts, images and objects moving through missionary networks, which allowed them to reframe their own identities, transforming notions of what it meant to be white, clean and civilised.

© The Author(s) 2023   157
L. M. Ratschiller Nasim, *Medical Missionaries and Colonial Knowledge in West Africa and Europe, 1885–1914*,
Cambridge Imperial and Post-Colonial Studies,
https://doi.org/10.1007/978-3-031-27128-1_4

4.1.1   Civilising Colonialism

Beginning in the 1870s, colonial powers entered a high imperial phase as they competed to formalise their imperial spheres of interest into colonial possessions. The Berlin Conference of 1884–1885 heralded the partition of Africa into formal European colonies. As a result of this, Europe's imperial powers monopolised the economic, legal and jurisdictional domains of African societies, while regional chiefs, who were willing to cooperate, were put in charge of local administration.[1] The increasing importance of the evangelical missionary movement over the course of the nineteenth century accompanied Europe's economic and political expansionism. However, the sheer diversity of missions in terms of regional backgrounds and denominational affiliations, as well as the multifarious arrangements with colonial governments and African authorities make it difficult to offer neat generalisations about attitudes to colonialism and empire during this phase of High Imperialism.[2]

In some cases, the Basel Mission directly participated in consolidating colonial rule by providing physical and strategic support to European governments in Africa. For example, the British repeatedly sought the advice and help of the Basel missionaries on the Gold Coast during their military campaigns against the Asante in 1874, 1896 and 1900. The Basel missionaries assisted them by gathering together people from their parishes in Akem villages to form what they called "Christian squadrons." The British government instructed the Swiss Federal Council in Berne to extend its special gratitude to the Committee in Basel for the strong support of these African Christians, who had rendered valuable service as porters and soldiers.[3] In his 1920 memoirs, the Basel missionary Otto Lädrach justified the military involvement of the Basel Mission on the

---

[1] Ulrike Schaper, Chieftaincy as a Political Resource in the German Colony of Cameroon, 1884–1916, in: Tanja Bührer/Flavio Eichmann/Stig Förster/Benedikt Stuchtey (eds), Cooperation and Empire. Local Realities of Global Processes, New York/ Oxford 2017, p. 194–222.

[2] Andrew Porter convincingly argued that we need to move beyond the definitions of Edward Said and the Comaroffs when we debate the cultural imperialism of missionaries. See Porter, 'Cultural Imperialism' and Protestant Missionary Enterprise; Ibid., Religion versus Empire? British Protestant Missionaries and Overseas Expansion, 1700–1914, Manchester 2004; Ibid., Missions and Empire, c. 1873–1914, in: Sheridan Gilley/ Brian Stanley (eds.), World Christianities c. 1815–c. 1914, Cambridge 2006, p. 560–575.

[3] Debrunner, Schweizer im kolonialen Afrika, p. 70.

Gold Coast as a necessity, "in order to preserve peace and promote the well-being of the African people."[4]

The histories of colonialism and Christian missions are intimately related, on both practical and ideological levels. The notion of colonialism—derived from the Latin "colonus" for farmer and termed "colonisation" before Albert Venn Dicey coined "colonialism" in relation to Ireland in 1886—carries within it a civilisational dimension, going beyond the settling of territory and economic exploitation to processes of cultural and religious transformation.[5] The idea of a civilising mission offered a common starting point for colonial states and mission societies to argue for the need for European expansionism. Although the exact meaning of a civilising mission was contested in ideological debates among and between political and religious protagonists, all agreed that Christian forces were needed when it came to the very heart of the whole colonial enterprise: the almost holy duty of civilising.[6]

Christian missions offered an overarching agenda, including literacy education, social discipline, economic arrangements, medical care and cultural values such as domesticity, dress and cleanliness that addressed both the mind and body. This has given rise to popular and scholarly caricatures of missionaries as cultural imperialists, racist patriarchal colonisers and agents of hegemonic globalising capitalism. More nuanced evaluation has been thwarted for decades due to historians' focus on missions as an extension of colonial ideology, rather than an analysis of them in their own right. To contribute to a critical understanding of the relationship between mission and colonial histories, it is crucial to examine the theological tenets and intellectual foundations upon which Christian missionaries based their civilising mission.[7]

---

[4] Otto Lädrach, Im Lande des Goldenen Stuhls. Erinnerungen aus Afrika, Basel 1920.

[5] Albert Venn Dicey, England's Case Against Home Rule, vol. 7, London 1886, p. 273.

[6] Jürgen Osterhammel, "The Great Work of Uplifting Mankind". Zivilisierungsmission und Moderne, in: Boris Barth/Jürgen Osterhammel (eds.), Zivilisierungsmissionen. Imperiale Weltverbesserung seit dem 18. Jahrhundert, Konstanz 2005, p. 363–426.

[7] Ryan Dunch, Beyond Cultural Imperialism: Cultural Theory, Christian Missions, and Global Modernity, in: History and Theory 41 (2002), p. 301–325; Thoralf Klein, Mission und Kolonialismus—Mission als Kolonialismus. Anmerkungen zu einer Wahlverwandtschaft, in: Claudia Kraft/Alf Lüdtke/Jürgen Martschukat (eds.), Kolonialgeschichten. Regionale Perspektiven auf ein globales Phänomen, Frankfurt a. M./New York 2010, p. 142–161.

Gustav Warneck, the initiator of German-speaking missiology, whose texts were used as part of the curriculum in the seminary in Basel, decried "the inconsiderate self-seeking which characterises the whole commercial and political intercourse of the Christian West with the non-Christian world." He acknowledged that "trade and colonial politics are opening the world's doors" but regretted that at the same time they were "closing the people's hearts to the Gospel; so that missions have liked best to seek their field of labour outside of the shadow of dispersed Christendom."[8] Missionary intellectuals cultivated transnational networks, met at interdenominational conferences and established correspondences and publications such as the influential *Allgemeine Missionszeitschrift*, edited by Warneck, which undercut their colonial loyalties and fostered a critical posture towards imperial projects perceived as detrimental to evangelisation.[9]

The Basel missionaries in West Africa, who came from Switzerland and Germany, worked on the Gold Coast, a British colony, and in Cameroon, a German colony. Although they accommodated certain German and British interests in their mission fields, the networks in which they operated transcended imperial boundaries. That is not to say that national affiliations and colonial sympathies were irrelevant, especially in the looming view of the First World War, but the Basel Mission considered and promoted itself as a supranational organisation.[10] The universalistic logic of Pietism and the global aspirations of the evangelical revival movement meant that most Basel missionaries refrained from expressions of overtly nationalistic enthusiasm.[11] The Basel Mission often stood in a tense and ambiguous relationship with colonial governments, particularly when the latter enforced the exploitation and dispossession of people in their mission areas. To be sure, the Basel missionaries, like most of

[8] Gustav Warneck, Outline of a History of Protestant Missions from the Reformation to the Present Time. A Contribution to Modern Church History, New York/Chicago/Toronto 1901, p. 345.

[9] Jeremy Best has shown that German Protestant missionaries promoted an internationalist Christian universalism that was "bent on the unification of people into a grand community of Protestant faith." See Jeremy Best, Heavenly Fatherland. German Missionary Culture and Globalization in the Age of Empire, Toronto 2020, p. 219.

[10] Feigk, Von Edinburgh nach Oegstgeest.

[11] Jeremy Best, Godly, International, and Independent: German Protestant Missionary Loyalties Before World War I, in: Central European History 47 (2014), p. 585–611, here p. 589.

their contemporaries, did not oppose colonial rule on principle, but they did seek to civilise it. And perhaps more fundamentally, as Dana Robert suggested, they sought to convert it.[12]

4.1.2   Basel's Colonial Entanglements

Basel became a hub of colonial entanglements by connecting people and money in Europe with trading, scientific, military and religious networks and institutions across the world during the colonial period. The city at the heart of the interregional triangle between Switzerland, Alsace and Wurttemberg drew on its long tradition of craftsmanship and manufacturing, financial and technological know-how and labour and capital surpluses to provide colonial powers and imperial ventures with personnel, expertise and funds, allowing them to advance their military, economic, civilisational and scientific goals. People from the region of Basel, and Switzerland more generally, served as mercenaries in colonial armies, held investments in the slave trade, participated in the evangelical missionary movement, initiated research expeditions and established trading companies in colonies all over the globe.[13]

In his seminal 2015 study on the scientists Paul and Fritz Sarasin, Bernhard C. Schär examined how the two cousins, originating from a Basel patrician family, contributed to knowledge about Celebes—known as Sulawesi in Indonesia nowadays—around 1900. Schär demonstrated that the Sarasins' research expeditions not only relied on the assistance of the Dutch colonial army but also helped to prepare the ground for the

---

[12] Dana L. Robert, Introduction, in: ibid. (ed.), Converting Colonialism: Visions and Realities in Mission History, 1706–1914, Grand Rapids 2008, p. 1–20.

[13] Philipp Krauer, Welcome to Hotel Helvetia! Friedrich Wüthrich's Illicit Mercenary Trade Network for the Dutch East Indies, 1858–1890, in: BMGN—Low Countries Historical Review 134 (2019) 3, p. 122–147; Lea Haller, Transithandel. Geld- und Warenströme im globalen Kapitalismus, Berlin 2019; Schär, From Batticaloa via Basel to Berlin; Béatrice Veyrassat, Histoire de la Suisse et des Suisses dans la marche du monde. XVIIe siècle—Première Guerre mondiale: Espaces—Circulations—Échanges, Neuchâtel 2018; Christof Dejung, Die Fäden des globalen Marktes. Eine Sozial- und Kulturgeschichte des Welthandels am Beispiel der Handelsfirma Gebrüder Volkart 1851–1999, Köln/Weimar/Wien 2013; Christian Koller, Die Fremdenlegion. Kolonialismus, Söldnertum, Gewalt 1831–1962, Paderborn 2013; Zangger, Koloniale Schweiz; Thomas David/Bouda Etemad/Janick Marina Schaufelbuehl, Schwarze Geschäfte. Die Beteiligung von Schweizern an Sklaverei und Sklavenhandel im 19. und 20. Jahrhundert, Zürich 2005.

formal colonisation of the island by the Netherlands in 1905.[14] Moreover, his book sheds light on the Sarasins' legacy in Switzerland, revealing how their colonial involvement in Southeast Asia shaped institutions such as the Natural History Museum, the Ethnological Museum and the Zoological Garden in Basel, as well as the Swiss Society for Natural Sciences and Switzerland's first national park in Grisons.[15]

Another striking example is that of the Basel patrician Carl Passavant. As a member of the Society for Natural Sciences in Basel, the young physician undertook two research expeditions to the west coast of Africa between 1883 and 1885 to complete a dissertation on "Craniological Studies of the Negro and the Negro peoples." Accompanied by a zoologist and an African assistant, he reached the territory known as the Cameroons, the coastal region around Douala, in 1883. From there, the research group repeatedly ventured inland to gather new information on people and places hitherto unknown to Europeans. This knowledge proved useful to German authorities that aspired to their own place in the imperial sun. The subsequent military interventions in Cameroon culminated in the first German colonial war in Africa.[16]

The more recent approach of colonial knowledge highlights how older definitions of colonialism as formalised territorial power relations limit the temporal scope and omit important forces of colonial history, such as private initiatives, non-governmental institutions and transimperial networks. This approach also reveals that colonial entanglements have changed bodies of knowledge, social conditions and cultural practices in Europe at least as much as they have affected former colonies. Passavant contributed to this process by leaving behind a rich visual legacy of 274 photographs, documenting his journey from Sierra Leone to Angola. The images of the Basel patrician venturing into tropical Africa allowed people

---

[14] Schär, Tropenliebe, p. 126–194.

[15] Ibid., p. 297–328.

[16] Stefanie Michels, Patrioten im Pulverdampf. Die Berichterstattung über die Kriegsereignisse vom Dezember 1884 in Kamerun, in: Jürg Schneider/Ute Röschenthaler/Bernhard Gardi (eds.), Fotofieber. Bilder aus West- und Zentralafrika. Die Reisen des Carl Passavant 1883–1885, Basel 2005, p. 83–96.

in Switzerland to visualise their own place in an increasingly interconnected world in the 1880s, revealing how Swiss people have perceived themselves and others since the colonial period.[17]

In fact, people from Switzerland, and from Basel particularly, had been involved in imperial activities in Africa since at least the early seventeenth century, long before European powers formalised their interests into colonial rule. In 1611, Samuel Braun from Basel first travelled to Amsterdam before boarding a merchant ship to the west coast of Africa. As a ship's surgeon, he participated in five of these journeys until 1620. The vessels he worked on traded cotton cloth, iron, glass beads and brass basins with gold, ivory and pepper.[18] Basel's upper class, such as Braun, invested in the West African trade, acquiring a fortune through these expeditions. Upon his return, Braun became a Member of Parliament and head surgeon of the hospital in Basel, applying his experience gained as a doctor in the tropics in the city's healthcare system. Braun is but one example of how people from Basel participated in the colonial trade and used their assets and expertise acquired abroad to gain influence at home.[19]

Throughout the eighteenth and nineteenth centuries, trading companies from Basel supplied slave ships leaving the ports of the Atlantic coast with industrial products. Studies on the merchant families Faesch und Burckhardt, for instance, have shown that they didn't content themselves with capitalising on freight but also directly invested in slave expeditions along the West African coast.[20] They did not shy away from operating illegally by continuing to equip slave ships after the European powers had

[17] Jürg Schneider/Barbara Lüthi, Carl Passavant (1854–1887): Eine Welt in Bildern, in: Traverse (2007) 3, p. 113–122.

[18] René Salathé, Basler und Baslerinnen auf Reisen. Eine Anthologie, Basel 2013, p. 24–26; Ralph Andreas Melzer, Samuel Braun (1590–1688), seefahrender Basler Wundarzt, in: Zürcher medizingeschichtliche Abhandlungen 268 (1996), p. 164.

[19] Schär, Tropenliebe, p. 61–77.

[20] Niklaus Stettler/Peter Haenger/Robert Labhardt, Baumwolle, Sklaven und Kredite. Die Basler Welthandelsfirma Christoph Burckhardt & Cie. in revolutionärer Zeit (1789–1815), Basel 2004; David/Etemad/Schaufelbuehl, Schwarze Geschäfte, p. 72–76; Peter Haenger/Robert Labhardt, Basel und der Sklavenhandel: Das Beispiel der Burkhardtschen Handelshäuser zwischen 1780 und 1815, in: Sandra Bott/Thomas David/Claude Lutzelschwab/Janick Marina Schaufelbuehl (eds.), Suisse—Afrique (18e–20e siècles): De la traite des Noirs à la fin du régime de l'apartheid/Schweiz—Afrika (18.–20. Jahrhundert): Vom Sklavenhandel zum Ende des Apartheid-Regimes, Münster 2005, p. 25–42.

formally banned the slave trade at the Congress of Vienna in 1815.[21] The Basel patricians accumulated considerable wealth during the age of slavery—whether they were directly involved with the slave trade or not—which paradoxically allowed them to finance the costly enterprise of training and sending missionaries abroad to compensate for the damages caused by the European slave trade.

Basel became a focal point of the revived interest in evangelism within German-speaking Protestantism, which contributed to its cosmopolitan character. By the second half of the nineteenth century, the city on the Rhine hosted one of the earliest and largest African communities in Europe, after Paris and London.[22] About 25 African women and men, some of whom were former slaves, joined the seminaries of the Basel Mission and the St. Chrischona Mission of Basel.[23] Their presence aroused public interest, which the mission societies tried to use to promote awareness for their cause across Europe by publishing biographies and photographs of their new fellows. Nearly half of them, however, succumbed to tuberculosis in the following years, eventually leading to the suspension of these training programmes.[24] Nevertheless, the history of the African community in nineteenth-century Basel illustrates how crucial mission societies were to early ideas of Africa and its people, particularly in Switzerland, a country without formal colonies.

4.1.3   The Popularity of Missionary Knowledge

Through their copious writings, missionaries conveyed stories, hopes and anxieties to readers in Europe, allowing them to imagine Africans and

---

[21] David/Etemad/Schaufelbuehl, Schwarze Geschäfte, p. 16; Hans Werner Debrunner, Basel und der Sklavenhandel: Fragmente eines wenig bekannten Kapitels der Basler Geschichte, in: Basler Stadtbuch 113 (1993), p. 95–101.

[22] Hans Werner Debrunner, Presence and Prestige: Africans in Europe. A History of Africans in Europe before 1918, Basel 1979, p. 301–323.

[23] The Chrischona Mission of Basel was founded by Pietists in 1840 and offered training that combined craftsmanship with missionary work. See John Schneid, Les Africains de Bâle au 19ème siècle, in: Sandra Bott/Thomas David/Claude Lutzelschwab/Janick Marina Schaufelbuehl (eds.), Suisse—Afrique (18e–20e siècles): De la traite des Noirs à la fin du régime de l'apartheid/Schweiz—Afrika (18–20. Jahrhundert): Vom Sklavenhandel zum Ende des Apartheid-Regimes, Münster 2005, p. 209–226.

[24] David/Etemad/Schaufelbuehl, Schwarze Geschäfte, p. 119–121.

other people around the globe and the distant countries they inhabited. These constructions were not, of course, all about otherness, but also about imagining the self, as authors and readers of such literature sought to make sense of their own identities in colonial contexts. The role of missionaries as brokers of colonial knowledge was particularly significant in Switzerland, which had no colonies of its own. Patrick Harries has demonstrated that mission societies "played an important role in shaping the way in which the Swiss—a people severely divided by language, religion, region and class—came to see themselves as a single community."[25]

The Basel Mission produced vast amounts of promotional material to raise awareness for their work, generate funds and recruit volunteers. The wide array of publications included specialised periodicals for children and women, popular tractates, collector card albums, missiology journals, calendars and magazines in German, French and English dealing with specific regions or fields of activity such as medicine. The most circulated periodical was *Der Evangelische Heidenbote* with roughly 25,000 copies monthly around 1900. The actual audience was presumably much higher than the official circulation figures indicate, since articles were passed on, read in public and discussed in prayer meetings, devotional hours, reading circles and in Sunday schools across German-speaking Europe.[26] Biographies and memoirs of individual missionaries aimed to create a personal connection between the evangelists in West Africa and the public at home by depicting their struggles and glorifying their accomplishments. The Basel Mission controlled a large media enterprise through which ordinary Swiss, Germans and other Europeans learned about people and places in the colonial world from the familiarity of their own home.[27]

---

[25] Harries, Butterflies and Barbarians, p. 4.

[26] Overview over the circulation of the mission periodicals, BMA, Q-24.3; Mack, Publikationen und Unterrichtsmaterialien, p. 120.

[27] For missionary media and their impact in Europe, see Felicity Jensz/Hanna Acke (eds.), Missions and Media. The Politics of Missionary Periodicals in the Long Nineteenth Century, Stuttgart 2013; Judith Becker/Katharina Stornig (eds.), Menschen—Bilder—Eine Welt. Ordnungen von Vielfalt in der religiösen Publizistik um 1900, Göttingen 2018.

Knowledge flowing through the Basel Mission's networks was particularly interactive and persuasive due to its rich visual and material nature.[28] The earliest photographs from the Gold Coast and Cameroon originated from Basel missionaries, who started using cameras in West Africa in 1860. Their pictures appeared in numerous local and regional newspapers, were reproduced on calendars and postcards, and were sold at missionary bazaars and fundraising events throughout Europe. They were used by itinerant preachers, missionaries on furlough and female collectors to illustrate their presentations. They were also assembled to form magic lantern shows to inform the rural populations at home about developments in the mission field abroad.[29]

With over 50,000 negatives, the Basel Mission archives hold a substantial body of sources with regard to the visual history of Africa.[30] In his introduction to the volume *Images and Empire*, Paul Landau highlighted why photographs were—and still are—pivotal to our knowledge of Africa in particular: "Unlike the discursive field that 'is' other parts of the imperial world—for instance, the Muslim Orient—the image-Africa lives on almost solely in picture form."[31] Considering that the European perception of the "Dark Continent" mainly consisted of visual images, the few photographs of West Africa that did exist around 1900 attracted a great deal of attention. The diffusion of pictures from the colonies reached a climax at the turn of the twentieth century due to new technical procedures that allowed for their reproduction on a large scale and the growing appetite of Europeans for images depicting the wider world. Through

[28] Linda Ratschiller, Material Matters: The Basel Mission in West Africa and Commodity Culture around 1900, in: ibid./Karolin Wetjen (eds.), Verflochtene Mission. Perspektiven auf eine neue Missionsgeschichte, Köln/Weimar/Wien 2018, p. 117–139; Ibid., Kranke Körper. Mission, Medizin und Fotografie zwischen der Goldküste und Basel 1885–1914, in: ibid./Siegfried Weichlein (eds.), Der schwarze Körper als Missionsgebiet. Medizin, Ethnologie, Theologie in Afrika und Europa 1880–1960, Köln/Weimar/Wien 2016, p. 41–72.

[29] Zusammenfassung der Referate. Reisepredigerkonferenz in Freundenstadt 1910, BMA, QH-14,1; Allgemeine Dienstanweisung für Reiseprediger der Basler Mission, 11.04.1911, BMA, QH-9,2.

[30] Paul Jenkins, The Earliest Generation of Missionary Photographers in West Africa and the Portrayal of Indigenous People and Culture in: History of Africa 20 (1993), p. 89–118.

[31] Paul S. Landau, Introduction. An Amazing Distance. Pictures and People in Africa, in: ibid./Deborah D. Kaspin (eds.), Images and Empires. Visuality in Colonial and Postcolonial Africa, Berkeley/Los Angeles/London 2002, p. 1–40, here p. 5.

their use in churches, schools, mass media and advertisement, depictions of Africa and Africans became part and parcel of everyday imagery and popular culture across European societies.[32]

The obsessive collecting of objects by mission societies and their material contributions to popular culture were also major factors that contributed to the popularity of missionary knowledge. The Basel Mission founded a "Museum of Ethnography and Natural History" as early as 1860, which makes it one of the oldest missionary collections on the European continent. The museum inventory grew rapidly over the following decades, since the Committee encouraged missionaries in West Africa, China and India to contribute ethnographic artefacts, natural specimens, illustrations and photographs to the collection.[33] These objects and images became widely accessible to the public through the Basel Mission's "Ethnographic Exhibitions," the first of which toured through Switzerland, Germany and France from 1908 to 1912.[34]

By labelling and promoting their display as an "Ethnographic Exhibition", the curators hoped to attract a wider audience, neither primarily concerned with evangelisation nor necessarily in favour of the Pietist cause. According to reports in the daily newspaper *Basler Nachrichten*,

---

[32] John Phillip Short, Magic Lantern Empire. Colonialism and Society in Germany, Ithaca/London 2012; David Ciarlo, Advertising Empire. Race and Visual Culture in Imperial Germany, London 2011; Jens Jäger, Plätze an der Sonne? Visualisierungen kolonialer Realitäten, in: Claudia Kraft/Alf Lüdtke/Jürgen Martschukat (eds.) Kolonialgeschichten. Regionale Perspektiven auf ein globales Phänomen, Frankfurt a. M./New York 2010, p. 162–184; Ibid., Bilder aus Afrika vor 1918. Zur visuellen Konstruktion Afrikas im europäischen Kolonialismus, in: Paul Gerhard (ed.), Visual History. Ein Studienbuch, Göttingen 2006, p. 134–148.

[33] Anweisung betreffs des Photographierens sowie des Sammelns von ethnographischen Gegenständen und Naturalien, in: Verordnungen und Mitteilungen für die Missionare der Basler Mission ("Amtsblatt"), herausgegeben vom Missionskomitee, XIII.–XX. (1901–1909), Basel 1909, BMA, Q-9,1a.

[34] Linda Ratschiller, "Die Zauberei spielt in Kamerun eine böse Rolle! " Die ethnografischen Ausstellungen der Basler Mission (1908–1912), in: Rebekka Habermas/Richard Hölzl (eds.), Mission global. Eine Verflechtungsgeschichte seit dem 19. Jahrhundert, Köln/Weimar/Wien 2014, p. 241–264.

the strategy paid off.[35] In 1910 alone, nearly 250,000 people in Switzerland, Alsace and six German cities visited the touring exhibition.[36] Parts of the collection then appeared in an exhibition in the Reichstag building in Berlin and at the Swiss National Exhibition in Berne in 1914. Until the last display in 1953, the Basel Mission's touring exhibition was presented in more than forty venues across Europe, illustrating that the appeal of their material collection extended far beyond evangelical circles and regional boundaries.[37] Missionary displays reached a much broader spectrum of the public than the ethnographic museums or even the colonial exhibitions of the period, as Annie E. Coombes has shown for Late Victorian and Edwardian England, by "taking articles, generally reserved for ethnographic collections, into a much more lively and equally controversial context."[38]

The Basel Mission also put together "mission valises" and sent them to regional support groups, schoolteachers and provincial museums in Switzerland, Wurttemberg, Alsace, Palatinate and Hessen. These boxes, weighing 15 kilograms each, contained annotated photographs, models, instruments, maps and artefacts, amounting to a DIY exhibition kit.[39] Crucially, the knowledge generated and disseminated by the Basel Mission also reached communities in the countryside. In a recent article, Rebekka Habermas has argued "that there was an entire rural world of colonial resonances that is still to be discovered."[40] She demonstrates how missionary networks created a colonial public sphere that also spoke to rural populations experiencing the dislocations of modernisation in Imperial Germany.

---

[35] Anonymous, Basler Missionsausstellung in der Kunsthalle, in: Basler Nachrichten, 21.10.1908; Anonymous, Zur ethnographischen Ausstellung der Basler Mission in Zürich. Korrespondenz, in: Basler Nachrichten, 11.03.1909.

[36] Georg Müller, Unsere Werbearbeit mit besonderer Berücksichtigung neuer Methoden. Referat an der Reisepredigerkonferenz in Freudenstadt 1912, p. 3, BMA, QH-14,1.

[37] Paul Jenkins/Guy Thomas, Die weite Welt rund um Basel: Mission, Medien und die regionale Vermittlung eines Afrikabildes im 19. und 20. Jahrhundert, in: Regio Basiliensis 45 (2004) 2, p. 99–107.

[38] Annie E. Coombes, Reinventing Africa. Museums, Material Culture and Popular Imagination in Late Victorian and Edwardian England, New Haven and London 1994, p. 174.

[39] Anonymous, Missionskoffer, in: Der Evangelische Heidenbote 77 (1904), p. 6.

[40] Habermas, Doing Mission in the Countryside, p. 503.

The Basel Mission's project in West Africa would have been doomed to failure from the beginning had it not been for the backing and enthusiasm of ordinary people in the Alemannic countryside.[41] People associated with the Basel Mission travelled endlessly through villages and small towns to address societies, schools and parishes, illustrating their lectures with images and objects. These visual and material sources provide tangible evidence as to how the Basel Mission shaped popular knowledge in the late nineteenth and early twentieth centuries. By offering a lens through which people in Basel and beyond could envision the colonial world, they allowed Europeans to retool their self-awareness to incorporate Africa and other parts of the earth into their religious, scientific and political frameworks. Colonial knowledge shaped deep-seated convictions and beliefs, which in the eyes of many contemporaries made colonisation a noble and necessary undertaking. Beyond and beneath the brutal facts of military, political and economic imperialism, the mobility of people and the circulation of knowledge during the colonial era fuelled identities of place and related senses of belonging.[42]

4.2   THE BASEL MISSION IN WEST AFRICA

The Basel Mission's claim to legitimacy in West Africa was based on their desire to create and sustain a Pietist presence and to bear witness against the ravages of the European slave trade and the economic exploitation that accompanied and followed this trade. In his instruction, the Inspector Christian Blumhardt described the mission to West Africa launching in 1828 as "a redemption for the injustice committed by Europeans, so that

---

[41] Marianne Bechhaus-Gerst has argued for the importance of analysing the local anchoring of colonialism in German regions, pointing to the fact that 80 to 90 percent of colonial personnel lived in Germany and not in overseas territories. Marianne Bechhaus-Gerst, Decolonize Germany? (Post)Koloniale Spurensuche in der Heimat zwischen Lokalgeschichte, Politik, Wissenschaft und "Öffentlichkeit", in: WerkstattGeschichte 75 (2017), p. 49–55.

[42] It has become mostly accepted by now that locality is produced socially and culturally, often in contexts of heightened mobility. See Arjun Appadurai, The Production of Locality, in: ibid. (ed.), Modernity at Large: Cultural Dimensions of Globalization, Minneapolis 1996, p. 178–199.

to some extent the thousands of bleeding wounds, caused by dirty greed-
iness and most cruel deceitfulness, can be healed."[43] The Committee's
fierce determination in condemning the institution of slavery, however,
was curbed by the ambivalent attitude of some Basel missionaries and the
deep roots of slavery in West African societies.[44]

4.2.1   Slavery and West Indian Christians on the Gold Coast

The first team of four Basel missionaries arrived at the colonial fort in
Christiansborg on the Gold Coast in 1828, at the invitation of the Danish
Crown and the Danish Lutheran Church. The beginnings of the Basel
Mission in West Africa were marked by high mortality rates among their
personnel and the failure to spread the gospel among the resident population. Three parties of missionaries were almost completely wiped out
by disease in the late 1820s and 1830s. The Committee recalled their
only surviving missionary in West Africa, Andreas Riis, in 1840, with the
intention of ending their mission on the Gold Coast just as they had
done earlier in Liberia.[45] By the mid-nineteenth century, mission societies in general were at the point of abandoning Africa as a viable mission
field altogether. The Basel Mission, however, launched a fresh start in
1843 and asked Riis to visit the Danish and British West Indies to recruit
former slaves. He returned to the Akuapem region on the Gold Coast
accompanied by 24 people from the West Indies.[46]

---

[43] Christian Blumhardt, Instruction for the brothers leaving for the Danish Gold Coast
in 1828, 15.09.1828, p. 1, BMA, D-10.3.3.

[44] Catherine Koonar, Using Child Labor to Save Souls: The Basel Mission in Colonial
Ghana, 1855–1900, in: Atlantic Studies 11 (2014) 4, p. 536–554; Cornelia Vogel-
sanger, Pietismus und afrikanische Kultur an der Goldküste. Die Einstellung der Basler
zur Haussklaverei, Zürich 1977. On the deep-rooted history of Christian slavery, see
Katharine Gerbner, Christian Slavery. Conversion and Race in the Protestant Atlantic
World, Philadelphia 2018. For a concise summary of slavery in West Africa, see Andreas
Eckert, Transatlantischer Sklavenhandel und Sklaverei in Westafrika, in: ibid./Ingeborg
Grau/Arno Sonderegger (eds.), Afrika 1500–1900. Geschichte und Gesellschaft, Wien
2010, p. 72–88.

[45] On Andreas Riis, see Seth Quartey, Missionary Practices on the Gold Coast, 1832–
1895. Discourse, Gaze and Gender in the Basel Mission in Pre-Colonial West Africa, New
York 2007, p. 41–74; Miller, Missionary Zeal, p. 129–135.

[46] Katja Füllberg-Stolberg, "Ein Sauerteig christlichen Lebens in der Masse afrikanischen Heidentums". Westindische Konvertiten an der Goldküste (1843–1850), in: Rebekka
Habermas/Richard Hölzl (eds.), Mission global. Eine Verflechtungsgeschichte seit dem

According to oral history, it was the chief of Akuapem—the so-called *Okuapehene*—Nana Addo Dankwa, that had encouraged Riis to bring West Indians to the Gold Coast by telling him: "When God created the world, He made a book (the Bible) for the white man and *abosom* (African gods) for the black man. But if you could show me a black man who reads the white man's book, then we would surely follow you."[47] The leaders of Akuapem had welcomed the Basel missionaries' presence, believing that they might contribute to the state's prosperity and development, but had remained critical of their faith.[48]

The Basel Mission assumed that West Indians, who were English-speaking Christians of African descent, would serve as a role model for the people they wished to convert on the Gold Coast. This strategy was used by a range of Protestant mission societies that collaborated with exponents of the abolitionist movement to establish Christian settlements in West Africa from the late eighteenth century onwards.[49] The recruitment of freed slaves from Jamaica and Antigua in the 1840s enabled a new generation of Basel missionaries and their wives to consolidate their work on the Gold Coast. The West Indians had to commit themselves contractually to work for the Basel Mission for at least five years before returning to their home countries. In 1854, *Der Evangelische Heidenbote* reported that "their settlement among their fellows marks a watershed in the history of this mission," noting that "the cases of death among

19. Jahrhundert, Köln/Weimar/Wien 2014, p. 31–58; Abraham Nana Opare Kwakye, Mission Impossible Becomes Possible: West Indian Missionaries as Actors in Mission in the Gold Coast, in: Interkulturelle Theologie 42 (2016) 2, p. 222–235; Peter A. Schweizer, Survivors on the Gold Coast. The Basel Missionaries in Colonial Ghana, Accra 2000, p. 50–53.

[47] Cited in: Kwakye, Mission Impossible Becomes Possible, p. 226.

[48] Abraham Nana Opare Kwakye, Encountering 'Prosperity' in Nineteenth Century Gold Coast: Indigenous Perceptions of Western Missionary Societies, in: Andreas Heuser (ed.), Pastures of Plenty: Tracing Religio-Scapes of Prosperity Gospel in Africa and Beyond, Frankfurt a. M. 2015, p. 217–228.

[49] Nemata Amelia Blyden, West Indians in West Africa, 1808–1880. The African Diaspora in Reverse, Rochester 2000; Horace O. Russell, The Missionary Outreach of the West Indian Chursmith Jamaican Baptist Missions to West Africa in the Nineteenth Century, New York 2000; David Killingray, The Black Atlantic Missionary Movement and Africa 1780s–1920, in: Journal of Religion in Africa 33 (2003) 1, p. 3–31; Jon F. Sensbach, Rebecca's Revival. Creating Black Christianity in the Atlantic World, Cambridge 2005.

our brothers have become extremely rare and the Negroes have begun to listen to the word of the cross."[50]

The Basel missionaries were instructed to diminish their manual work load to prevent exhaustion and disease following the arrival of the West Indian Christians. Besides providing hard manual labour on the Basel Mission's construction sites and plantations, noticeably reducing the mortality rate among European missionaries, the West Indians also helped to clear the doubts and suspicions that the Akuapem leaders had about the Basel Mission. The people of Akuapem started sending their children to the Basel Mission school in Akropong, which was set up by Riis and the West Indian Alexander Clerk in 1843. Catherine Mulgrave, originating from the West Indies, and her husband, the Liberian teacher George Peter Thompson, established a second school at Christiansborg that same year.[51]

Soon after the opening of the school in Akropong, Riis purchased a plantation and slaves for labour, triggering anger and sanctions from the mission board in Basel.[52] Not only were missionaries not supposed to own private property but he had also acted against a founding principle of the Basel Mission: the abolitionist cause. Time and again, the question of slavery provoked bitter disputes between the Committee in Basel and the missionaries in West Africa, who gathered at regional conferences to voice their views towards the leadership in Switzerland. An internal investigation in 1862 revealed that 23 mission members, most of whom were African catechists, owned a total of 242 slaves on the Gold Coast. The Committee responded to these findings by ordering that the slaves had to be freed within two years while guaranteeing that the owners would receive compensation.[53]

Most Basel missionaries, by contrast, feared that the Committee's total ban of slavery would not only discourage Africans from joining the mission but also undermine the social cohesion of their parishes. They perceived the interference in a West African institution, which they considered to be very different from the transatlantic slave trade run by

---

[50] Anonymous, Westindische Missionsgeschwister, in: Der Evangelische Heidenbote 27 (1854), p. 80–81.

[51] Sill, Encounters in Quest of Christian Womanhood, p. 109–132.

[52] Quartey, Missionary Practices on the Gold Coast, p. 67–74.

[53] Schlatter, Geschichte der Basler Mission, vol. 3, p. 78.

Europeans, as a social, economic and moral dilemma.[54] They argued that the type of domestic slavery practised in Akuapem conceived of slaves as family members, and advocated instead for a transitional solution, invoking the complexity of West African societies that relied on intricate structures of interdependency and diverse forms of slavery.[55] The Basel missionaries had arrived on the Gold Coast soon after the transatlantic slave trade had been officially abolished. The British government enacted the 1834 Slave Emancipation Act at the coastal forts but did not decree the liberation of slaves inland until the Gold Coast became a Crown Colony in 1874. The question of slavery continued to preoccupy the Basel Mission in West Africa until 1914, despite the radical stance of the leadership in Basel.[56]

Most West Indians decided to return home after their five-year stay on the Gold Coast, no doubt put off by their huge workload, low pay and the presumptuous behaviour of the Basel missionaries towards them.[57] Despite their relatively short stay, the Basel Mission would have probably quit the Gold Coast for good had it not been for their engagement. They crucially contributed to the foundation of numerous new stations and schools, most importantly the Teacher Training Institute in 1848. Graduates of the Institute included descendants of the West Indians who had stayed on the Gold Coast, as well as the first generation of Akuapem

[54] Koonar, Using Child Labor to Save Souls; Vogelsanger, Pietismus und afrikanische Kultur an der Goldküste.

[55] David/Etemad/Schaufelbuehl, Schwarze Geschäfte, p. 110–113; Peter Haenger, Pioniere wider Willen: Die missionsinterne Sklavenbefreiung an der Golkdüste, in: Christine Christ-von Wedel/Thomas K. Kuhn (eds.), Basler Mission. Menschen, Geschichte, Perspektiven 1815–2015, Basel 2015, p. 101–106.

[56] Raymond E. Dumett, Traditional Slavery in the Akan Region in the Nineteenth Century: Sources, Issues, and Interpretations, in: David Henige/T.C. McCaskie (eds.), West African Economic and Social History. Studies in Memory of Marion Johnson, Madison 1990, p. 7–22; Andreas Eckert, Slavery in Colonial Cameroon, 1880s to 1930s, in: Martin Klein/Suzanne Miers (eds.), Slavery and Colonial Rule in Africa, London 1999, p. 133–148; Peter Haenger, Slaves and Slave Holders on the Gold Coast: Towards an Understanding of Social Bondage in West Africa, Basel 2000; Rebecca Shumway/Trevor R. Getz (eds.), Slavery and its Legacy in Ghana and the Diaspora, London et al. 2018.

[57] Füllberg-Stolberg, "Ein Sauerteig christlichen Lebens in der Masse afrikanischen Heidentums", p. 48–51.

converts, often sons of regional authorities who could not rule in a matrilineal society.[58]

The marriage preferences of the West Indians, whose children frequently married into African merchant families, were another important factor in contributing to both the spread of Christianity and the fostering of economic ties on the Gold Coast. The second generation of West Indians laid the foundation for the present-day Presbyterian Church of Ghana, while their economic impact was particularly clear in the agricultural sector.[59] They had brought with them coffee, tobacco, cocoyam, mango, pear and breadfruit as possible cash crops suitable for the soil and climate in Akuapem.[60] The expansion and intensification of cash crop production on the Gold Coast created new workplaces for African converts, boosting the Basel Mission's appeal among the resident population, and increased the society's revenue. The Basel Mission opened their first trading post in Christiansborg in 1854, where coffee from Akropong was sold for export.[61]

4.2.2   Cooperation and Conflict in German Cameroon

Cameroon was different from the Basel Mission's other mission fields, in that they were invited to start work there because Cameroon had become a German "protectorate" in 1884 and they were perceived as a German organisation in the *Kaiserreich*.[62] The first evangelical missionaries to

---

[58] C.K. Graham, The History of Education in Ghana. From the Earliest of Times to the Declaration of Independence, Kumasi 2013, p. 54–56.

[59] Noel Smith, The History of the Presbyterian Church in Ghana, 1835–1960, Accra 1966, p. 35–44.

[60] Anthony A. Beeko, The Trail Blazers. Fruits of 175 Years of the Presbyterian Church of Ghana (1828–2003), Accra 2004.

[61] The missionary Hermann Ludwig Rottmann, the first accountant and prospective director of the Basel Mission Trading Company, arrived on the Gold Coast that same year. See Miescher, Hermann Ludwig Rottmann.

[62] For a general overview of Cameroon under German colonial rule, see Martin Njeuma (ed.), Introduction to the History of Cameroon. Nineteenth and Twentieth Centuries, London 1989; Stefanie Michels, Imagined Power Contested: Germans and Africans in the Upper Cross River Area of Cameroon, 1887–1916, Berlin/Münster 2004; Florian Hoffmann, Okkupation und Militärverwaltung in Kamerun. Etablierung und Inszenierung des kolonialen Gewaltmonopols 1891–1914, Göttingen 2007; Ulrike Schaper, Koloniale Verhandlungen. Gerichtsbarkeit, Verwaltung und Herrschaft in Kamerun 1884–1916, Frankfurt a. M. 2012.

settle in Cameroon worked for the English Baptist Missionary Society. They gained a foothold on the island of Fernando Po in 1841 and reached Victoria on the mainland in 1845, where they remained until this English enclave became part of the German colony of Cameroon. The German authorities were suspicious of the British Baptists and thus encouraged the German-speaking Pietists from Basel, who had been working on the Gold Coast since 1828, to assume mission work in the region. The Baptist Missionary Society quit Cameroon in 1885, blaming the unfavourable climate as a reason for their departure.[63]

The support groups of the Basel Mission based in southern Germany endorsed the idea of establishing mission stations in a German colony, whereas the Committee was reluctant due to Cameroon's size and the population's heterogeneity.[64] These initial reservations soon faded for reasons that the Committee member Adolf Sarasin openly addressed in 1914: "We came to recognise that no German mission was capable of putting themselves forward, and to refuse to assume this task meant to surrender the whole colony to the sole influence of the Catholic mission."[65] Resentments against Catholics, and Catholic proselytising more specifically, were a key feature of the evangelical missionary movement, which constantly tried to curb the influence of Catholic missions.[66] The Order of Pallottines, founded by Vincenz Pallotti in 1835, fuelled the Committee's fear of the growing influence of Catholicism in Africa. The Pallottines, however, saw themselves clearly disadvantaged by the *Kulturkampf* in Bismarck's Germany. They had to wait until 1890 to receive approval for missionary work in Cameroon from the Foreign Office.[67]

---

[63] Carl Mirbt, Die Eigenart der deutschen Mission. Vortrag auf der Weltmissionskonferenz in Edinburgh, Basel 1910, p. 51; Eckart, Medizin und Kolonialimperialismus, p. 234; Ralph A. Austen/Jonathan Derrick, Middlemen of the Cameroons Rivers. The Duala and their Hinterland c. 1600–c. 1960, Cambridge 1999, p. 122.

[64] Horst Gründer, Christliche Mission und deutscher Imperialismus. Eine politische Geschichte ihrer Beziehung während der deutschen Kolonialzeit (1884–1914) unter besonderer Berücksichtigung Afrikas und Chinas, Paderborn 1982, p. 135–137.

[65] Adolf Sarasin, La mission de Bâle au Caméroun, Bâle 1914, p. 15–16.

[66] Helmut Walser Smith, German Nationalism and Religious Conflict: Culture, Ideology, Politics, 1870–1914, Princeton 1995; Christopher Clark/Wolfram Kaiser (eds.), Culture Wars. Secular-Catholic Conflict in Nineteenth-Century Europe, Cambridge 2003.

[67] Heinrich Vieter, "Die Jugend ist unsere Zukunft". Chronik der katholischen Mission Kamerun 1890–1913, Friedberg 2011.

The Basel Mission succeeded the British Baptists in 1886 by purchasing the stations Bethel and Victoria located on the coast with the help of the German Foreign Office. Their mission field in the southwest of German Cameroon covered approximately 40,000 square meters and was home to half a million people.[68] Gottlieb Munz, who the Committee had entrusted with the management of the mission in Cameroon, soon found himself in conflict with the African parishes. Baptist congregations rebelled against the Basel Mission and set up their own independent parishes, culminating in the creation of the Native Baptist Church in March of 1888, still in existence today.[69]

The Basel Mission tried to prevent the proliferation of the Native Baptists with the help of the colonial government, albeit with little success.[70] They faced fierce competition in the conversion market, not only from Catholics and African Christians but also from other evangelical missionary societies. In 1890, the Basel Mission had to concede part of their parishes to the German Baptists, who settled at six locations in the southwest.[71] The American Presbyterians moved from Ogowe in Gabon to the southeast of Cameroon in 1889, where they established five mission stations. In the face of this heterogenous group of serious competitors, the Basel Mission's Inspector Walter Oettli declared in 1911 that Cameroon was a "battle ground" on which various powers "collide, mutually promote, inhibit and feud each other," thereby creating a "peculiar mental fermentation process."[72]

---

[68] Jaap van Slageren, Les origines de l'église évangélique du Cameroun. Missions européennes et christianisme autochtone, Leiden 1972, p. 44–72.

[69] Jean-Paul Messina/Jaap van Slageren, Histoire du christianisme au Cameroun. Des originies à nos jours, Paris/Yaoundé 2005, p. 36–46; Bengt Sundkler/Christopher Steed, A History of the Church in Africa, Cambridge 2000, S. 259–273.

[70] The missionary Karl Stolz vividly described how the opposition of the Cameroonian Baptists impaired the plans of the Basel Mission. Karl Stolz, Neue Nachrichten aus Kamerun, in: Der Evangelische Heidenbote 67 (1894), p. 17–18, here p. 18. See further Thorsten Altena, "Ein Häuflein Christen mitten in der Heidenwelt des dunklen Erdteils." Zum Selbst- und Fremdverständnis protestantischer Missionare im kolonialen Afrika 1884–1918, Münster 2003, p. 40–43.

[71] Mirbt, Die Eigenart der deutschen Mission, p. 52–53; Gründer, Christliche Mission und deutscher Imperialismus, p. 138–139; Eckart, Medizin und Kolonialimperialismus, p. 234.

[72] Walter Oettli, Gegenwärtige Missionsprobleme der Basler Mission in Kamerun, Basel 1911, p. 24, BMA, E. 28.

Upon their arrival, the Basel missionaries assessed that Cameroon was home to some 250 different linguistic groups. The population at the time of formal colonisation was estimated at around 3 to 3.5 million with different Bantu groups living in coastal and forest areas.[73] Inhabitants on Cameroon's coast had been in contact with Europeans, Americans, Asians and other Africans for centuries, and were therefore familiar with different Christian denominations. In contrast, the Fulbe and Sudanese communities, who lived in the grasslands in northern Cameroon, remained under Muslim influence during the German colonial era.[74] Until the takeover of Cameroon by the British and French in 1914, the Basel Mission operated through 16 main stations and 246 secondary stations with a total number of 15,112 parishioners.[75] On the Gold Coast, the Basel Mission recorded 11 main stations and 185 outposts with a total of 25,042 parishioners across two main districts, Ga and Twi, in 1914. Official mission publications estimated that one-fifth of the total population of these two districts were Basel parishioners.[76]

African mission members ran most of the Basel Mission's secondary stations in West Africa. The statistics in the Basel Mission's annual reports show that the number of these "indigenous workers" more than quadrupled between 1885 and 1914, from an initial 134 to more than 650. In the same period, the total annual number of European male missionaries residing in West Africa lay between 25 and 140, approximately half of whom were accompanied by their wives. Meanwhile, the number of single female missionaries—referred to as "maidens" in the statistics—remained marginal.[77]

The Basel missionaries often performed minor administrative tasks in West African colonies, as assessors in court proceedings, for example,

[73] They included the Duala at the Cameroon basin, the Bakwiri at Mount Cameroon as well as the Bakoko at the lower course of the Sanaga and Lokundje.

[74] Sebastian Gottschalk, Kolonialismus und Islam. Deutsche und britische Herrschaft in Westafrika (1900–1914), Frankfurt a. M. 2017. On images of Islam within the Basel Mission, see Melanie Stempfel, Islambilder der Basler Mission. Eine Untersuchung anhand der Text- und Bildpublizistik zwischen 1906 und 1938, Master Thesis, University of Fribourg, 2012; Friedrich Würz, Die mohammedanische Gefahr in Westafrika, Basel 1904.

[75] Evangelische Missionsgesellschaft zu Basel (ed.), Neunundneunzigster Jahresbericht, Basel 1914, p. 8.

[76] Schlatter, Geschichte der Basler Mission, vol. 3, p. 155.

[77] Compiled with the statistics in the Basel Mission's annual reports. See Evangelische Missionsgesellschaft zu Basel (ed.), Jahresberichte, Basel 1885–1914.

while their civilising mission made them tolerated or welcome in many places. In the case of German Cameroon, the collaboration of the Basel Mission with the colonial government played an important role in Germany's expansion into northern Cameroon. While the Basel Mission relied on stable political conditions, including military repression, the colonial administration valued the consolidating influence of the Basel missionaries in recently acquired territories.[78] However, despite a symbiotic relationship, Thorsten Altena forcefully demonstrated that the leaders of the Basel Mission did not conceive of their mission in Cameroon as a patriotic act, regularly finding themselves at odds with German colonial politics.[79] At the end of 1898, an open and protracted dispute broke out between the Basel Mission and the German administration over missionary property on Mount Cameroon and in the Buea district and, more importantly, the ill-treatment and expropriation of Cameroonians.[80]

German colonial policy in Cameroon encouraged the development of large plantations for tea, cacao, coffee and oil palms. For this purpose, laws were passed that enabled the government to deprive the resident population of most of their land and to sell it cheaply to European plantation companies. Furthermore, Cameroonians were ordered to pay taxes, which meant they were forced to find new sources of income, such as working on these plantations.[81] From 1900, the Basel missionaries openly defied the government's measures in Cameroon, arguing that Africans were perfectly capable of growing the new colonial crops and

---

[78] Edward Forcha Lekunze, Chieftaincy and Christianity in Cameroon 1886–1926. A Historical and Comparative Analysis of the Evangelistic Strategy of the Basel Mission, Ann Arbor 1988; Jonas N. Dah, Missionary Motivations and Methods. A Critical Examination of the Basel Mission in Cameroon 1886–1914, Basel 1983.

[79] Altena, "Ein Häuflein Christen mitten in der Heidenwelt des dunklen Erdteils", p. 39.

[80] Horst Gründer/Paul Jenkins/Mary Njikam, Mission und Kolonialismus. Die Basler Mission und die Landfrage in Deutsch-Kamerun, Basel 1986; Jürg Schneider, Haarrisse der Macht: Aspekte regionaler Kolonialgeschichte am Mount Cameroon, Licentiate Thesis, University of Basel, 2001; Gründer, Christliche Mission und deutscher Imperialismus, p. 141–153.

[81] Andreas Eckert, Grundbesitz, Landkonflikte und kolonialer Wandel. Douala 1880 bis 1960, Stuttgart 1999.

that they should be permitted to farm their own land under their own management.[82]

4.2.3 Economics, Linguistics and Education

The Basel Mission's appeal for the creation of an independent class of African farmers in Cameroon was part of a set of three strategies that were aimed at transforming African societies socially and economically, deemed paramount for achieving evangelical goals. Firstly, the Basel Mission maintained the importance of establishing autonomous Christian villages, which they called "salems," where African parishioners could build an independent economic existence outside of the dominant colonial economy.[83] Colonial governments in West Africa promoted foreign-controlled plantation economies that destroyed communal life and reduced many Africans to landless and often itinerant agrarian proletarians.[84] As a response to this development, the Basel Mission supported the creation of independent family-run cacao and coffee farms.[85] Tetteh Quarshie, a Ga speaker who had trained as a smith in the Basel Mission workshop in Christiansborg, became one of the most successful cacao farmers on the Gold Coast in the late nineteenth century.[86]

[82] Gründer/Jenkins/Njikam, Mission und Kolonialismus; Schneider, Haarrisse der Macht.

[83] Karl Renntisch, Mission und wirtschaftliche Entwicklung, Basel 1975, p. 349–352; Erik Halldén, The Culture Policy of the Basel Mission in the Cameroons 1886–1905, Lund 1968.

[84] Emmanuel Kwaku Akyeampong et al. (eds.), Africa's Development in Historical Perspective, Cambridge 2014; Martin Lynn, Commerce and Economic Change in West Africa. The Palm Oil Trade in the Nineteenth Century, Cambridge 1997; Robin Law (ed.), From Slave Trade to 'Legitimate' Commerce. The Commercial Transition in Nineteenth-Century West Africa, Cambridge 1993; Anthony C. Hopkins, An Economic History of West Africa, New York 1973.

[85] Karl Rennstich, Handwerker-Theologen und Industrie-Brüder als Botschafter des Friedens. Entwicklungshilfe der Basler Mission im 19. Jahrhundert, Stuttgart 1985, p. 67–70; Hans Werner Debrunner, A History of Christianity in Ghana, Accra 1967, p. 252–253; Schlatter, Geschichte der Basler Mission, vol. 3, p. 87–88, 115, 191.

[86] Franc, Wie die Schweiz zur Schokolade kam, p. 77–79.

Secondly, the Basel Mission's strategy crucially depended on preaching the gospel in African languages.[87] This approach was rooted in the belief, traceable to Martin Luther, that an individual's mother tongue was the only effective medium for the insight that produced conversion and salvation. The Basel missionaries were required to master the languages spoken in their mission areas, in contrast to English and American mission societies that used interpreters to communicate with the resident population.[88] Their efforts initially concentrated on administering church life, including service and catechism, in regional languages, since this promised greater evangelisation success. Over the years, the Basel missionaries translated the Bible into numerous languages they had learnt in West Africa.[89]

The vernacularisation of the Bible required a degree of sensitivity, openness and adaptability on the part of the Basel missionaries, which fundamentally changed the Bible itself. "Missionary adoption of the vernacular" was, as Lamin Sanneh insisted, "tantamount to adopting indigenous cultural criteria for the message, a piece of radical indigenization far greater than the standard portrayal of mission as Western cultural imperialism."[90] The translation process was always an exercise in mutual transformation. John Peel's study of Anglican Church missionaries among the Yoruba demonstrated how Bible translations induced shifts in theological meaning. He showed that because missionaries and their translators among the Yoruba had to seek out vernacular expressions for their concepts, they "often ended up using terms which Muslims had introduced."[91] In an environment where Christian missionaries had to work between their own theological heritage, Yoruba beliefs and Islam, difficult conceptual choices had to be made.

---

[87] Erika Eichholzer, Missionary Linguistics on the Gold Coast: Wrestling with Language, in: Patrick Harries/David Maxwell (eds.), The Spiritual in the Secular. Missionaries and Knowledge about Africa, Grand Rapids/Cambridge 2012, p. 72–99, here p. 98.

[88] Christian Blumhardt, Instruction for the brothers leaving for the Danish Gold Coast in 1828, 15.09.1828, p. 1, BMA, D-10.3.3.

[89] Sara Pugach, Africa in Translation. A History of Colonial Linguistics in Germany and Beyond, 1814–1945, Ann Arbor 2012, p. 21–48.

[90] Lamin Sanneh, Translating the Message: The Missionary Impact on Culture, Marynoll 1998, p. 3.

[91] John D. Y. Peel, Religious Encounter and the Making of the Yoruba, Bloomington 2003, p. 189.

Several members of the Basel Mission gained wide recognition for their expertise as translators and linguists. Johann Gottlieb Christaller and Johannes Zimmermann, who worked on the Gold Coast, put together dictionaries of the Twi and Ga-Adangme languages that are still in use to this day.[92] The Basel Mission extended their language policy in West Africa to their schools, which conflicted with colonial policies on education. The British and German administrations in the region planned to replace African tongues with their respective national languages.[93] The Basel missionary Adolf Mohr reported in 1901 that the British Governor on the Gold Coast, Matthew Nathan, had told him that "vernaculars should become extinct and interpreters rendered superfluous," upon which he allegedly replied: "Hopefully our mission will succeed in keeping them alive."[94] Although the Basel Mission integrated English into their curricula on the Gold Coast from the mid-nineteenth century, a concession to colonial realities, regional languages remained the main medium of teaching and linguistics continued to form one of their key preoccupations.[95]

Thirdly, the Basel Mission pursued an ambitious literacy and education strategy since their ideal of a spiritual rebirth required people to be able to experience the Word directly for themselves in the language of

---

[92] Johann Gottlieb Christaller, A Dictionary of the Asante and Fante Language Called Tshi, Basel 1881; Ibid., Twi Mmebusem Mpensa-Ahansia Mmoaano. A Collection of Three Thousand and Six Hundred Tshi Proverbs, Basel 1879; Ibid., Grammar of the Asante and Fante Language called Tshi, Based on the Akuapem Dialect, Basel 1875; Johannes Zimmermann, A Dictionary, English, Tshi (Asante), Akra, Basel 1874; Ibid., A Grammatical Sketch of the Akra- or Ga- Language, with Some Specimens of it from the Mouth of the Natives and a Vocabulary of the Same with an Appendix on the Adanme-Dialect, Stuttgart 1858.

[93] Kenneth J. Orosz, Religious Conflict and the Evolution of Language Policy in German and French Cameroon, 1885–1939, New York et al. 2008; Ibid., An African Kulturkampf. Religious Conflict and Language Policy in German Cameroon, 1885–1914, in: Sociolinguistica 25 (2011) 1, p. 81–93; Cyrelene Amoah Boampong, Rethinking British Colonial Policy in the Gold Coast: The Language Factor, in: Transactions of the Historical Society of Ghana 15 (2013), p. 137–157.

[94] Adolf Mohr, Letter to Committee, 04.02.1901, BMA, D-1.74.24.

[95] See, for instance, the publications by the Basel Mission doctor Rudolf Fisch. Rudolf Fisch, Grammatik der Dagomba-Sprache, gesprochen in Nord-Togo und den nördlichen Bezirken der Goldküste (Dagbane), Berlin 1912; Ibid., Wörtersammlung Dagbáne-Deutsch, Berlin 1913; Ibid., Dagbane-Sprachproben. Mitteilungen veröffentlicht vom Seminar für Kolonialsprachen in Hamburg, Hamburg 1913.

their birth.[96] Independent Bible study was central to Pietist faith, which is why the Basel Mission published a large range of so-called primers— literacy training books—in African languages. Primers were small in size and had a simple layout, which made them cheap to reproduce. The Basel Mission's own publishing house in Basel and their printing plants on the ground in West Africa also produced tractates, Bible translations, song- and hymnbooks in regional languages. While these types of publications were not new to West Africa, the scale of their production was unprece- dented, forming a vital resource for the popularisation of Christianity in the region.[97]

The majority of the Basel Mission's funds were allocated to the devel- opment of schooling. They ran a comprehensive school system in the Twi and Ga regions on the Gold Coast, from primary schools in villages to teachers' training colleges.[98] The annual report for 1914 recorded that a total of 7,819 pupils on the Gold Coast attended one of the 157 Basel Mission schools. In Cameroon, it was a total of 22,818 pupils in 384 Basel Mission schools, most of whom were instructed by African teachers.[99] The syllabus focused on religious instruction but also included "ele- ments of European science," reading, writing, arithmetic, handicraft and hygiene. In the Basel Mission's boarding schools and seminaries, classes further comprised German, history and geography.[100] Many people in West Africa associated converting to Christianity with the prospect of a European school education. Christianity and literacy were considered to be synonymous terms, which is illustrated by the moniker they gave to the Basel missionaries: "Europeans of the Books."[101]

---

[96] Martin Göhring, Kameruner Schulbilder, in: Der Evangelische Heidenbote 74 (1901), p. 78–79.

[97] Clark/Ledger-Lomas, The Protestant International, p. 30.

[98] Graham, The History of Education in Ghana, p. 54–56; Sonia Abun-Nasr, Von der "Umbildung heidnischer Landessprachen zu christlichen". Die Anfänge von Schrift und Schriftlichkeit in Akuapem, Goldküste, in: Reinhard Wendt (ed.), Wege durch Babylon. Missionare, Sprachstudien und interkulturelle Kommunikation, Tübingen 1998, p. 181–220.

[99] Evangelische Missionsgesellschaft zu Basel (ed.), Neunundneunzigster Jahresbericht, Basel 1914, p. 8.

[100] Oettli, Gegenwärtige Missionsprobleme der Basler Mission in Kamerun, p. 28–32, BMA, E. 28.

[101] Jakob Keller, Im Hinterland von Kamerun, in: Evangelisches Missionsmagazin 49 (1905), p. 27–36, here p. 32.

The Basel missionaries' decisions as to which languages were recorded, translated and used in the mission schools harboured considerable potential for conflict. One language was not chosen over another simply because it was more popular or widespread. Rather, it depended on the geographical position of mission stations or the quality of the relationship between individual missionaries and regional authorities. The process of fixing, defining and demarcating a language not only divided previously related linguistic groups but missionaries also commonly created, or arguably invented, new languages by merging several into one.[102] Notwithstanding that missionary linguistics constituted a source of disruption, they also represented a powerful means of expression and communication, empowering people in West Africa to challenge and oppose colonial policies and imperial exploitation. Tony Ballantyne showed, for example, that "literacy and the Bible provided successive generations of Māori leaders with new skills and knowledge that could be turned against colonization."[103]

The Basel Mission's economic, linguistic and educational policies had a profound impact on the regions in which they operated. They were not, however, simply implemented rigidly according to the Basel Mission's preconceived plans but rather they grew organically through interaction with African translators, intermediaries and authorities.[104] Since farming, translating and teaching crucially involved dialogue with African people and adoption of their frame of reference, the Basel Mission's strategies were fundamentally shaped by these people's concepts and willingness to cooperate. This was not least because it was usually West African Christians who introduced their fellow citizens to the Basel Mission's

[102] Paul S. Landau, Language, in: Norman Etherington (ed.), Missions and Empire, Oxford 2005, p. 194–215; Fabian, Time and the Work Anthropology, ch. 7, p. 131–150; Harries, Butterflies and Barbarians, p. 155–181; Tony Ballantyne, Paper, Pen, and Print: The Transformation of the Kai Tahu Knowledge Order, in: Comparative Studies in Society and History 53 (2011) 2, p. 232–260.

[103] Ballantyne, Entanglements of Empire, p. 4.

[104] Benjamin N. Lawrance/Emily Lynn Osborn/Richard L. Roberts (eds.), Intermediaries, Interpreters, and Clerks. African Employees in the Making of Colonial Africa, Madison 2006; Rebekka Habermas, Intermediaries, Kaufleute, Missionare, Forscher und Diakonissen, in: ibid./Alexandra Przyrembel (eds.), Von Käfern, Märkten und Menschen. Kolonialismus und Wissen in der Moderne, Göttingen 2013, p. 27–48; Gilbert Dotsé Yigbe, Von Gewährsleuten zu Gehilfen und Gelehrigen. Der Beitrag afrikanischer Mitarbeiter zur Entstehung einer verschrifteten Kultur in Deutsch-Togo, in: Rebekka Habermas/Richard Hölzl (eds.), Mission global. Eine Verflechtungsgeschichte seit dem 19. Jahrhundert, Köln/Weimar/Wien 2014, p. 159–175.

economics, linguistics and education, adapting and reinterpreting them as they did so. By appropriating these three pillars of the Basel Mission's strategy into their own frameworks, West African actors triggered the development of new narratives and ways of living, allowing for the reformulation of individual futures and collective histories.[105]

4.3   MISSION MEDICINE
AND HEALTH IN THE COLONIES

By the time the first institutions of tropical medicine saw the light of day in European metropolises around 1900, the Basel Mission had acquired more than 70 years of knowledge about health in tropical colonies. The British schools for tropical medicine and the *Institut für Schiffs- und Tropenkrankheiten* sought to train colonial doctors to protect the health of officials, traders and settlers, providing space for laboratory research as well as practical training before they were sent to colonial posts.[106] European powers were not initially interested in providing medical services to the general population in their colonies. Their focus lay on the acclimatisation and well-being of European personnel as well as the prevention of epidemic outbreaks. Colonial doctors generally worked in urban areas and overviewed large-scale measures such as soil decontamination, vaccination campaigns and segregation projects. The health care provided by the Basel Mission, in contrast, spread out into rural regions and focussed on the treatment of individual patients, including both Europeans and Africans.[107]

---

[105] For an example of how African Christians, connected to the Basel Mission, recorded and elaborated historical and cultural narratives, see Tomas C. McCaskie, Local Knowledge: An Akuapem Twi History of Asante, in: History in Africa 38 (2011), p. 169–192.

[106] Deborah J. Neill, Science and Civilizing Missions. Germans and the Transnational Community of Tropical Medicine, in: Bradley Naranch/Geoff Eley (eds.), German Colonialism in a Global Age, Durham/London 2014, p. 74–92, here p. 76.

[107] Sources outlining the different roles of government physicans and mission doctors include Alexander Lion, Die Volkshygiene für Eingeborene in ihren Beziehungen zur Kolonialwirtschaft und Kolonialverwaltung, in: Koloniale Rundschau 2 (1910), p. 772–774; Gottlob Haussleiter, Die Bedeutung der ärztlichen Mission in den deutschen Kolonien, in: Die ärztliche Mission 6 (1911), p. 5–16.

4.3.1   The Basel Medical Mission in West Africa

Rudolf Fisch, the first scientifically trained Basel Mission doctor in West Africa, arrived in Aburi on the Gold Coast with two chests of instruments and drugs in 1885. The hill station in Aburi, about 25 miles inland from Accra and 1,450 feet above sea level, formed the headquarters of the Basel medical mission. The Committee selected Aburi due to its geographical position, centrally located between the main stations of Abokobi, Akropong and Odumase/Krobo, on the cool plateau of the Akuapem Mountain Range. Aburi was home to the first European medical facility away from the coastal towns in the entire Gold Coast Colony. During his research expedition, Mähly had assessed that Aburi was "without any doubt" the healthiest place in the mission area, mainly due to its fresh source water, compact soil and air circulation.[108] From March 1886, there was a telegraph connection between Aburi and Accra, meaning that the mission doctor could be notified in case of any medical emergencies on the coast.[109] This line was expanded to other mission stations in the following years. The medical centre in Aburi initially comprised of a sanatorium for European missionaries, housed in a two-storey building with eight patient rooms, and an outpatient clinic for African patients.[110]

Fisch swiftly implemented daily consultation hours from 2 to 5 pm. According to him, these were widely attended by "all classes of Africans from the local 'royal' family to the poorest, expelled leper, from the smart fetish masters to the mentally ill."[111] In his first annual account, the mission doctor reported that he had treated more than 600 African patients, some of whom had walked for 20 hours to consult with him.[112] The early years of the medical mission in Aburi show that the population was quite willing to listen to and accept the medical missionary among them. Nevertheless, conversions remained rare. The

---

[108] Ernst Mähly, The hygienic conditions of the African mission area, p. 19–20, BMA, D-1.39.K.

[109] Station chronicle Aburi, 1856–1916, p. 66, BMA, D-5.10; Alfred Eckhardt, Letter to Committee, 09.06.1889, BMA, D-1.48.66.

[110] Fischer, Der Missionsarzt Rudolf Fisch, p. 237.

[111] Rudolf Fisch, Vierzig Jahre ärztliche Mission auf der Goldküste, in: Deutsches Institut für ärztliche Mission Tübingen (ed.), Die deutsche evangelische ärztliche Mission nach dem Stand des Jahres 1928, Stuttgart 1928, p. 16–27, here p. 17.

[112] Rudolf Fisch, Annual report for 1885, 30.01.1886, BMA, D-1.43.26.

Basel Mission attributed the lack of evangelising success to adverse social influences, such as the patriarchal power of elders.[113] The construction of a mission hospital, where patients were confined and possibly underwent a life-changing experience, was thus seen as an important step in the advancement of the mission as a whole. The mission hospital in Aburi, comprising of a surgery room, four patient rooms and an attached clay house to host additional patients and families, was completed in 1900.[114]

The first year of the hospital in Aburi saw 22 inpatients while 1644 outpatients came to see Fisch in his practice. The number of patients grew rapidly over the next years, partially because Fisch started travelling and offering consultation hours at mission stations throughout the Gold Coast. In 1902, Fisch saw 4002 outpatients and 36 inpatients in Aburi while covering more than 3000 kilometres with his bicycle on 30 different medical tours.[115] By 1906, the number of outpatients in Aburi had reached 7,891 and the hospital hosted 62 patients, which caused Fisch to appeal to the Committee for the expansion of the existing facilities and the dispatch of additional medical missionaries.[116] The growing demand for mission medicine was indicative of broader economic and social shifts at the turn of the twentieth century, including the expansion of cacao cultivation, the operation of gold mines and the building of roads and railways.[117]

A crucial factor for the mounting success of the Basel medical mission was the training and employment of African assistants. Their tasks included the laborious treatment of wounds and the time-consuming operation of dispensaries. Medicines imported from Europe had to be weighed out, ointments had to be mixed and pills had to be rolled.[118] Most of the early medical assistants were former patients who had become Basel Mission parishioners. Later, most of the medical staff was recruited

---

[113] Schlatter, Geschichte der Basler Mission, vol. 3, p. 49.

[114] Rudolf Fisch, Annual report for 1900, 31.01.1901, BMA, D-1.73.12.

[115] Rudolf Fisch, Annual report for 1902, 06.02.1903, BMA, D-1.77.19.

[116] Hermann Feldmann, Das ärztliche Missionswerk der deutschen Missionsgesellschaften, in: Die ärztliche Mission 1 (1906), p. 1–3, 17–20, here p. 17.

[117] Karl David Patterson, Health in Colonial Ghana. Disease, Medicine, and Socio-Economic Change, 1900–1955, Waltham 1981, p. 1–9.

[118] Alfred Eckhardt, Annual report for 1889, 07.05.1890, BMA, D-1.50.96.

from the graduate pool of the Basel Mission schools.[119] Medical assistants played a crucial role in popularising mission medicine in their communities of origin, as David Hardiman and David Arnold have shown.[120] The Basel Mission also offered basic medical training to African pastors and schoolteachers at the hospital in Aburi, so that they could provide medical care in the villages in which they worked.[121]

The Committee sent a second mission doctor to the Gold Coast in 1887. Alfred Eckhardt first assisted Fisch in Aburi and then practised at the Basel Mission station in Christiansborg. In 1891, he moved to Odumase, where he opened a new hospital together with a nurse, the deaconess Klara Finckh, whom he had met during his home leave in Berlin.[122] Finckh, a pastor's daughter from the Wurttemberg region who had trained at the deaconessate in Hall, was the first nurse to be employed by the Basel Mission.[123] She provided medical care in Odumase, where more than one thousand patients sought her help in 1892, assisted Eckhardt during operations, regularly visited mission members in other parishes and sold "truly incredible quantities of wound medication," according to Eckhardt.[124]

Just two years after their arrival in Odumase, both Eckhardt and Finckh passed away in the space of five months of each other. Fisch reported that his fellow mission doctor succumbed to a liver abscess in April while the deaconess died of black water fever in September 1893.[125] Following Eckhardt's sudden death, a new Basel Mission doctor named Friedrich Hey started practising in Aburi in 1895 and soon moved to the hospital

[119] Schlatter, Geschichte der Basler Mission, vol. 3, p. 94–97.

[120] Hardiman, The Mission Hospital 1880–1960, p. 208; David Arnold, Introduction. Disease, Medicine and Empire, in: ibid. (ed.), Imperial Medicine and Indigenous Societies, Manchester 1988, p. 1–26, here p. 2.

[121] Fischer, Der Missionsarzt Rudolf Fisch, p. 208–213.

[122] Alfred Eckhardt, Annual report for 1892, 15.01.1893, BMA, D-1.56.132.

[123] Basler Missionskomitee (ed.), An die Freunde des Ärztlichen Zweiges der Basler Mission, Basel 1892, p. 4; Gabriela Hofstetter, "Gehet hin und pfleget." Basler Missionarinnen im Dienst der Ärztlichen Mission in Asien und Afrika (1892–1945), Zürich 2002, p. 51–52.

[124] Alfred Eckhardt, Annual report for 1892, 15.01.1893, BMA, D-1.56.132; Ibid., Ein Arbeitsjahr in Odumase (Goldküste), in: An die Freunde des Ärztlichen Zweiges der Basler Mission, Basel 1893, p. 5–11, here p. 9.

[125] Rudolf Fisch, Letter to Committee, 10.10.1893, BMA, D-1.59.36.

in Odumase. Originating from the Palatinate region, Hey had trained as an orderly before joining the seminary in Basel. The Basel Mission's house doctor, Adolf Hägler, recognised Hey's potential as a mission doctor, recommending him as a suitable candidate to the Committee. Thereupon, Hey began a medical degree alongside his missionary training in the seminary by taking lectures at the University of Basel and assisting at the surgical department of the *Bürgerspital*, the city's public hospital. Despite not having completed secondary school, Hey graduated in October of 1891 thanks to the support of the Rector of the University of Basel, Professor Julius Kollmann.[126]

Five years after Hey's arrival in West Africa, the Committee decided to transfer him to Bonaku in Cameroon, where he became the first Basel Mission doctor to practise from November 1900. Hey soon found himself in conflict with his fellow missionaries and patients to the point that a continuation of his medical work seemed impossible.[127] Disagreements arose over the prophylactic intake of quinine, which Hey encouraged and many missionaries refused, and alcohol, which the mission doctor condemned but many of his non-medical colleagues and parishioners consumed. Hey complained in a letter to the Inspector that "many missionaries would still be alive if they had led a more reasonable life."[128] Following a heated exchange of allegations between Bonaku and Basel, Hey and his wife left Cameroon in April of 1902. Hey subsequently worked for several trading companies on the Gold Coast between 1904 and 1908, where he also temporarily served as a representative British government physician.[129]

The first Basel Mission hospital in Cameroon was completed in the spring of 1902 in Douala. In the absence of a mission doctor, it was nurses, African assistants, ordinary missionaries and their spouses who

---

[126] Christine Wolters, Dr. Friedrich Hey (1864–1960), Missionsarzt und Bückeburger Unternehmer, in: Hubert Höing (ed.), Strukturen und Konjunkturen. Faktoren in der schaumburgischen Wirtschaftsgeschichte, Bielefeld 2004, p. 328–366.

[127] Friedrich Hey, Annual report about the medical mission in Cameroon, Bonaku, December 1901, p. 20, BMA, E-2.14.141; Karl Eugen Schuler, Letter to Inspector, 03.03.1902, BMA, E-2.15.38.

[128] Friedrich Hey, Letter to Inspector, 20.11.1902, Personal File Friedrich Hey, BMA, BV 1261.

[129] Eckart, Medizin und Kolonialimperialismus, p. 248.

administered drugs, saw to the comfort of the patients and gave spiritual advice to the ill and dying. Every major station in West Africa had an outpatient clinic, where people associated with the Basel Mission found themselves strenuously engaged in medical work, drawing on their basic knowledge while explicitly acting according to the tenets of biblical healing.[130] A number of Basel missionaries in West Africa had taken a ten and a half-month long course at the German Institute for Medical Mission in Tübingen.[131] Others with an interest in health care proceeded on their own initiative. The Principal of the Basel Mission's Girls' Institute in Douala, for instance, dedicated herself to birth assistance and maternal health for African women from 1904.[132]

The medical mission with academically trained physicians in Cameroon was resumed in 1907, when the Committee employed Arthur Häberlin on a three-year contract. Once again, however, quarrels between veteran missionaries and the mission doctor prevented the stabilisation of the

---

[130] Johannes Kopp, Der Missionar als Arzt an der Goldküste, in: An die Freunde des Ärztlichen Zweiges der Basler Mission, Basel 1892, p. 25–32; Jakob Stutz, Bericht aus Bonaku, in: Verein für ärztliche Mission (ed.), Bericht über das 5. Geschäftsjahr 1903, p. 32–34; Jonathan Striebel, Krankheitsbilder aus Bali, in: Verein für ärztliche Mission (ed.), Bericht über das 11. Geschäftsjahr 1909, p. 26–29; Anna Merkle, Bericht aus Bali, in: Verein für ärztliche Mission (ed.), Bericht über das 13. Geschäftsjahr 1910–1911, p. 7–10; Jakob Stutz, Aus meiner ärztlichen Praxis, in: Verein für ärztliche Mission in Stuttgart (ed.), Mitteilungen aus der ärztlichen Mission 10 (1911), p. 4–7; Niklaus Wöll, Der Missionar als Arzt, in: Verein für ärztliche Mission in Stuttgart (ed.), Mitteilungen aus der ärztlichen Mission 10 (1911), p. 7–8; Christiane Gutekunst, Bericht von der Station Bonaku, in: Verein für ärztliche Mission (ed.), Bericht über das 14. Geschäftsjahr 1911–1912, p. 8–11; Karl Stolz, Auf Vorposten in Kamerun, in: Verein für ärztliche Mission (ed.), Bericht über das 15. Geschäftsjahr 1912–1913, p. 32; Johannes Flogaus, Der Missionar als Arzt in Kamerun, in: Verein für ärztliche Mission (ed.), Bericht über das 16. Geschäftsjahr 1913–1914, p. 32–36; Milla Roos, Die ärztliche Mission in Bali, in: Verein für ärztliche Mission (ed.), Bericht über das 16. Geschäftsjahr 1913–1914, p. 36–37.

[131] In 1914 they included Eduard Lewerenz in Bali (Cameroon), Johannes Flogaus in Bonaku (Cameroon), Niklaus Wöll in Douala (Cameroon) as well as Emil Nothwang in Anum (Gold Coast).

[132] Eckart, Medizin und Kolonialimperialismus, p. 248. The Basel missionaries in Cameroon also stared a leper colony in Ossidinge in 1913. See BMA, E-2.40.45.

medical mission in Cameroon.[133] The Committee did not renew Häberlin's contract in May of 1910. Nonetheless, Basel Mission members based in Cameroon ensured that medical care was widely available in the areas where they operated.[134] Meanwhile on the Gold Coast, the medical mission with scientifically trained staff was further consolidated with the arrival of young and well-qualified physicians and nurses. Hermann Vortisch, who had studied in Basel, Tubingen and Munich, and practised at hospitals in Berne and Basel, filled in for Fisch in Aburi, while he was on home leave from 1903 to 1905.[135]

Sophie Hertlein, who had completed a nursing course offered by the Association for Women's Mission in Basel and taken anaesthesia classes with Professor Paul Niehans in Berne, joined Fisch upon his return to Aburi in 1905.[136] Fisch's medical team was further strengthened in 1909 with the employment of Theodor Müller. Born to Basel missionaries from Wurttemberg, Müller had trained in Munich, Heidelberg and Karlsruhe, before joining the military as a doctor. He recalled being inspired to become a mission doctor by Fisch, who he had heard of as a child. The arrival of Müller, who was familiar with the latest developments in surgery, and two additional nurses, Emma Metzger and Berta Öchsler, led to a significant increase in operations in the hospital in Aburi.[137] The staff in Aburi now performed approximately 24,000 ambulatory treatments, including on their medical tours, and over 400 surgical interventions each year between 1909 and 1914.[138] Given the overcrowded hospital, the

---

[133] Arthur Häberlin, Letter to Inspector Theodor Oehler, Douala, 04.08.1908, BMA, E-2.27.141; Ibid., Letter to Pastor Friedrich Würz, Douala, 11.08.1908, BMA, E-2.27.143; Friedrich Würz, Letter to Committee, 20.03.1909, BMA, E-27.29.79; Theodor Oehler, Letter to Arthur Häberlin, 07.06.1909, BMA, E-27.29.81.

[134] Eckart, Medizin und Kolonialimperialismus, p. 241–254.

[135] Hermann Vortisch, Bericht von Aburi, in: Verein für ärztliche Mission (ed.), Bericht über das 6. Geschäftsjahr 1904, p. 17–19; Ibid., Bericht von Aburi, in: Verein für ärztliche Mission (ed.), Bericht über das 7. Geschäftsjahr 1905, p. 25–31.

[136] Committee report, 15.02.1905, BMA, Komitee-Protokoll 1905, §157.

[137] Emma Metzger, Blick in ein afrikanisches Missionsspital, in: Verein für ärztliche Mission (ed.), Bericht über das 15. Geschäftsjahr 1912–1913, p. 29–31.

[138] Theodor Müller, Jahresbericht der Station Aburi, in: Verein für ärztliche Mission (ed.), Bericht über das 16. Geschäftsjahr 1913–1914, p. 7–13, here p. 8.

patients often had to find a place to stay in the village, even though the original four beds in 1900 had been increased to twelve.[139]

In light of the developments in Aburi, the Committee decided upon the construction of a new, considerably larger and more modern hospital, including X-ray equipment. The Basel Mission Trading Company, which had made enormous gains in the cacao business on the Gold Coast in recent years, donated 250,000 Swiss Francs for this project.[140] In the spring of 1914, the Committee additionally commissioned the mission doctor Karl Huppenbauer, who was born in Akropong on the Gold Coast and had trained in medicine in Tubingen, to work at the hospital in Aburi. The outbreak of the First World War, however, abruptly ended Huppenbauer's engagement and the reconstruction of the mission hospital in Aburi. The Basel Mission's plans were finally executed in 1928 with the establishment of a mission hospital inland in Agogo, which remains one of the major hospitals in southern Ghana to date.[141]

The Basel Mission shunned engagement with scientific medicine until the 1880s, viewing it as a costly diversion from true evangelisation. By 1900, however, the Committee had incorporated medical training, methods and technologies into their agenda, enthusiastically endorsing medical work as a key to the hearts and minds of potential converts. This was partially due to their growing confidence in the effectiveness of scientific medicine during this period, or as Christoffer H. Grundmann expressed it: "Physicians now could cure diseases previously considered fatal, thereby allowing Christian doctors to reconsider the scriptural charge of being sent by their Lord and Master to heal."[142] Significant innovations in the conceptualisation and design of medical instruments, such as the stethoscope, pharmacological advances in drug therapy, improvements in surgery, the development of sera and vaccines, and the understanding of aetiologies at the end of the nineteenth century gave new impetus to the medical missionary venture.[143]

---

[139] Theodor Müller, Annual report for 1911, 18.03.1912, BMA, D-1.97.22.

[140] Wanner, Die Basler Handels-Gesellschaft A.G., p. 629; Schlatter, Geschichte der Basler Mission, vol. 1, p. 377; Ibid., Geschichte der Basler Mission, vol. 3, p. 188–189.

[141] Schmid, Medicine, Faith and Politics in Agogo.

[142] Christoffer H. Grundmann, Mission and Healing in Historical Perspective, in: International Bulletin of Missionary Research 32 (2008) 4, p. 185–187, here p. 186.

[143] Jennings, "Healing of Bodies, Salvation of Souls", p. 27.

The Basel Mission doctors portrayed their medical activities as a living example of Christ's own work. They believed that they were able to access African communities through their medical work and hoped that people who had been indifferent to the gospel would start seeking their help for medical treatment, thereby providing an avenue of opportunity for evangelising work. Rudolf Fisch defined the medical mission as "the pursuit of our Lord's Great Commission through physicians appointed for this purpose. The medical art is thereby put into the service of God's Kingdom."[144] The Basel Mission built up a network of health services in certain regions on the Gold Coast and in Cameroon that stretched into rural communities. With the employment of medical missionaries from the 1880s, the training of medical assistants and nurses, and the establishment of mission hospitals and outpatient clinics throughout their mission areas, the Basel Mission ensured that the resident population were exposed to the possibility of healing via scientific medicine.

4.3.2   Growing Interest in "Indigenous Hygiene"

The involvement of the Basel Mission in delivering health care to the African population on the Gold Coast and in Cameroon was increasingly valued by imperial policy-makers, who attached more and more importance to the physical well-being of their subjects in tropical colonies. There was a marked shift in the period between 1885 and 1914 from an initial emphasis on the health and survival of white colonists to the teaching of hygiene to the resident population in the colonies, ostensibly for their own benefit. The improvement of "indigenous hygiene"—as it was referred to during the colonial period before World War I—became a key concern of colonial governments in Africa around 1900, for both economic and cultural reasons. Reflecting their increasing involvement in public health at home, European authorities now advocated extending preventive medical measures to the colonies.[145]

---

[144] Rudolf Fisch, Die ärztliche Mission unter den Negern. Ansprache am Jahresfest der Basler Mission am 3. Juli 1895, in: Evangelisches Missionsmagazin 39 (1895), p. 371–377, here p. 372.

[145] Alison Bashford, Medicine, Gender and Empire, in: Philippa Levine (ed.), Gender and Empire, Oxford 2004, p. 112–133.

In the British Empire, medical services remained disorganised and catered mostly to European settlers and colonisers until Joseph Chamberlain became the Colonial Secretary in 1895. He defined the British expansion in Africa as "constructive imperialism," which was based on the idea that imperialism was for the benefit of the colonised people and for the rational utilisation of colonial resources. Medicine, alongside formal education and economic changes, was thus seen as an essential component of both bringing progress to Africans and serving Britain's imperial interests. Chamberlain made the Colonial Office an important pillar of British colonial governance and extended colonial medicine to include healthcare for African subjects.[146]

The West African Medical Service, created in 1902, received particular attention under Chamberlain. Closely administrated from the Colonial Office in London, which controlled recruitment, pay, promotions and postings, it remained racial in its recruitment pattern and metropolitan in its administration.[147] Chamberlain was convinced that disease control and medical intervention were indispensable elements of Britain's imperial mission. He appointed Patrick Manson as the Colonial Office's first medical adviser and put government opinion and resources behind Manson's efforts to establish the School of Tropical Medicine in London.[148] Chamberlain, whose political and economic support propelled the institutionalisation of tropical medicine in Great Britain, elaborated on the constructive aims of tropical medicine in 1905:

> I cannot myself think of any subject of scientific research and philanthropic enterprise which is more interesting, and the duty of supporting is one, which we owe to the Empire, and from which we cannot divest ourselves whatever our political opinions may be. This duty to which I refer has increased in recent years with the continual extension of our territory, with

---

[146] Anna Crozier, Practising Colonial Medicine: The Colonial Medical Service in British East Africa, London/New York 2007, p. 3–4.

[147] Ryan Johnson, "An All-White Institution": Defending Private Practice and the Formation of the West African Medical Staff, in: Medical History 54 (2010), p. 237–254; Ibid., The West African Medical Staff and the Administration of Imperial Tropical Medicine, 1902–1914, in: The Journal of Imperial and Commonwealth History 38 (2010) 3, p. 419–439.

[148] Mark Harrison, Tropical Medicine in Nineteenth-Century India, in: The British Journal for the History of Science 25 (1992) 3, p. 299–318; Worboys, Manson, Ross and Colonial Medical Policy.

the increase of our scientific knowledge, and our opportunities, and also with what I may call the awakening of our Imperial conscience. We owe this duty to the vast population for which we have gradually made ourselves responsible.[149]

Chamberlain's address at the festival dinner in aid of the London School of Tropical Medicine is indicative of the way in which tropical medicine came to be seen as integral to imperial progress. There was often a disconnect, however, between the rhetoric of colonial medical policy and what was achieved in practice. Scholars examining the complexity of public health measures in British colonies have demonstrated how fractured they remained. Regardless of the grand hopes and ambitions of imperial medical discourse, the actual workings of medical policy were always contingent on regional specificities and conditions on the ground. In terms of both practice and formulation, they relied on the agency of African or Asian intermediaries and subordinate workers.[150]

German colonialism flourished in the very same period in which scientific medicine emerged as a dominating force in the 1880s. The health of colonised peoples, however, was not a priority of imperial policy until the early twentieth century, when the colonial agenda saw a significant reorientation after protracted, costly and controversial wars. In 1904, German troops started brutal actions to repress colonial protests and retaliate against the Herero, Nama and other communities in German South-West Africa. One year later, they started the so-called Maji Maji War in German East Africa as a response to the rebellion of several population groups there.[151] This ruthless warfare led to a political crisis in Berlin and federal elections in 1907, coined the "Hottentot elections" by contemporaries. The restructuring of colonial bureaucracy and the appointment of Bernhard Dernburg as head of the German colonial administration in 1907 are generally considered turning points in Germany's colonial history.[152]

---

[149] Joseph Chamberlain, Address at the festival dinner in aid of the London School of Tropical Medicine, 10.05.1905, cited in: Chakrabarti, Medicine and Empire, p. 153.

[150] Amna Khalid/Ryan Johnson, Introduction, in: ibid. (eds.), Public Health in the British Empire. Intermediaries, Subordinates and the Practice of Public Health, 1850–1960, London 2011, p. 1–31.

[151] Susanne Kuss, German Colonial Wars and the Context of Military Violence, Cambridge/London 2017, p. 37–75.

[152] Hermann J. Hiery, Die Kolonialverwaltung, in: Horst Gründer/Hermann Hiery (eds.), Die Deutschen und ihre Kolonien. Ein Überblick, Berlin 2017, p. 179–200.

Dernburg, a left-liberal banker, became the State Secretary for Colonial Affairs in the newly created German Imperial Colonial Office. He emphasised the necessity of reforming economic, legal and social policies, including questions of health and medicine, with regard to the colonies: "While one used to colonise by means of destruction, one can now colonise by means of preservation, which encompasses the missionary as well as the doctor, the railway as well as the machine, the advanced theoretical and applied sciences in all fields."[153] Research in tropical medicine was to serve this reorientation in colonial policy and German authorities began to recognise the economic, political and cultural value of a hygiene mission among the population in the colonies. Dernburg deplored that there had not been "an organised study of tropical diseases affecting the natives" since most physicians in the colonies served the military. He argued that this deficiency had to be eradicated urgently by studying the "sanitary conditions of Negroes."[154]

One of the most prominent figures in this new era of German colonial medicine was the physician Ludwig Külz, who was a member of the medical services in Togo and Cameroon between 1902 and 1912. He noted that "the Negro" had been "the object of fervent discussions, anthropologists study his body, missionaries address his soul" but that "his capital value" had not "gained enough importance for our practical action yet."[155] In a piece for the *Archiv für Schiffs- und Tropenhygiene* in 1911, Külz summarised Germany's new colonial goals in a nutshell: "The colonial economy should make use of the Negroes' arms; hygiene should keep them strong and increase their numbers."[156] The welfare of the African population ascended in the list of official priorities mainly because it was seen to be a prerequisite for economic development and growth.[157]

---

[153] Bernhard Dernburg, Zielpunkte des Deutschen Kolonialwesens. Zwei Vorträge, Berlin 1907, p. 9.

[154] Handwritten excerpt of Dernburg's speech to the budget commission of the Reichstag, 18.02.1908, cited in: Eckart, Medizin und Kolonialimperialismus, p. 58.

[155] Ludwig Külz, Grundzüge der kolonialen Eingeborenenhygiene, in: Beihefte zum Archiv für Schiffs- und Tropenhygiene 15 (1911), p. 386–475, here p. 402.

[156] Ibid.

[157] Walter Bruchhausen/Volker Roelcke, Categorising 'African Medicine': The German Discourse on East African Healing Practices, 1885–1918, in: Waltraud Ernst (ed.), Plural

While demographic discourses in European societies were characterised by growing Malthusian fears of overpopulation, a mercantilist concept of population continued to exist in the colonies, where a large population was seen as the basis for, and expression of, economic strength and imperial power.[158] Külz argued that "sanitary pedagogics" and the implementation of "colonial racial hygiene" were to support what he coined the *koloniale Menschenökonomie*—"colonial human economy."[159] According to him, "natives should not only be seen as the main producers of export assets and consumers of imported goods" but particularly as the most important "source of labour supply for all European companies" since Europeans were seemingly unable to permanently acclimatise in the tropics.[160] This concern for human resources was one of the driving forces of German colonial medicine, alongside missionary enthusiasm and scientific and medical ambitions.

The growing interest in "indigenous hygiene" was closely linked to the *Kaiserreich's* ever growing demand for able-bodied, disciplined workers. Sebastian Conrad has shown that, from the mid-1880s, the so-called workers' question became an urgent problem of colonial policy in the German colonies. The project of educating subjects for work, however, focused just as much on the inhabitants of the colonies as on the so-called work-shy—a collective term used for all unemployed and homeless persons—in Wilhelmine Germany.[161] Crucially, it was institutions of the *Innere Mission* and mission societies operating in the German colonies that took up the task of creating workers' colonies both at home and

Medicine, Tradition and Modernity, 1800–2000, London/New York 2002, p. 76–94, here p. 79.

[158] Heinrich Hartmann, Tropical Soldiers? New Definitions of Military Strength in the Colonial Context (1884–1914), in: Martin Lengwiler/Nigel Penn/Patrick Harries (eds.), Science, Africa and Europe. Processing Information and Creating Knowledge, London/New York 2019, p. 125–149.

[159] Ludwig Külz, Beiträge zum Bevölkerungsproblem unserer tropischen Kolonien, in: Archiv für Rassen- und Gesellschafts-Biologie 7 (1910), p. 533–563; Ibid., Die Volkshygiene für Eingeborene in ihren Beziehungen zur Kolonialwirtschaft und Kolonialverwaltung, in: Deutsches Kolonialblatt (1910), p. 12–21.

[160] Külz, Grundzüge der kolonialen Eingeborenenhygiene, p. 394.

[161] Sebastian Conrad, "Education for Work" in Colony and Metropole. The Case of Imperial Germany, c. 1880–1914, in: Harald Fischer-Tiné/Susanne Gehrmann (eds.), Empires and Boundaries. Rethinking Race, Class and Gender in Colonial Settings, New York/London 2009, p. 23–40.

abroad. The project of education for work only promised sustained success in conjunction with a Christian work ethic.[162]

The scientific, political and religious concerns for "indigenous hygiene" were shared across imperial boundaries. In the British case, a 1912 publication by the physician Francis Fremantle emphasised the need to secure "the utmost physical efficiency and therefore welfare for the 400,000,000 inhabitants of the British Empire" since "the health of the people is the supreme law."[163] The British Governmental Commission for Education in the Colonies even demanded that hygiene should take precedence over all other teaching subjects in the curriculum. It became a compulsory subject in primary and secondary schools in Britain's African colonies at the turn of the century. Special attention was given to girls and young women in order to tackle the high mortality rate in children. The Basel Mission schools on the Gold Coast introduced teaching materials on hygiene published by the British government in 1906.[164]

Hygiene no longer existed solely to preserve Europeans' health but increasingly came to be seen as part of the civilising mission. Hans Ziemann, head of the civilian and military medical service in Cameroon from 1908, emphasised that economic, social and cultural progress of the German colonial territories was only conceivable in connection with the "hygienic conquest of Africa."[165] According to him, doctors working in the colonies had a crucial role to play in the advancement of the colonial project. Likewise, Külz saw it as their duty not only "to preserve the full capacity of the indigenous people," who represented "the colonial main value," "the most valuable possession" and "the actual organic capital stock" of colonial power, "but also to lift them as far as possible."[166] This statement reflected the colonial dual mandate, the coupling of economic

---

[162] Paul Jenkins, Land und Arbeit als vergessene Werte in der Mentalität von Baseler MissionarInnen um 1900. Ein Essay mit Bildquellen, in: Inge Mager (ed.), Christentum und Kirche vor der Moderne. Industrialisierung, Historismus und die Deutsche Evangelische Kirche. Zweites Symposium der deutschen Territorialgeschichtsvereine, 9. bis 11. Juni 1995, Hannover 1995, p. 137–147.

[163] Francis Fremantle, Health and Empire, London 1912, p. 348–349, 368.

[164] Lectures on Health Subjects. A Series of Lectures Issued by the Gold Coast Government for Use in Government Schools for Educational Purpose, London 1906, BMA, D.II.c.88.

[165] Hans Ziemann, Wie erobert man Afrika für die weisse und farbige Rasse? in: Beihefte zum Archiv für Schiffs- und Tropenhygiene 11 (1907), p. 235–259.

[166] Külz, Volkshygiene, p. 12.

interest with moralistic altruism, characteristic of this period in colonial history.[167]

Since metropolitan policy-makers strived for economic gains and cultural improvement with minimal metropolitan investment, medical missions came to play a key role in the hygiene mission in tropical colonies. The State Secretary for Colonial Affairs Dernburg recognised that mission societies and their medical facilities offered a valuable foundation for the realisation of his vision of colonialism by means of preservation. In 1907, he wrote a confidential letter to the Councillor of the Higher Administrative Court in Berlin, Max Berner, who served as a middleman for the German mission societies, in which he expounded that the new appreciation for tropical medicine was "a very rewarding field opening up for the missions," arguing that when the "Negro is delivered from his physical ailments and gains trust, then his mind opens up for influences of a higher nature."[168]

The first director of the Institute for Medical Mission in Tubingen, Max Fiebig, a former medical officer in the Royal Netherlands East Indies Army for over twenty years, emphasised that the cooperation of his institution with the *Institut für Schiffs- und Tropenkrankheiten* served "general patriotic interests" through "Christianisation, cultivation and hygienic uplift of the colonial peoples."[169] Fiebig's declaration highlights that the institutionalisation of tropical medicine and hygiene stemmed from scientific as well as political changes taking place in the late nineteenth century. While the growing supremacy of bacteriology and parasitology triggered a profound shift in medical research practices—most notably, the rise of the laboratory—the colonial expansion of European powers in Africa proved no less constitutive for the new discipline.

By the time colonial governments began to intensify their medical efforts towards their colonial subjects, many mission societies had already established themselves as a vital element of health care in the colonies,

---

[167] Bruchhausen, Medizin zwischen den Welten, p. 434–451.

[168] Bernhard Dernburg, Letter to Max Berner, 24.11.1907, cited in: Eckart, Medizin und Kolonialimperialismus, p. 58.

[169] Max Fiebig, Warum das Deutsche Institut für ärztliche Mission in Tübingen und nicht in Hamburg errichtet wird, p. 7, BMA, QH-3.1.

serving those excluded by the colonial state.[170] While the British and German governments in West Africa set up separate healthcare services for Europeans and Africans respectively, the Basel Mission insisted on offering healing to both.[171] It is likely, therefore, as argued by Megan Vaughan, that Africans saw missionaries differently from either the colonising forces or government medical officers, due to the wider and more integrated role that missionaries played in their societies.[172] The Basel Mission doctors used their unique position as both missionaries and medical men in tropical colonies to contribute to religious, scientific and colonial bodies of knowledge. Their role as intermediaries of hygiene between West Africa and Europe, however, highlights that the meanings and practices of purity, health and cleanliness grew out of continual and contentious negotiation processes both abroad and at home.

References

Sonia Abun-Nasr, Von der "Umbildung heidnischer Landessprachen zu christlichen". Die Anfänge von Schrift und Schriftlichkeit in Akuapem, Goldküste, in: Reinhard Wendt (ed.), Wege durch Babylon. Missionare, Sprachstudien und interkulturelle Kommunikation, Tübingen 1998, p. 181–220.

Emmanuel Kwaku Akyeampong et al. (eds.), Africa's Development in Historical Perspective, Cambridge 2014.

Thorsten Altena, "Ein Häuflein Christen mitten in der Heidenwelt des dunklen Erdteils." Zum Selbst- und Fremdverständnis protestantischer Missionare im kolonialen Afrika 1884–1918, Münster 2003.

Anonymous, Westindische Missionsgeschwister, in: Der Evangelische Heidenbote 27 (1854), p. 80–81.

Anonymous, Missionskoffer, in: Der Evangelische Heidenbote 77 (1904), p. 6.

---

[170] Yolana Pringle, Crossing the Divide: Medical Missionaries and Government Service in Uganda, 1897–1940, in: Anna Greenwood (ed.), Beyond the State. The Colonial Medical Service in British Africa, Manchester 2016, p. 19–38; Markku Hokkanen, The Government Medical Service and British Missions in Colonial Malawi, c. 1891–1940: Crucial Collaboration, Hidden Conflicts, in: Anna Greenwood (ed.), Beyond the State. The Colonial Medical Service in British Africa, Manchester 2016, p. 39–63.

[171] On the division of state-run medical services along racial lines in West African colonies, see Neill, Networks in Tropical Medicine, p. 98–102.

[172] Megan Vaughan, Healing and Curing: Issues in the Social History and Anthropology of Medicine in Africa, in: Social History of Medicine 7 (1994) 2, p. 283–295, here p. 294–295.

Anonymous, Basler Missionsausstellung in der Kunsthalle, in: Basler Nachrichten, 21.10.1908

Anonymous, Zur ethnographischen Ausstellung der Basler Mission in Zürich. Korrespondenz, in: Basler Nachrichten, 11.03.1909.

Arjun Appadurai, The Production of Locality, in: ibid. (ed.), Modernity at Large: Cultural Dimensions of Globalization, Minneapolis 1996.

David Arnold, Introduction. Disease, Medicine and Empire, in: ibid. (ed.), Imperial Medicine and Indigenous Societies, Manchester 1988, p. 1–26.

Ralph A. Austen/Jonathan Derrick, Middlemen of the Cameroons Rivers. The Duala and their Hinterland c. 1600– c. 1960, Cambridge 1999.

Tony Ballantyne, Paper, Pen, and Print: The Transformation of the Kai Tahu Knowledge Order, in: Comparative Studies in Society and History 53 (2011) 2, p. 232–260.

Tony Ballantyne, Entanglements of Empire. Missionaries, Māori, and the Question of the Body, Durham/London 2014.

Alison Bashford, Medicine, Gender and Empire, in: Philippa Levine (ed.), Gender and Empire, Oxford 2004, p. 112–133.

Basler Missionskomitee (ed.), An die Freunde des Ärztlichen Zweiges der Basler Mission, Basel 1892.

Marianne Bechhaus-Gerst, Decolonize Germany? (Post)Koloniale Spurensuche in der Heimat zwischen Lokalgeschichte, Politik, Wissenschaft und "Öffentlichkeit", in: WerkstattGeschichte 75 (2017), p. 49–55.

Judith Becker/Katharina Stornig (eds.), Menschen—Bilder—Eine Welt. Ordnungen von Vielfalt in der religiösen Publizistik um 1900, Göttingen 2018.

Anthony A. Beeko, The Trail Blazers. Fruits of 175 Years of the Presbyterian Church of Ghana (1828–2003), Accra 2004.

Jeremy Best, Godly, International, and Independent: German Protestant Missionary Loyalties Before World War I, in: Central European History 47 (2014), p. 585–611.

Jeremy Best, Heavenly Fatherland. German Missionary Culture and Globalization in the Age of Empire, Toronto 2020.

Nemata Amelia Blyden, West Indians in West Africa, 1808–1880. The African Diaspora in Reverse, Rochester 2000.

Cyrelene Amoah Boampong, Rethinking British Colonial Policy in the Gold Coast: The Language Factor, in: Transactions of the Historical Society of Ghana 15 (2013), p. 137–157.

Walter Bruchhausen, Medizin zwischen den Welten. Geschichte und Gegenwart des medizinischen Pluralismus im südöstlichen Tansania, Göttingen 2006.

Walter Bruchhausen/Volker Roelcke, Categorising 'African Medicine': The German Discourse on East African Healing Practices, 1885–1918, in:

Waltraud Ernst (ed.), Plural Medicine, Tradition and Modernity, 1800–2000, London/New York 2002, p. 76–94.

Pratik Chakrabarti, Medicine and Empire, 1600–1960, Basingstoke 2014.

Johann Gottlieb Christaller, Grammar of the Asante and Fante Language called Tshi, Based on the Akuapem Dialect, Basel 1875.

Johann Gottlieb Christaller, Twi Mmebusem Mpensa-Ahansia Mmoaano. A Collection of Three Thousand and Six Hundred Tshi Proverbs, Basel 1879.

Johann Gottlieb Christaller, A Dictionary of the Asante and Fante Language Called Tshi, Basel 1881.

David Ciarlo, Advertising Empire. Race and Visual Culture in Imperial Germany, London 2011.

Christopher Clark/Wolfram Kaiser (eds.), Culture Wars. Secular-Catholic Conflict in Nineteenth-Century Europe, Cambridge 2003.

Christopher Clark/Michael Ledger-Lomas, The Protestant International, in: Abigail Green/Vincent Viaene (eds.), Religious Internationals in the Modern World. Globalization and Faith Communities since 1750, Basingstoke 2012, p. 23–52.

Sebastian Conrad, "Education for Work" in Colony and Metropole. The Case of Imperial Germany, c. 1880–1914, in: Harald Fischer-Tiné/Susanne Gehrmann (eds.), Empires and Boundaries. Rethinking Race, Class and Gender in Colonial Settings, New York/London 2009, p. 23–40.

Annie E. Coombes, Reinventing Africa. Museums, Material Culture and Popular Imagination in Late Victorian and Edwardian England, New Haven and London 1994.

Anna Crozier, Practising Colonial Medicine: The Colonial Medical Service in British East Africa, London/New York 2007.

Jonas N. Dah, Missionary Motivations and Methods. A Critical Examination of the Basel Mission in Cameroon 1886–1914, Basel 1983.

Thomas David/Bouda Etemad/Janick Marina Schaufelbuehl, Schwarze Geschäfte. Die Beteiligung von Schweizern an Sklaverei und Sklavenhandel im 19. und 20. Jahrhundert, Zürich 2005.

Hans Werner Debrunner, A History of Christianity in Ghana, Accra 1967.

Hans Werner Debrunner, Presence and Prestige: Africans in Europe. A History of Africans in Europe before 1918, Basel 1979.

Hans Werner Debrunner, Schweizer im kolonialen Afrika, Basel 1991.

Hans Werner Debrunner, Basel und der Sklavenhandel: Fragmente eines wenig bekannten Kapitels der Basler Geschichte, in: Basler Stadtbuch 113 (1993), p. 95–101.

Christof Dejung, Die Fäden des globalen Marktes. Eine Sozial- und Kulturgeschichte des Welthandels am Beispiel der Handelsfirma Gebrüder Volkart 1851–1999, Köln/Weimar/Wien 2013.

Bernhard Dernburg, Zielpunkte des Deutschen Kolonialwesens. Zwei Vorträge, Berlin 1907.

Albert Venn Dicey, England's Case Against Home Rule, vol. 7, London 1886.

Raymond E. Dumett, Traditional Slavery in the Akan Region in the Nineteenth Century: Sources, Issues, and Interpretations, in: David Henige/T.C. McCaskie (eds.), West African Economic and Social History. Studies in Memory of Marion Johnson, Madison 1990, p. 7–22.

Ryan Dunch, Beyond Cultural Imperialism: Cultural Theory, Christian Missions, and Global Modernity, in: History and Theory 41 (2002), p. 301–325.

Wolfgang U. Eckart, Medizin und Kolonialimperialismus. Deutschland 1884–1945, Paderborn 1997.

Andreas Eckert, Grundbesitz, Landkonflikte und kolonialer Wandel. Douala 1880 bis 1960, Stuttgart 1999.

Andreas Eckert, Slavery in Colonial Cameroon, 1880s to 1930s, in: Martin Klein/Suzanne Miers (eds.), Slavery and Colonial Rule in Africa, London 1999, p. 133–148.

Andreas Eckert, Transatlantischer Sklavenhandel und Sklaverei in Westafrika, in: ibid./Ingeborg Grau/Arno Sonderegger (eds.), Afrika 1500–1900. Geschichte und Gesellschaft, Wien 2010, p. 72–88.

Alfred Eckhardt, Ein Arbeitsjahr in Odumase (Goldküste), in: An die Freunde des Ärztlichen Zweiges der Basler Mission, Basel 1893, p. 5–11.

Erika Eichholzer, Missionary Linguistics on the Gold Coast: Wrestling with Language, in: Patrick Harries/David Maxwell (eds.), The Spiritual in the Secular. Missionaries and Knowledge about Africa, Grand Rapids/Cambridge 2012, p. 72–99.

Evangelische Missionsgesellschaft zu Basel (ed.), Jahresberichte, Basel 1885–1914.

Evangelische Missionsgesellschaft zu Basel (ed.), Neunundneunzigster Jahresbericht, Basel 1914.

Johannes Fabian, Time and the Work of Anthropology. Critical Essays 1971–1991, Chur et al. 1991.

Matthäus Feigk, Von Edinburgh nach Oegstgeest. Die transnationalen missionarischen Netzwerke Europas am Beispiel der Basler Mission 1910–1920, in: Linda Ratschiller/Karolin Wetjen (eds.), Verflochtene Mission. Perspektiven auf eine neue Missionsgeschichte, Köln/Weimar/Wien 2018, p. 45–64.

Hermann Feldmann, Das ärztliche Missionswerk der deutschen Missionsgesellschaften, in: Die ärztliche Mission 1 (1906), p. 1–3, 17–20.

Rudolf Fisch, Die ärztliche Mission unter den Negern. Ansprache am Jahresfest der Basler Mission am 3. Juli 1895, in: Evangelisches Missionsmagazin 39 (1895), p. 371–377.

Rudolf Fisch, Grammatik der Dagomba-Sprache, gesprochen in Nord-Togo und den nördlichen Bezirken der Goldküste (Dagbane), Berlin 1912.

Rudolf Fisch, Dagbane-Sprachproben. Mitteilungen veröffentlicht vom Seminar für Kolonialsprachen in Hamburg, Hamburg 1913.

Rudolf Fisch, Vierzig Jahre ärztliche Mission auf der Goldküste, in: Deutsches Institut für ärztliche Mission Tübingen (ed.), Die deutsche evangelische ärztliche Mission nach dem Stand des Jahres 1928, Stuttgart 1928, p. 16–27.

Friedrich Hermann Fischer, Der Missionsarzt Rudolf Fisch und die Anfänge medizinischer Arbeit der Basler Mission an der Goldküste (Ghana), Herzogenrath 1991.

Johannes Flogaus, Der Missionar als Arzt in Kamerun, in: Verein für ärztliche Mission (ed.), Bericht über das 16. Geschäftsjahr 1913–1914, p. 32–36.

Andrea Franc, Wie die Schweiz zur Schokolade kam. Der Kakaohandel der Basler Handelsgesellschaft mit der Kolonie Goldküste (1893–1960), Basel 2008.

Francis Fremantle, Health and Empire, London 1912.

Katja Füllberg-Stolberg, "Ein Sauerteig christlichen Lebens in der Masse afrikanischen Heidentums". Westindische Konvertiten an der Goldküste (1843–1850), in: Rebekka Habermas/Richard Hölzl (eds.), Mission global. Eine Verflechtungsgeschichte seit dem 19. Jahrhundert, Köln/Weimar/Wien 2014, p. 31–58.

Katharine Gerbner, Christian Slavery. Conversion and Race in the Protestant Atlantic World, Philadelphia 2018.

Martin Göhring, Kameruner Schulbilder, in: Der Evangelische Heidenbote 74 (1901), p. 78–79.

Sebastian Gottschalk, Kolonialismus und Islam. Deutsche und britische Herrschaft in Westafrika (1900–1914), Frankfurt a. M. 2017.

C. K. Graham, The History of Education in Ghana. From the Earliest of Times to the Declaration of Independence, Kumasi 2013.

Horst Gründer, Christliche Mission und deutscher Imperialismus. Eine politische Geschichte ihrer Beziehung während der deutschen Kolonialzeit (1884–1914) unter besonderer Berücksichtigung Afrikas und Chinas, Paderborn 1982.

Horst Gründer/Paul Jenkins/Mary Njikam, Mission und Kolonialismus. Die Basler Mission und die Landfrage in Deutsch-Kamerun, Basel 1986.

Christoffer H. Grundmann, Mission and Healing in Historical Perspective, in: International Bulletin of Missionary Research 32 (2008) 4, p. 185–187.

Christiane Gutekunst, Bericht von der Station Bonaku, in: Verein für ärztliche Mission (ed.), Bericht über das 14. Geschäftsjahr 1911–1912, p. 8–11.

Rebekka Habermas, Intermediaries, Kaufleute, Missionare, Forscher und Diakonissen, in: ibid./Alexandra Przyrembel (eds.), Von Käfern, Märkten und Menschen. Kolonialismus und Wissen in der Moderne, Göttingen 2013, p. 27–48.

Rebekka Habermas, Colonies in the Countryside: Doing Mission in Imperial Germany, in: Journal of Social History 50 (2017), p. 502–517.

Peter Haenger, Slaves and Slave Holders on the Gold Coast: Towards an Understanding of Social Bondage in West Africa, Basel 2000.

Peter Haenger, Pioniere wider Willen: Die missionsinterne Sklavenbefreiung an der Golkdüste, in: Christine Christ-von Wedel/Thomas K. Kuhn (eds.), Basler Mission. Menschen, Geschichte, Perspektiven 1815–2015, Basel 2015, p. 101–106.

Peter Haenger/Robert Labhardt, Basel und der Sklavenhandel: Das Beispiel der Burkhardtschen Handelshäuser zwischen 1780 und 1815, in: Sandra Bott/ Thomas David/Claude Lutzelschwab/Janick Marina Schaufelbuehl (eds.), Suisse—Afrique (18e-20e siècles): De la traite des Noirs à la fin du régime de l'apartheid/Schweiz—Afrika (18.–20. Jahrhundert): Vom Sklavenhandel zum Ende des Apartheid-Regimes, Münster 2005, p. 25–42.

Erik Halldén, The Culture Policy of the Basel Mission in the Cameroons 1886–1905, Lund 1968.

Lea Haller, Transithandel. Geld- und Warenströme im globalen Kapitalismus, Berlin 2019.

David Hardiman, The Mission Hospital 1880–1960, in: Mark Harrison/ Margaret Jones/Helen Sweet (eds.), From Western Medicine to Global Medicine. The Hospital Beyond the West, Hyderabad 2009, p. 198–220.

Patrick Harries, Butterflies and Barbarians. Swiss Missionaries and Systems of Knowledge in South-East Africa, Oxford 2007.

Mark Harrison, Tropical Medicine in Nineteenth-Century India, in: The British Journal for the History of Science 25 (1992) 3, p. 299–318.

Heinrich Hartmann, Tropical Soldiers? New Definitions of Military Strength in the Colonial Context (1884–1914), in: Martin Lengwiler/Nigel Penn/ Patrick Harries (eds.), Science, Africa and Europe. Processing Information and Creating Knowledge, London/New York 2019, p. 125–149.

Gottlob Haussleiter, Die Bedeutung der ärztlichen Mission in den deutschen Kolonien, in: Die ärztliche Mission 6 (1911), p. 5–16.

Hermann J. Hiery, Die Kolonialverwaltung, in: Horst Gründer/Hermann Hiery (eds.), Die Deutschen und ihre Kolonien. Ein Überblick, Berlin 2017, p. 179–200.

Florian Hoffmann, Okkupation und Militärverwaltung in Kamerun. Etablierung und Inszenierung des kolonialen Gewaltmonopols 1891–1914, Göttingen 2007.

Gabriela Hofstetter, "Gehet hin und pfleget." Basler Missionarinnen im Dienst der Ärztlichen Mission in Asien und Afrika (1892–1945), Zürich 2002.

Markku Hokkanen, The Government Medical Service and British Missions in Colonial Malawi, c. 1891–1940: Crucial Collaboration, Hidden Conflicts, in: Anna Greenwood (ed.), Beyond the State. The Colonial Medical Service in British Africa, Manchester 2016, p. 39–63.

Anthony C. Hopkins, An Economic History of West Africa, New York 1973.

Jens Jäger, Bilder aus Afrika vor 1918. Zur visuellen Konstruktion Afrikas im europäischen Kolonialismus, in: Paul Gerhard (ed.), Visual History. Ein Studienbuch, Göttingen 2006, p. 134–148.

Jens Jäger, Plätze an der Sonne? Visualisierungen kolonialer Realitäten, in: Claudia Kraft/Alf Lüdtke/Jürgen Martschukat (eds.) Kolonialgeschichten. Regionale Perspektiven auf ein globales Phänomen, Frankfurt a. M./New York 2010, p. 162–184.

Paul Jenkins, Land und Arbeit als vergessene Werte in der Mentalität von Baseler MissionarInnen um 1900. Ein Essay mit Bildquellen, in: Inge Mager (ed.), Christentum und Kirche vor der Moderne. Industrialisierung, Historismus und die Deutsche Evangelische Kirche. Zweites Symposium der deutschen Territorialgeschichtsvereine, 9. bis 11. Juni 1995, Hannover 1995, p. 137–147.

Paul Jenkins, The Earliest Generation of Missionary Photographers in West Africa and the Portrayal of Indigenous People and Culture in: History of Africa 20 (1993), p. 89–118.

Paul Jenkins/Guy Thomas, Die weite Welt rund um Basel: Mission, Medien und die regionale Vermittlung eines Afrikabildes im 19. und 20. Jahrhundert, in: Regio Basiliensis 45 (2004) 2, p. 99–107.

Michael Jennings, "Healing of Bodies, Salvation of Souls". Missionary Medicine in Colonial Tanganyika, 1870s–1939, in: Journal of Religion in Africa 38 (2008), p. 27–56.

Felicity Jensz/Hanna Acke (eds.), Missions and Media. The Politics of Missionary Periodicals in the Long Nineteenth Century, Stuttgart 2013.

Ryan Johnson, "An All-White Institution": Defending Private Practice and the Formation of the West African Medical Staff, in: Medical History 54 (2010), p. 237–254.

Ryan Johnson, The West African Medical Staff and the Administration of Imperial Tropical Medicine, 1902–1914, in: The Journal of Imperial and Commonwealth History 38 (2010) 3, p. 419–439.

Jakob Keller, Im Hinterland von Kamerun, in: Evangelisches Missionsmagazin 49 (1905), p. 27–36.

Amna Khalid/Ryan Johnson, Introduction, in: ibid. (eds.), Public Health in the British Empire. Intermediaries, Subordinates and the Practice of Public Health, 1850–1960, London 2011, p. 1–31.

David Killingray, The Black Atlantic Missionary Movement and Africa 1780s–1920, in: Journal of Religion in Africa 33 (2003) 1, p. 3–31.

Thoralf Klein, Mission und Kolonialismus—Mission als Kolonialismus. Anmerkungen zu einer Wahlverwandtschaft, in: Claudia Kraft/Alf Lüdtke/Jürgen Martschukat (eds.), Kolonialgeschichten. Regionale Perspektiven auf ein globales Phänomen, Frankfurt a. M./New York 2010, p. 142–161.

Christian Koller, Die Fremdenlegion. Kolonialismus, Söldnertum, Gewalt 1831–1962, Paderborn 2013.

Catherine Koonar, Using Child Labor to Save Souls: The Basel Mission in Colonial Ghana, 1855–1900, in: Atlantic Studies 11 (2014) 4, p. 536–554.

Johannes Kopp, Der Missionar als Arzt an der Goldküste, in: An die Freunde des Ärztlichen Zweiges der Basler Mission, Basel 1892, p. 25–32.

Philipp Krauer, Welcome to Hotel Helvetia! Friedrich Wüthrich's Illicit Mercenary Trade Network for the Dutch East Indies, 1858–1890, in: BMGN—Low Countries Historical Review 134 (2019) 3, p. 122–147.

Ludwig Külz, Beiträge zum Bevölkerungsproblem unserer tropischen Kolonien, in: Archiv für Rassen- und Gesellschafts-Biologie 7 (1910), p. 533–563.

Ludwig Külz, Die Volkshygiene für Eingeborene in ihren Beziehungen zur Kolonialwirtschaft und Kolonialverwaltung, in: Deutsches Kolonialblatt (1910), p. 12–21.

Ludwig Külz, Grundzüge der kolonialen Eingeborenenhygiene, in: Beihefte zum Archiv für Schiffs- und Tropenhygiene 15 (1911), p. 386–475.

Susanne Kuss, German Colonial Wars and the Context of Military Violence, Cambridge/London 2017.

Abraham Nana Opare Kwakye, Encountering 'Prosperity' in Nineteenth Century Gold Coast: Indigenous Perceptions of Western Missionary Societies, in: Andreas Heuser (ed.), Pastures of Plenty: Tracing Religio-Scapes of Prosperity Gospel in Africa and Beyond, Frankfurt a. M. 2015, p. 217–228.

Abraham Nana Opare Kwakye, Mission Impossible Becomes Possible: West Indian Missionaries as Actors in Mission in the Gold Coast, in: Interkulturelle Theologie 42 (2016) 2, p. 222–235.

Otto Lädrach, Im Lande des Goldenen Stuhls. Erinnerungen aus Afrika, Basel 1920.

Paul S. Landau, Introduction. An Amazing Distance. Pictures and People in Africa, in: ibid./Deborah D. Kaspin (eds.), Images and Empires. Visuality in Colonial and Postcolonial Africa, Berkeley/Los Angeles/London 2002, p. 1–40.

Paul S. Landau, Language, in: Norman Etherington (ed.), Missions and Empire, Oxford 2005, p. 194–215.

Robin Law (ed.), From Slave Trade to 'Legitimate' Commerce. The Commercial Transition in Nineteenth-Century West Africa, Cambridge 1993.

Benjamin N. Lawrance/Emily Lynn Osborn/Richard L. Roberts (eds.), Intermediaries, Interpreters, and Clerks. African Employees in the Making of Colonial Africa, Madison 2006.

Edward Forcha Lekunze, Chieftaincy and Christianity in Cameroon 1886–1926. A Historical and Comparative Analysis of the Evangelistic Strategy of the Basel Mission, Ann Arbor 1988.

Alexander Lion, Die Volkshygiene für Eingeborene in ihren Beziehungen zur Kolonialwirtschaft und Kolonialverwaltung, in: Koloniale Rundschau 2 (1910), p. 772–774.

Martin Lynn, Commerce and Economic Change in West Africa. The Palm Oil Trade in the Nineteenth Century, Cambridge 1997.

Tomas C. McCaskie, Local Knowledge: An Akuapem Twi History of Asante, in: History in Africa 38 (2011), p. 169–192.

Ralph Andreas Melzer, Samuel Braun (1590–1688), seefahrender Basler Wundarzt, in: Zürcher medizingeschichtliche Abhandlungen 268 (1996), p. 164.

Anna Merkle, Bericht aus Bali, in: Verein für ärztliche Mission (ed.), Bericht über das 13. Geschäftsjahr 1910–1911, p. 7–10.

Jean-Paul Messina/Jaap van Slageren, Histoire du christianisme au Cameroun. Des origines à nos jours, Paris/Yaoundé 2005.

Emma Metzger, Blick in ein afrikanisches Missionsspital, in: Verein für ärztliche Mission (ed.), Bericht über das 15. Geschäftsjahr 1912–1913, p. 29–31.

Stefanie Michels, Imagined Power Contested: Germans and Africans in the Upper Cross River Area of Cameroon, 1887–1916, Berlin/Münster 2004.

Stefanie Michels, Patrioten im Pulverdampf. Die Berichterstattung über die Kriegsereignisse vom Dezember 1884 in Kamerun, in: Jürg Schneider/ Ute Röschenthaler/Bernhard Gardi (eds.), Fotofieber. Bilder aus West- und Zentralafrika. Die Reisen des Carl Passavant 1883–1885, Basel 2005, p. 83–96.

Giorgio Miescher, Hermann Ludwig Rottmann. Zu den Anfängen der Basler Missions-Handels-Gesellschaft in Christiansborg (Ghana), in: Lilo Roost Vischer/Anne Mayor/Dag Henrichsen (eds.), Werkschau Afrikastudien, vol. 2: Brücken und Grenzen, Münster 1999, p. 345–362.

Jon Miller, Missionary Zeal and Institutional Control. Organizational Contradictions in the Basel Mission on the Gold Coast, 1828–1917, London/New York 2003.

Carl Mirbt, Die Eigenart der deutschen Mission. Vortrag auf der Weltmissionskonferenz in Edinburgh, Basel 1910.

Theodor Müller, Jahresbericht der Station Aburi, in: Verein für ärztliche Mission (ed.), Bericht über das 16. Geschäftsjahr 1913–1914, p. 7–13.

Deborah J. Neill, Networks in Tropical Medicine. Internationalism, Colonialism, and the Rise of a Medical Specialty, 1890–1930, Stanford 2012.

Deborah J. Neill, Science and Civilizing Missions. Germans and the Transnational Community of Tropical Medicine, in: Bradley Naranch/Geoff Eley (eds.), German Colonialism in a Global Age, Durham/London 2014, p. 74–92.

Martin Njeuma (ed.), Introduction to the History of Cameroon. Nineteenth and Twentieth Centuries, London 1989.

Kenneth J. Orosz, Religious Conflict and the Evolution of Language Policy in German and French Cameroon, 1885–1939, New York et al. 2008.

Kenneth J. Orosz, An African Kulturkampf. Religious Conflict and Language Policy in German Cameroon, 1885–1914, in: Sociolinguistica 25 (2011) 1, p. 81–93.

Jürgen Osterhammel, "The Great Work of Uplifting Mankind". Zivilisierungsmission und Moderne, in: Boris Barth/Jürgen Osterhammel (eds.), Zivilisierungsmissionen. Imperiale Weltverbesserung seit dem 18. Jahrhundert, Konstanz 2005, p. 363–426.

Karl David Patterson, Health in Colonial Ghana. Disease, Medicine, and Socio-Economic Change, 1900–1955, Waltham 1981.

John D. Y. Peel, Religious Encounter and the Making of the Yoruba, Bloomington 2003.

Andrew Porter, 'Cultural Imperialism' and Protestant Missionary Enterprise, 1780–1914, in: The Journal of Imperial and Commonwealth History 25 (1997) 3, 367–391.

Andrew Porter, Religion versus Empire? British Protestant Missionaries and Overseas Expansion, 1700–1914, Manchester 2004.

Andrew Porter, Missions and Empire, c.1873–1914, in: Sheridan Gilley/Brian Stanley (eds.), World Christianities c. 1815–c. 1914, Cambridge 2006, p. 560–575.

Yolana Pringle, Crossing the Divide: Medical Missionaries and Government Service in Uganda, 1897–1940, in: Anna Greenwood (ed.), Beyond the State. The Colonial Medical Service in British Africa, Manchester 2016, p. 19–38.

Sara Pugach, Africa in Translation. A History of Colonial Linguistics in Germany and Beyond, 1814–1945, Ann Arbor 2012.

Seth Quartey, Missionary Practices on the Gold Coast, 1832–1895. Discourse, Gaze and Gender in the Basel Mission in Pre-Colonial West Africa, New York 2007.

Linda Ratschiller, "Die Zauberei spielt in Kamerun eine böse Rolle!" Die ethnografischen Ausstellungen der Basler Mission (1908–1912), in: Rebekka Habermas/Richard Hölzl (eds.), Mission global. Eine Verflechtungsgeschichte seit dem 19. Jahrhundert, Köln/Weimar/Wien 2014, p. 241–264.

Linda Ratschiller, Kranke Körper. Mission, Medizin und Fotografie zwischen der Goldküste und Basel 1885–1914, in: ibid./Siegfried Weichlein (eds.), Der schwarze Körper als Missionsgebiet. Medizin, Ethnologie, Theologie in Afrika und Europa 1880–1960, Köln/Weimar/Wien 2016, p. 41–72.

Linda Ratschiller, Material Matters: The Basel Mission in West Africa and Commodity Culture around 1900, in: ibid./Karolin Wetjen (eds.), Verflochtene Mission. Perspektiven auf eine neue Missionsgeschichte, Köln/Weimar/Wien 2018, p. 117–139.

Karl Renntisch, Mission und wirtschaftliche Entwicklung, Basel 1975.

Karl Rennstich, Handwerker-Theologen und Industrie-Brüder als Botschafter des Friedens. Entwicklungshilfe der Basler Mission im 19. Jahrhundert, Stuttgart 1985.

Dana L. Robert, Introduction, in: ibid. (ed.), Converting Colonialism: Visions and Realities in Mission History, 1706–1914, Grand Rapids 2008, p. 1–20.

Milla Roos, Die ärztliche Mission in Bali, in: Verein für ärztliche Mission (ed.), Bericht über das 16. Geschäftsjahr 1913–1914, p. 36–37.

Horace O. Russell, The Missionary Outreach of the West Indian Chursmith Jamaican Baptist Missions to West Africa in the Nineteenth Century, New York 2000.

René Salathé, Basler und Baslerinnen auf Reisen. Eine Anthologie, Basel 2013.

Lamin Sanneh, Translating the Message: The Missionary Impact on Culture, Marynoll 1998.

Adolf Sarasin, La mission de Bâle au Caméroun, Bâle 1914.

Ulrike Schaper, Koloniale Verhandlungen. Gerichtsbarkeit, Verwaltung und Herrschaft in Kamerun 1884–1916, Frankfurt a. M. 2012.

Ulrike Schaper, Chieftaincy as a Political Resource in the German Colony of Cameroon, 1884–1916, in: Tanja Bührer/Flavio Eichmann/Stig Förster/Benedikt Stuchtey (eds), Cooperation and Empire. Local Realities of Global Processes, New York/Oxford 2017, p. 194–222.

Bernhard C. Schär, Tropenliebe. Schweizer Naturforscher und niederländischer Imperialismus in Südostasien um 1900, Frankfurt a. M./New York 2015.

Bernhard C. Schär, From Batticaloa via Basel to Berlin. Transimperial Science in Ceylon and Beyond around 1900, in: The Journal of Imperial and Commonwealth History 48 (2020) 2, p. 230–262, DOI: https://doi.org/10.1080/03086534.2019.1638620.

Wilhelm Schlatter, Geschichte der Basler Mission 1815–1915, 3 vol., Basel 1916.

Pascal Schmid, Medicine, Faith and Politics in Agogo: A History of Health Care Delivery in Rural Ghana, ca. 1925 to 1980, Wien/Zürich 2018.

John Schneid, Les Africains de Bâle au 19ème siècle, in: Sandra Bott/Thomas David/Claude Lutzelschwab/Janick Marina Schaufelbuehl (eds.), Suisse—Afrique (18e–20e siècles): De la traite des Noirs à la fin du régime de l'apartheid/Schweiz—Afrika (18.–20. Jahrhundert): Vom Sklavenhandel zum Ende des Apartheid-Regimes, Münster 2005, p. 209–226.

Jürg Schneider, Haarrisse der Macht: Aspekte regionaler Kolonialgeschichte am Mount Cameroon, Licentiate Thesis, University of Basel, 2001.

Jürg Schneider/Barbara Lüthi, Carl Passavant (1854–1887): Eine Welt in Bildern, in: Traverse (2007) 3, p. 113–122.

Peter A. Schweizer, Survivors on the Gold Coast. The Basel Missionaries in Colonial Ghana, Accra 2000.

Jon F. Sensbach, Rebecca's Revival. Creating Black Christianity in the Atlantic World, Cambridge 2005.

John Phillip Short, Magic Lantern Empire. Colonialism and Society in Germany, Ithaca/London 2012.

Rebecca Shumway/Trevor R. Getz (eds.), Slavery and its Legacy in Ghana and the Diaspora, London et al. 2018.

Ulrike Sill, Encounters in Quest of Christian Womanhood: The Basel Mission in Pre- and Early Colonial Ghana, Leiden/Boston 2010.

Helmut Walser Smith, German Nationalism and Religious Conflict: Culture, Ideology, Politics, 1870–1914, Princeton 1995.

Noel Smith, The History of the Presbyterian Church in Ghana, 1835–1960, Accra 1966.

Melanie Stempfel, Islambilder der Basler Mission. Eine Untersuchung anhand der Text- und Bildpublizistik zwischen 1906 und 1938, Master Thesis, University of Fribourg, 2012.

Niklaus Stettler/Peter Haenger/Robert Labhardt, Baumwolle, Sklaven und Kredite. Die Basler Welthandelsfirma Christoph Burckhardt & Cie. in revolutionärer Zeit (1789–1815), Basel 2004.

Karl Stolz, Neue Nachrichten aus Kamerun, in: Der Evangelische Heidenbote 67 (1894), p. 17–18.

Karl Stolz, Auf Vorposten in Kamerun, in: Verein für ärztliche Mission (ed.), Bericht über das 15. Geschäftsjahr 1912–1913, p. 32.

Jonathan Striebel, Krankheitsbilder aus Bali, in: Verein für ärztliche Mission (ed.), Bericht über das 11. Geschäftsjahr 1909, p. 26–29.

Jakob Stutz, Bericht aus Bonaku, in: Verein für ärztliche Mission (ed.), Bericht über das 5. Geschäftsjahr 1903, p. 32–34.

Jakob Stutz, Aus meiner ärztlichen Praxis, in: Verein für ärztliche Mission in Stuttgart (ed.), Mitteilungen aus der ärztlichen Mission 10 (1911), p. 4–7.

Bengt Sundkler/Christopher Steed, A History of the Church in Africa, Cambridge 2000.

Jaap van Slageren, Les origines de l'église évangélique du Cameroun. Missions européennes et christianisme autochtone, Leiden 1972.

Megan Vaughan, Healing and Curing: Issues in the Social History and Anthropology of Medicine in Africa, in: Social History of Medicine 7 (1994) 2, p. 283–295.

Béatrice Veyrassat, Histoire de la Suisse et des Suisses dans la marche du monde. XVIIe siècle—Première Guerre mondiale: Espaces—Circulations—Échanges, Neuchâtel 2018.

Heinrich Vieter, "Die Jugend ist unsere Zukunft". Chronik der katholischen Mission Kamerun 1890–1913, Friedberg 2011.

Cornelia Vogelsanger, Pietismus und afrikanische Kultur an der Goldküste. Die Einstellung der Basler zur Haussklaverei, Zürich 1977.

Hermann Vortisch, Bericht von Aburi, in: Verein für ärztliche Mission (ed.), Bericht über das 6. Geschäftsjahr 1904, p. 17–19.

Hermann Vortisch, Bericht von Aburi, in: Verein für ärztliche Mission (ed.), Bericht über das 7. Geschäftsjahr 1905, p. 25–31.

Gustav Wanner, Die Basler Handels-Gesellschaft A.G. 1859–1959, Basel 1959.

Gustav Warneck, Outline of a History of Protestant Missions from the Reformation to the Present Time. A Contribution to Modern Church History, New York/Chicago/Toronto 1901.

Niklaus Wöll, Der Missionar als Arzt, in: Verein für ärztliche Mission in Stuttgart (ed.), Mitteilungen aus der ärztlichen Mission 10 (1911), p. 7–8.

Christine Wolters, Dr. Friedrich Hey (1864–1960), Missionsarzt und Bückeburger Unternehmer, in: Hubert Höing (ed.), Strukturen und Konjunkturen. Faktoren in der schaumburgischen Wirtschaftsgeschichte, Bielefeld 2004, p. 328–366.

Michael Worboys, Manson, Ross and Colonial Medical Policy: Tropical Medicine in London and Liverpool, 1899–1914, in: Roy MacLeod/Milton Lewis (eds.), Disease, Medicine, and Empire. Perspectives on Western Medicine and the Experience of European Expansion, London/New York 1988, p. 21–37.

Friedrich Würz, Die mohammedanische Gefahr in Westafrika, Basel 1904.

Gilbert Dotsé Yigbe, Von Gewährsleuten zu Gehilfen und Gelehrigen. Der Beitrag afrikanischer Mitarbeiter zur Entstehung einer verschrifteten Kultur in Deutsch-Togo, in: Rebekka Habermas/Richard Hölzl (eds.), Mission global. Eine Verflechtungsgeschichte seit dem 19. Jahrhundert, Köln/Weimar/Wien 2014, p. 159–175.

Andreas Zangger, Koloniale Schweiz. Ein Stück Globalgeschichte zwischen Europa und Südostasien (1860–1930), Bielefeld 2011.

Hans Ziemann, Wie erobert man Afrika für die weisse und farbige Rasse? in: Beihefte zum Archiv für Schiffs- und Tropenhygiene 11 (1907), p. 235–259.

Johannes Zimmermann, A Grammatical Sketch of the Akra- or Ga- Language, with Some Specimens of it from the Mouth of the Natives and a Vocabulary of the Same with an Appendix on the Adanme-Dialect, Stuttgart 1858.

Johannes Zimmermann, A Dictionary, English, Tshi (Asante), Akra, Basel 1874.

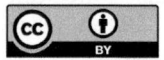

PART II

Negotiations of Hygiene "on the Margins" 1885–1914

CHAPTER 5

Locating Filth: Sin, Syphilis and the Path to Purity

Hygiene became a key issue in the advancement of the civilising mission in the late nineteenth century as ideas of a healthy body and cultural progress fused with each other. New meanings of hygiene were negotiated on the alleged margins of colonial society, where norms were called into question and boundaries constantly transgressed. The rationale behind the civilising mission implied that the Basel medical missionaries were operating on the frontier of civilisation, where people still lived in sin, dirt and disease. Hygiene appeared as the new colonial crusade, bringing together religious, scientific and political stakeholders and their interests, which allowed the Basel Mission doctors to reinforce the significance of their mission. The core objective of their hygiene mission in West Africa, however, was to raise awareness for the individual's inherent sinfulness by promoting a Pietist path to purity.

5.1   On a Hygiene Mission in West Africa

Regarding the prospects of a medical mission, the members of the Committee recorded in 1880 that "combining bodily and spiritual healing" constituted "a valid thought" since "sin and disease (death) are

© The Author(s) 2023   215
L. M. Ratschiller Nasim, *Medical Missionaries and Colonial Knowledge in West Africa and Europe, 1885–1914*,
Cambridge Imperial and Post-Colonial Studies,
https://doi.org/10.1007/978-3-031-27128-1_5

closely linked."[1] Hermann Prätorius, the Basel Mission's Inspector for Africa, who accompanied Mähly on his medical research expedition in 1882–1883, confirmed that "the physical misery, the disease misery" prevalent in Africa was "sadly, in many cases" associated with the "misery of sin" in an article printed in the monthly magazine *Der Evangelische Heidenbote*. He concluded that "in the heathen land it becomes terribly clear that sin is the cause of human decay."[2] Twelve years later, the Basel Mission doctor Alfred Eckhardt maintained that "on the Gold Coast, it is particularly obvious that sin frequently and directly results in disease."[3]

The longstanding Pietist interpretation of disease as a distorted relationship with God still held true for the Basel Mission doctors, who frequently explained physical suffering with reference to a sinful way of life. The first issue of the Basel Mission's medical magazine in 1891 reported: "Our doctors are under the impression of the horrible bodily misery of the heathens every day, which is a true reflection of the reign of sin and estrangement from God among these people."[4] Although they identified pathogens under the microscope, the Basel Mission doctors believed that physical processes were closely intertwined with spiritual causes. In their view, body and mind were united through the soul, at the centre of which stood the heart.[5] To keep one's body and mind clean and healthy, therefore, was not an end in itself but a prerequisite for the evolution of the soul and the purification of the heart.

For the Basel Mission doctors, healing always had an incorporeal connotation and complete cure could only be achieved through spiritual cleansing and adopting a Christian way of life. They were not interested in a purely physical healing process, since medical treatments such as surgery or drugs did not address what they considered to be the

---

[1] Committee report, 28.04.1880, BMA, Komitee-Protokoll 1880, §158.

[2] Prätorius, Mittheilungen aus der afrikanischen Visitationsreise, p. 26.

[3] Alfred Eckhardt, Land, Leute und ärztliche Mission auf der Goldküste, Basel 1894, p. 27. In the Basel Mission's medical magazine he stated similarly: "Often the disease is a fully obvious consequence of sin!" Alfred Eckhardt, Ärztliche Missionsarbeit in Christiansborg, in: An die Freunde des Ärztlichen Zweiges der Basler Mission, Basel 1891, p. 8–19, here p. 16.

[4] Basler Missionskomitee (ed.), An die Freunde des Ärztlichen Zweiges der Basler Mission, Basel 1891, p. 4.

[5] The Basel Mission doctors elaborated on the connection between body, mind and soul in their reports and publications. For the latter, see selectively Hey, Der Tropenarzt, 1st ed., p. 41–66; Vortisch, Die Nervosität als Störung zwischen Seele und Geist, p. 15–21.

true cause of disease: sin. The essential sinfulness of traditional African society was therefore stressed and the connection between sin and disease was a central feature of medical missionary ideology. In a report from 1891, Fisch—upset about the low numbers of conversions in Aburi at the time—highlighted this point:

> All the help for the body alone is merely a drop in the sea of heathen misery. Only when a great, true community of the Lord takes root here, can misery be controlled. If a significant share of the people is not converting, then not even 10,000 mission doctors can save the people from doom.[6]

The Basel Mission doctors interpreted discomfort, pain and disease as means through which God communicated his will to individual people. They considered illness to be a time of reflection, a chance for critical self-examination of one's way of life and faith, and, ultimately, an opportunity to purify one's heart and (re-)connect with God.[7] This aspect was stressed in efforts to gain financial and ideological support from evangelicals back home. In the specialised journal *An die Freunde des Ärtzlichen Zweiges der Basler Mission*, Inspector Theodor Oehler described to potential supporters and benefactors that:

> [...] in the heathen world, the connection between disease and sin comes to light with frightening clarity. In thousands of cases, the physical disease is the sharp rod in God's hands to reawaken a long muted conscience and to make a sinner aware of the impending retaliation.[8]

To promote this connection between disease and sin, the Basel Mission doctors operated as "itinerant preachers with subsequent medical advice."[9] Using their bicycles to reach surrounding villages and more remote areas in West Africa, they travelled from station to station to hold consultation hours and offer their guidance. Rudolf Fisch was the first

---

[6] Rudolf Fisch, Second quarterly report for 1891, 02.09.1891, BMA, D-1.55.13.

[7] Hey, Wegweiser für den Christen über Leiden, Krankheit, Heilung, p. 14–27. On the meaning of pain for Basel Pietism in general, see Hebeisen, Leidenschaftlich fromm, p. 209–215.

[8] Theodor Oehler, An die Freunde des Ärztlichen Zweiges der Basler Mission, Basel 1892, p. 1–5, here p. 1.

[9] Friedrich Hey, Annual report for 1896, 05.02.1897, BMA, D-1.64.167.

to introduce the bicycle to the Gold Coast in 1892, thereby challenging the longstanding practice of Europeans being carried in hammocks by African porters. Fisch's fellow missionaries were at first appalled that he had broken this established taboo. They believed that journeys on foot or on a bike had to be avoided at all costs in order not to overexert and endanger one's health. In their view, Fisch was acting against tested and proven principles of tropical hygiene that he himself had advocated for many years.[10]

The Basel missionaries' initial reluctance in replacing the hammock with the bicycle demonstrates how strongly hygiene norms dominated their daily lives in West Africa. Over the years, however, the bicycle became an inherent part of the Basel Mission on the Gold Coast, as the picture of the missionaries leaving the General Conference in Aburi in 1900 illustrates (Fig. 5.1).[11] The hammock had never been a particularly popular mode of travel among the Basel missionaries, who regularly complained about how difficult it was to find reliable and affordable porters, but it continued to be seen as the most hygienic means of transport in West Africa, especially for women.[12]

The bicycle allowed the Basel Mission doctors to increase the scope of their work far beyond hospital walls. On their extended tours, they not only preached the gospel but also gave lectures on modes of infection, prophylactic measures and methods of treatment.[13] By promoting a preventive programme for both spiritual and physical health, their medical mission comprised more than basic first aid and curative care. In 1902, Fisch started writing circular letters in African languages to promote

---

[10] Rudolf Fisch, Das Klima der Westküste von Afrika. Manuskript zur Anleitung für ausziehende Missionare von Januar 1890, BMA, D-1.53.8; Alfred Eckhardt, Annual report for 1892, 15.01.1893, BMA, D-1.56.132; Correspondenzblatt der Basler Missionare, 17.04.1895.

[11] Rudolf Fisch, The Missionaries leaving the General Conference, 1893/1906, BMA, D-30.09.023.

[12] See, for instance, Alfred Eckhardt, Letter to Committee, 02.10.1887, BMA, D-1.47.10; Rudolf Fisch, Annual report for 1900, 31.01.1901, BMA, D-1.73.12. On the role of porters in colonial history more generally, see Sonja Malzner/Anne D. Peiter (eds.), Der Träger. Zu einer "tragenden" Figur der Kolonialgeschichte, Bielefeld 2018.

[13] Rudolf Fisch's handwritten diary contains entries between 1908 and 1911. Rudolf Fisch, Diary, BMA, D-10-24. Here: Rudolf Fisch, Diary Entry on 25–26.08.1910, BMA, D-10.24.

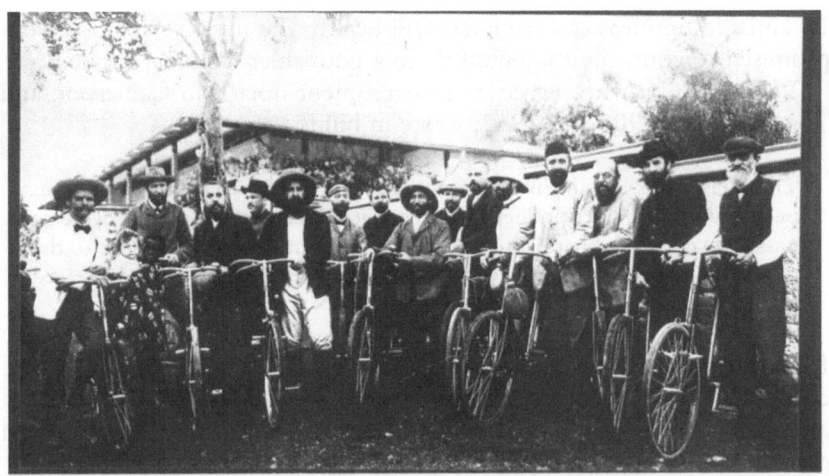

Fig. 5.1 Rudolf Fisch, The Missionaries leaving the General Conference, 1893/1906, BMA, D-30.09.023

what he thought were the "most fundamental rules of hygiene."[14] These guidelines, including recommendations on childbirth and the treatment of wounds, were sent to all the rulers in the areas in which the Basel Mission had established stations.[15] The Basel Mission doctors believed that new values and behaviours of hygiene would make people in West Africa more aware of the close connection between sin and disease.

Over the years, the Basel Mission doctors not only complemented their circulars to regional authorities with information on the most common diseases and ways to treat them but also translated general textbooks on health and hygiene into African languages.[16] Their efforts were increasingly valued by colonial doctors, politicians and a general public interested in the economic and cultural development of the colonies. In Germany, a growing circle of colonial enthusiasts, who were not necessarily supporters of mission societies due to their oftentimes differing agendas, acknowledged that missionaries had a crucial role to play in the civilising mission.

[14] Rudolf Fisch, Annual report for 1902, 06.02.1903, BMA, D-1.77.19.

[15] Fischer, Der Missionsarzt Rudolf Fisch, p. 183–185.

[16] They included Ngus' a Malea (Hygiene and sanitation), BMA, E.I.g.34; Maboa ma bekombo ba wie (About diseases in the tropics), BMA, EI.g.35.

By embedding ideas of cleanliness and health, the mission doctors' work promised to contribute significantly to a flourishing colonial society.[17]

Ludwig Külz, who served as a government doctor in Cameroon and Togo between 1902 and 1912, wrote in hindsight:

> The German colonial physicians noticed everywhere that the indigenous people who had been influenced by missionaries stepped out of hygienic passivity very soon, that baptised mothers brought their sick children to the physician far more than the others, that the value of the child increased and its active care was noticeable.[18]

Külz, who was generally very critical of the missionary movement, conceded in this article, printed in *Anthropos* in 1919–1920, that missionaries had been the driving forces behind the spread of hygienic norms and practices in the colonies. In a time when scientific medicine and the colonial state increasingly appeared as empirical and secular enterprises, the Basel Mission doctors appealed to medical scientists and colonial stakeholders by promising to locate and root out allegedly indecent body practices and irrational beliefs. The medical missionaries used manifold networks and media to depict immorality and disease among the people they wished to convert, thereby emphasising the need for their work to both their supporters at home and a wider audience beyond evangelical circles.

In 1889, Theodor Christlieb published a study on medical missions, in which he expounded: "Medical attendance best illustrates to half-civilised and barbaric people alike that Christian science is superior to heathen ignorance and that Christian love and philanthropy are superior to heathen selfishness and ferocity."[19] By putting scientific medicine and hygienic knowledge to the service of evangelisation, the Basel Mission doctors hoped to demonstrate that their belief and health system was superior both conceptually and morally to West African cosmologies of faith and healing. Medicine and hygiene were believed to assume what

---

[17] Fabian, Time and the Work of Anthropology, ch. 8, p. 155–169.

[18] Ludwig Külz, Die Abhängigkeit der geistigen und kulturellen Rückständigkeit der Naturvölker von ihren endemischen Krankheiten, in: Anthropos 14/15 (1919/1920) 1/3, p. 33–45, here p. 44–45.

[19] Theodor Christlieb, Ärztliche Missionen, Gütersloh 1889, p. 85.

Walter Bruchhausen has called a "pacemaker function" by leveraging colonial expansion and the civilising mission.[20]

Public approval of the hygiene mission in West Africa emboldened the Basel Mission to underline the role of hygiene as an uncontroversial yet potent component in the making of civilised communities. In contrast to the abstract and internal process of conversion, hygiene offered clear evidence of transformation, visible on individual bodies. As Jean and John Comaroff have shown for missionary rhetoric in nineteenth-century South Africa, "the blighted body served as a graphic symptom of moral disorder."[21] Hygiene with its alleged capacity not only to prevent disease but also remove moral disorder came to epitomise civilisational progress. Africa appeared indecent rather than merely unwashed, since ideas of hygiene were rooted in religious conceptions of purity and always entailed social and moral implications.

Beyond and beneath its promotional value, however, the hygiene discourse also reveals that missionaries, and Europeans more generally, were desperately looking for ways to make sense of the perceived chaos around them. The foods, smells and bodily practices that Europeans encountered and commented upon in many sources from the late nineteenth and early twentieth centuries indicate that hygiene appeared as a way to order the unfamiliarity of their African environment. Detailed rules of order and cleanliness purported that they were in control of colonial subjects and places. The preaching of hygiene attenuated their feelings of insecurity by establishing seemingly clear boundaries of purity and thus lent ideological support to Europeans in the colonial world.

5.2 THE INSISTENCE ON SYPHILIS

The diagnosis of syphilis offered clear evidence for the pressing need and concrete benefit of the Basel medical mission in West Africa. As early as 1882, Mähly had assessed that a significant number of Africans suffered from venereal diseases, primarily syphilis. Syphilis continued to present a prevalent diagnosis in health reports from the Gold Coast with the arrival of the Basel medical missionaries from 1885. Fisch's annual reports continually stated that 70 to 80 per cent of his patients suffered from

---

[20] Bruchhausen, Die "hygienische Eroberung" der Tropen, p. 213.

[21] Comaroff/Comaroff, Of Revelation and Revolution, vol. 2, p. 324.

what he called *"Lustseuche"*—desire epidemic—referring to syphilis.[22] His yearly statistical surveys implied that the venereal disease was a permanent feature of the people on the Gold Coast: "This is the unspeakably miserable moral state of these poor people, expressed in numbers."[23]

In the Basel Mission's diverse media, syphilis represented the epitome of heathen immorality and uncontrolled sexuality in West Africa. The epidemic proportions of syphilis called for urgent action. Healing of the body alone, however, did not promise improvement, particularly in the case of sexually transmitted diseases, as long as their apparent cause—the sexually promiscuous behaviour of Africans—had not been eliminated. Africans thus had to be educated about the true cause of the disease: their sinful way of life that triggered the condition.[24] In a speech at the annual Basel Mission Festival on 3 July 1895, Rudolf Fisch deployed the threat of syphilis to remind his audience of the desolate moral and sanitary conditions on the Gold Coast:

> Physicians are used to see all sorts of terrible diseases but it is not without shuddering that we see these walking revelations of God's wrath upon all the sins of mankind, these awfully disfigured faces, these bodies diffusing the smell of death covered with terrible wounds, these people stricken with syphilis, who waste away for years.[25]

Syphilitic Africans embodied the apparent sinfulness of African societies and the imperative need for the medical mission, which paid attention to both the body and the soul. The condition called *fwempow* in the Twi language—meaning "big nose"—caused salient changes in physical appearance and thus proved particularly suited to advertise the

[22] See, for example Fisch's annual report for 1892: "On average, 70,8 per cent of my patients suffer from syphilis. This percentage is about the same every year. It gives a deep insight into the misery and shame that have come upon our poor people." Rudolf Fisch, Annual report for 1892, 14.01.1893, BMA, D-1.57.48.

[23] Rudolf Fisch, Annual report for 1890, 06.02.1891, BMA, D-1.53.39.

[24] Megan Vaughan, Syphilis in Colonial East and Central Africa: The Social Construction of an Epidemic, in: Terence Ranger/Paul Slack (eds.), Epidemics and Ideas. Essays on the Historical Perception of Pestilence, Cambridge 1992, p. 269–302, here p. 273.

[25] The speech was printed in the *Evangelisches Missionsmagazin* that same year. Fisch, Die ärztliche Mission unter den Negern, p. 374.

medical mission.[26] The Basel Mission doctors disseminated photographs of afflicted Africans in their handbooks and articles, showing the typical features of the disease: the *Gundu*—a thickening and broadening of the nose—as well as the distortion of the forearms and lower legs.[27] Since colonial discourse on African people was fundamentally fixated on their bodies, these images aroused interest beyond the medical community.

The campaign to combat syphilis became a key indicator of the progress of the Basel Mission as a whole. The missionaries, who advocated Christian monogamy and heavily condemned polygamy as well as extra-marital and premarital sexual relations, felt vindicated in their struggle by the supposed enormous occurrence of a sexually transmitted disease. They went out of their way to encourage West Africans to embrace their marriage and family model as the basis for sexual, social and economic order. As many studies have demonstrated, the colonial discourse on African people was thoroughly sexualised and the implementation of monogamous patriarchal matrimony was one of the core concerns of the civilising mission.[28] Most cases of deviant behaviour, as recorded in the Basel Mission's parish council protocols, were concerned with the infringement of Christian sexual morals.[29]

In contrast to most missionaries, who saw African sexuality as inherently uncontrolled and excessive, some European observers believed that it was the social and economic changes of colonialism that had spoiled the supposedly primitive and reassuringly innocent sexuality of

[26] Hermann Vortisch, Erfahrungen über einige spezifische Krankheiten an der Gold-küste, in: Archiv für Schiffs- und Tropenhygiene 10 (1906), p. 537–539.

[27] Rudolf Fisch, Über die Behandlung der Amöbendysenterie und einige andere tropen-medizinische Fragen, in: Archiv für Schiffs- und Tropenhygiene 8 (1904), p. 207–212.

[28] See selectively Natasha Erlank, Missionary Views on Sexuality in Xhosaland in the Nineteenth Century, in: Le Fait Missionaire 11 (2001), p. 9–43; Ibid., Strange Bedfellows. The International Missionary Council, the International African Institute, and Research into African Marriage and Family, in: Patrick Harries/David Maxwell (eds.), The Spiritual in the Secular. Missionaries and Knowledge about Africa, Grand Rapids 2012, p. 267–292; Comaroff/Comaroff, Home-made Hegemony; Patricia Grimshaw, Faith, Missionary Life, and the Family, in: Philippa Levine (ed.), Gender and Empire, Oxford 2004, p. 260–280; Manktelow, Missionary Families; Maxwell, The Missionary Home.

[29] On the use of parish council protocols as sources, see Karolin Wetjen, Gemeinde im Laboratorium. Aushandlungsprozesse des Christentums und Kirchenzucht in der Mission am Beginn des 20. Jahrhunderts, in: Linda Ratschiller/Karolin Wetjen (eds.), Verflochtene Mission. Perspektiven auf eine neue Missionsgeschichte, Köln/Weimer/Wien 2018, p. 89–116.

pre-colonial Africans.[30] British officials on the Gold Coast, for instance, argued that the weakening of chiefly male control and the abolition of previously severe punishments for sexual offences had facilitated both the emancipation of women and the syphilis epidemic. Despite their differing perceptions of African sexuality, British administrators advocated for the extension of Christian morality as the only solution for re-establishing social and moral order.[31] African authorities also participated in the discourse on how to combat syphilis, using it as an argument to extend their influence and tighten their control over their communities, particularly their female subjects.[32]

It was certainly no coincidence that most photographs of patients suffering from syphilis in the Basel Mission doctors' publications depicted women. It was female rather than male sexuality that was taken to be the problem.[33] Uncontrolled female sexuality was seen to bring sterility, depopulation and eventually what scientists of the time called "degeneration." Fisch was convinced that the syphilis epidemic would result in the extinction of whole villages, inevitably leading to the doom of African societies: "It is a wonder to me that these poor people still exist, yes even proliferate, at least in certain places. However, there are a number of villages, in my opinion, that will perish of this disease soon."[34] Although mortality rates did not support his apprehension, Fisch maintained that syphilis was both the cause and consequence of degeneration.[35]

In 1910, Theodor Müller, a young mission doctor who had joined Fisch in Aburi a year earlier, openly questioned his colleagues' diagnosis: "Experienced tropical doctors report that over 50 per cent of their

[30] Vaughan, Curing Their Ills, p. 129.

[31] Stephen Addae, The Evolution of Modern Medicine in a Developing Country: Ghana 1880–1960, Durham 1997, p. 355–360; Deborah Pellow, Sex, Disease, and Culture Change in Ghana, in: Philip W. Setel/Milton Lewis/Maryinez Lyons (eds.), Histories of Sexually Transmitted Diseases and HIV/AIDS in Sub-Saharan Africa, Westport/London 1999, p. 17–41.

[32] Vaughan, Syphilis in Colonial East and Central Africa, p. 277–278.

[33] Sander Gilman has shown that the image of the African woman was equated with that of the prostitute, both implying uninhibited sexuality. See Sander Gilman, Difference and Pathology: Stereotypes of Sexuality, Race and Madness, Ithaca 1985, p. 89–101, 109–111.

[34] Rudolf Fisch, Annual report for 1890, 06.02.1891, BMA, D-1.53.39.

[35] Fisch also associated syphilis with a high infant mortality rate on the Gold Coast. See Fisch, Die ärztliche Mission unter den Negern, p. 374.

patients suffer from syphilis. In reality, I only very rarely catch sight of fresh syphilis."[36] He observed that the symptoms of the disease under scrutiny often differed from those of syphilis: the progressive paralysis of the nervous system occurring in syphilitic patients in Europe did not occur on the Gold Coast.[37] He suggested instead that the ailment that his predecessors had identified as syphilis for over 25 years was in effect yaws—a non-venereal, infectious skin disease.[38] Müller's assertion was nothing short of revolutionary as it not only contradicted a well-established diagnosis but also unsettled the theoretical foundation of the medical mission, since the widespread disease could no longer be attributed to sinful behaviour.[39]

So why then had the Basel medical missionaries failed to acknowledge that the disease they lamented for so many years was actually yaws and not syphilis? From a scientific perspective, although the disease agents could be identified microscopically from 1905, it was still not possible to distinguish the pathogens of yaws and syphilis under the microscope.[40] The scientific difficulty in telling apart syphilis from yaws also led famous tropical doctors, such as Heinrich Botho Scheube and Carl Mense, to be under the mistaken belief that African societies suffered from a syphilis epidemic around 1900.[41] Moreover, the tenacity of this medical myth was certainly aided by the fact that the drugs used to treat syphilis also

---

[36] Theodor Müller, Quarterly report for 1910, 15.09.1910, BMA, D-1.95.19.

[37] Theodor Müller, Annual report for 1911, 18.03.1912, BMA, D-1.97.22.

[38] Yaws is a chronic infectious disease occurring in warm and humid areas of Africa, South America and Asia, whose pathogens are closely related to the ones of syphilis. It is transmitted by smear infection, mostly among children living in poor sanitary conditions. Like syphilis, the disease is divided in three stages. Yet unlike syphilis, damage to the central nervous system or the internal organs does not occur in the case of yaws in the tertiary stage. Instead, the skin and skeletal system are affected. Addae, The Evolution of Modern Medicine in a Developing Country, p. 361–368.

[39] Theodor Müller, Annual report for 1911, 18.03.1912, BMA, D-1.97.22.

[40] Vaughan, Syphilis in Colonial East and Central Africa, p. 281.

[41] Heinrich Botho Scheube, Krankheiten der warmen Länder, 1st ed., Jena 1896, p. 228; Carl Mense, Syphilis und venerische Krankheiten in den neu der Kultur erschlossenen Ländern besonders in Afrika, in: Archiv für Schiffs- und Tropenhygiene 4 (1900), p. 86–109.

proved effective in dealing with yaws.[42] Fisch reported in 1891 that his treatment of syphilis was popular among the people on the Gold Coast:

> When a few syphilitics come from one place, I am certain that many more patients will visit me from there in the near future. Why this is the case is of course easy to see. With iodine or mercury preparations, even very serious cases of syphilis can easily be transferred to a latent illness.[43]

In contrast to many other conditions, the Basel Mission doctors appeared fairly successful in treating what they thought was syphilis with medical preparations, wound care and occasionally also surgery. In 1905, the medical missionary Hermann Vortisch described syphilitic patients as "the best promotion for the medical mission."[44] The diagnosis and successful treatment of syphilis offered a valuable promotional tool for the Basel Mission on the Gold Coast over many years, providing visible evidence for the validity of their medical procedures.

On a cultural level, the longstanding assumption that Africans were sexually hyperactive certainly obscured the identification of a non-venereal disease.[45] The diagnosis of syphilis confirmed what the Basel Mission doctors expected to find in West Africa all along. Missionaries, colonial authorities and scientists paid obsessive attention to the sexuality of Africans.[46] Their preoccupation with sexual practices, family constellations and initiation rites mirrored developments in Europe, where the sexuality of the working classes, and of women in particular, was a major concern. Syphilis was already a dreaded disease in Europe for centuries

---

[42] Theodor Müller, Annual report for 1911, 18.03.1912, BMA, D-1.97.22; Albert Neisser, Sind Syphilis und Frambösie verschiedene Krankheiten? in: Archiv für Schiffs-und Tropenhygiene 12 (1908), p. 173–179, here p. 175.

[43] Rudolf Fisch, Annual report for 1890, 06.02.1891, BMA, D-1.53.39.

[44] Hermann Vortisch, Letter to the Committee, 26.04.1905, BMA, D-1.84.11.

[45] This had been a common stereotype in Europe since the eighteenth century. See Desiree Lewis, Representing African Sexualities, in: Sylvia Tamale (ed.), African Sexualities. A Reader, Cape Town et al. 2011, p. 199–216; Gilman, Difference and Pathology.

[46] Ann Laura Stoler, Race and the Education of Desire. Foucault's History of Sexuality and the Colonial Order of Things, Durham/London 1995; Daniel J. Walther, Sex and Control. Venereal Disease, Colonial Physicians, and Indigenous Agency in German Colonialism, 1884–1914, New York/Oxford 2005, Ibid., Sex and Control in Germany's Overseas Possessions: Venereal Disease and Indigenous Agency, in: Nina Berman/Klaus Mühlhahn/Patrice Nganang (eds.), German Colonialism Revisited. African, Asian, and Oceanic Experiences, Ann Arbor 2014, p. 71–84.

before city missionaries started associating the condition with the lower social strata and their promiscuous behaviour in the nineteenth century.[47]

From a Pietist point of view, uncontrolled sexual desire entailed punishment through disease. This belief, derived from an Old Testament statement "that by what things a man sins, by these he is punished," got in the way of a swift revision of the diagnosis of syphilis.[48] As late as 1909, Fisch stated in his annual report that the high occurrence of syphilis on the Gold Coast was "God's punishment for sinful acts."[49] This controversial interpretation, however, increasingly lost ground and became untenable in light of new scientific evidence and growing public criticism. The German dermatologist and psychiatrist Iwan Bloch, for instance, sharply condemned the Christian syphilis theory in his 1901 publication *Der Ursprung der Syphilis*.[50] In the fourth edition of *Tropische Krankheiten* in 1912, Fisch, who had returned to Basel that same year for retirement, finally revised his diagnosis, changing the chapter on syphilis into a chapter on yaws.[51]

Another factor that supported the misdiagnosis of syphilis was the nature of missionary discourse, in which sexually transmitted diseases were rarely explicitly named. Fisch's early reports from the Gold Coast do not address syphilis directly. He merely alludes to the condition in brief and convoluted sentences describing his surroundings as a place "where the flesh reigns"[52] or reporting on the "successful treatment of a certain disease very widely spread here like at home."[53] This type of account was characteristic for missionary publications, which often did not label

[47] Roger Davidson/Lesley A. Hall (eds.), Sex, Sin and Suffering. Venereal Disease and European Society since 1870, London/New York 2001; Lutz Sauerteig, Krankheit, Sexualität, Gesellschaft. Geschlechtskrankheiten und Gesundheitspolitik in Deutschland im 19. und frühen 20. Jahrhundert, Stuttgart 1999; Frevert, Professional Medicine and the Working Classes in Imperial Germany. On the history of syphilis in Europe and beyond, see the classic study by Claude Quétel, Le mal de Naples. Histoire de la syphilis, Paris 1986.

[48] The Bible quotation is taken from the Book of Wisdom 11:16.

[49] Rudolf Fisch, Annual report for 1909, 31.12.1909, BMA, D-1.93.24.

[50] Iwan Bloch, Der Ursprung der Syphilis. Eine medizinische und kulturgeschichtliche Untersuchung, vol. 1, Jena 1901, p. 15–21.

[51] Fisch, Tropische Krankheiten, 4th ed., p. 225–258.

[52] Rudolf Fisch, Second quarterly report for 1886, 03.07.1886, BMA, D-1.45.6.

[53] Fisch's report was amended with the word "evil" between "certain" and "disease" in red pencil. Rudolf Fisch, Annual report for 1886, 08.01.1887, BMA, D-1.45.9.

venereal diseases by name but merely alluded to them as their ravages came to represent the fundamental evils against which the missionaries were battling. The puritan taboo surrounding sexuality initially impeded the Basel Mission doctors in taking a closer look at the condition in front of them.

Finally, the Basel medical missionaries accepted the diagnosis of syphilis so willingly because they constantly felt pressured to justify themselves to evangelicals who rejected this form of missionary work as proselytising.[54] The notion of "proselytising" gained currency in nineteenth-century Europe when Protestant media used the term with decidedly negative connotations to describe Catholic conversion practices—a tendency further reinforced by the Culture Wars. Protestant authors proposed a mission at once more thorough, more effective and more liberal than the one allegedly pursued by the Catholic Church. From their perspective, quality could only be obtained by addressing an individual's conscience, ensuring that he or she knew and understood the basic tenets of Protestantism and imparting to him or her the message of salvation.[55]

Evangelical critics of medical missions disputed the validity of medicine as a missionary tool, accusing medical missionaries of "luring heathens and Mohammedans to Christianity by means of a dose of castor oil or Epsom salt."[56] They reiterated that the initiative to convert had to come from the individual rather than from the missionary. Protestant missionary endeavours were framed as prioritising personal awakening over formal conversion to differentiate them from Catholic missionary activities.[57] The Basel Mission doctors emphasised time and again that their medical work was subordinate to their role as evangelists, pointing to the fact that a person affected by disease was more responsive to the message of Christ than a healthy person, as Hermann Vortisch expounded in 1905:

---

[54] Fisch, Die ärztliche Mission unter den Negern, p. 371–372.

[55] Gustav Warneck, Blicke in die römische Missionspraxis, in: Allgemeine Missionszeitschrift 10 (1885), p. 1–29, 49–66, here p. 13–14; Carl Mirbt, Die Missionsmethode der römisch-katholischen Kirche, in: Allgemeine Missionszeitschrift 28 (1901), p. 257–276, here p. 266–267.

[56] Gottlieb Olpp, Die ärztliche Mission, ihre Begründung, Arbeitsmethode und Erfolge, 2nd ed., Barmen 1918, p. 34.

[57] Hauser, German Religious Women in Late Ottoman Beirut, p. 138–140.

A lot of heathens are receptive to evangelisation when they come to see the physician, and that is indeed the wish and the aim of the mission doctor; that not only the body, but also the mind, the heart and the soul of the black man receives medicine and gets cured.[58]

The diagnosis of syphilis unequivocally linked disease to sin and allowed the Basel Mission doctors to emphasise that their medical mission addressed the individual as a whole, including body, mind, soul and heart. Their misinterpretation of yaws as a venereal disease persisted for so long because it served their own interests. The apparent popularity of their syphilis treatment offered a point of entry to address essential tenets of Pietist faith with their African patients. The Basel medical missionaries tried to convince them that syphilis was an indicator of apostasy, providing clear evidence for the deep sinfulness of their heathen beliefs and practices. In line with Pietist notions of healing, they maintained that an effective cure to any medical problem could only come about through conversion, even claiming that this was "the actual purpose of disease."[59]

5.3 Bodily Knowledge, Individualism and Spiritual Rebirth

The overarching goal of the Basel Mission, as well as of the medical mission in particular, was individual conversion. The Pietist concept of a spiritual rebirth was imagined as a result of inner conflicts and unrests, an individual's personal experience with God.[60] The Basel missionary Ferdinand Ernst, who worked in Cameroon from 1897 to 1909, captured this in a nutshell: "Christianity is not a matter that can be taught or instilled but rather has to be experienced."[61] This view of conversion as an individual experience, however, was hardly reconcilable with the dominant view in West African societies, where humans' bodies and metaphysical

---

[58] Hermann Vortisch, Der Arzt im Urwald, in: Der Feierabend, Nr. 19, Hannover 1905, p. 74–75, here p. 74.

[59] Endre Zsindely, Krankheit und Heilung im älteren Pietismus, Zürich/Stuttgart 1962, p. 64.

[60] Gestrich, Pietismus und ländliche Frömmigkeit, p. 349, 355–356; Becker, Conversio im Wandel.

[61] Cited in: Hauss, Der Pionier der Balimission, p. 16.

essence existed through their complex correlations with ancestors, the family unit and the village collective.[62]

The Basel Mission doctors believed that the teaching of hygiene was an effective method to dissociate potential converts from their communities of origin by increasing personal responsibility for health, strengthening individualism in social matters and providing the mental disposition necessary for a conversion to Christianity. They argued that the promotion of bodily knowledge encouraged practices of self-examination, thereby paving the way for a spiritual rebirth. They assigned accountability for physical and spiritual well-being to the individual person, using their medical work to raise awareness of sin and repentance. The missionary intellectual Gustav Warneck asserted that:

> [...] when Christianity has awakened the consciousness of sin, civilising impulses follow regarding clothing, housing and work for example, because then shamelessness, impurity, laziness and greed are recognised as vices that are incompatible with Christian life.[63]

Based on Warneck's notion that acknowledgement of sin entailed far-reaching social and cultural transformations, the Basel Mission doctors declared recognition of one's sinful heart as the most important condition for medical and civilisational progress. They tried to instil in their patients notions of self-awareness and practices of introspection by merging Pietist tenets of purity with concepts of health and cleanliness. Born-again Christians were expected to give outward expression to their spiritual rebirth by renouncing bodily practices deemed incompatible with their new beliefs and adopting a new code of conduct. To the Basel Mission doctors, hygiene reflected one's dedication to a pious life and indicated proximity to God, serving as the prime marker of difference with respect to the allegedly heathen environment.

---

[62] Emmanuel Kwaku Akyeampong, Disease in West African History, in: ibid. (ed.), Themes in West Africa's History, Athens/Oxford/Accra 2006, p. 186–207; Steven Feierman/John M. Janzen (eds.), The Social Basis of Health and Healing in Africa, Berkeley et al. 1992; Vaughan, Curing Their Ills; Norman Etherington, Missionary Doctors and African Healers in Mid-Victorian South Africa, in: South African Historical Journal 19 (1987), p. 77–92.

[63] Gustav Warneck, Evangelische Missionslehre. Ein missionstheoretischer Versuch, ed. by Friedemann Knödler, Bonn 2015, p. 498.

Moreover, the Basel Mission doctors valued hygiene as a means to promote "rational scientific views on cause and effect."[64] In an article on the significance of the medical mission for German colonies, the missiologist Gottlob Haussleiter commented in 1911: "More necessary than the training of the mind, the heathen needs the purification of his reason."[65] The medical missionaries argued that knowledge of hygiene played an essential part in this purification process by encouraging rationality, responsibility and the formation of a logical mind. They viewed Africans as people of the body while defining themselves as people of the mind. This longstanding opposition at the heart of imperial ideology presumed that Africans were less intellectual and more emotional while Europeans were more logical and self-controlled.[66] Therefore, they sought to access the conceptual world of Africans through bodily practices.

While the Basel Mission addressed their message to the individual, they conceived of a vertical and horizontal circulation of Christian ideas and practices from African teachers and mission-educated children to the larger community.[67] Hygiene became a main subject in the Basel Mission's schools from 1892, improving their standing in the eyes of colonial authorities.[68] The mission schools had been controversial for supposedly encouraging Africans to question the colonial government, especially through their emphasis on literacy.[69] On the Gold Coast, British administrators took several steps to legally restrict the nature of the education offered to African pupils with their successive education

---

[64] Rudolf Fisch, Annual report for 1902, 06.02.1903, BMA, D-1.77.19.

[65] Haussleiter, Die Bedeutung der ärztlichen Mission in den deutschen Kolonien, p. 13.

[66] Ratschiller/Weichlein (eds.), Der schwarze Körper als Missionsgebiet; Paul S. Landau, Explaining Surgical Evangelism in Colonial Southern Africa. Teeth, Pain and Faith, in: The Journal of African History 37 (1996) 2, p. 261–281.

[67] The Basel Mission's annual report for 1913 emphasised the importance of hygiene classes, where "children are to learn how to best protect themselves against diseases and what has to happen in houses and villages to improve health conditions." Evangelische Missionsgesellschaft zu Basel (ed.), Neunundachtzigster Jahresbericht, Basel 1913, p. 90.

[68] Elementary Hygiene for Primary Schools, 1st ed., 1892, BMA, C.II.c.177; Teaching Plan for the Elementary-Schools of the Basel Mission on the Gold Coast, 1895, BMA, D-10.004.12.

[69] Anonymous, Ein Wort zu Gunsten der Missionsschulen, in: Evangelisches Missionsmagazin 29 (1885), p. 234–240.

ordinances.[70] They stipulated that one of the first and foremost duties of education was to teach habits of cleanliness, discipline and hygiene.[71]

Patrick Manson, an eminent figure of tropical medicine, gave a speech at Livingstone College in 1908, in which he underlined that mission schools were the most important institutions of tropical medicine, hygiene and sanitation since they had access to "native children."[72] Livingstone College in London had been established in 1893 by a conference of doctors sponsored by the Church Missionary Society for the instruction of missionaries in the elements of surgery, basic physiology, tropical diseases and hygiene.[73] It remained a unique institution in Europe until 1906, when the German Institute for Medical Mission was established in Tubingen. By then, the institution had already drawn hundreds of missionaries from countries around the world for elementary medical training. It attracted support from influential representative of the Church of England, the medical community and the universities.[74]

The nine-month course at Livingstone College was designed for non-medical missionaries, who were expected "to teach the hygiene required in tropical climates, and to deal scientifically with outbreaks of epidemics."[75] In his address on the College's Commemoration Day in 1908, Manson advised the 299 missionaries who had completed the course so far: "Train up a child in the way he should walk, and when he is grown he will not only benefit personally but he will assist at all events in propagating the doctrines of hygiene, which the European teacher is

[70] Gold Coast Colony Educational Department (ed.), Rules, London 1887; Ibid. (ed.), Code of Regulations with Schedules and Appendices, London 1894; Ibid. (ed.), Education Rules, Accra 1910; Ibid. (ed.), Imperial Education Conference Papers, London 1914.

[71] Lectures on Health Subjects. A Series of Lectures Issued by the Gold Coast Government for Use in Government Schools for Educational Purpose, London 1906, BMA, D.II.c.88.

[72] Patrick Manson, Tropical Research in its Relation to the Missionary Enterprise, Being an Address Delivered at Livingstone College on Commemoration Day, June 29, 1908, London 1909; Anonymous, Livingstone College Commemoration Day, in: Journal of Tropical Medicine and Hygiene 11, 15.07.1908, p. 218.

[73] Good, The Steamer Parish, p. 41–42.

[74] Anonymous, Livingstone College: Report for 1905–6, in: Journal of Tropical Medicine and Hygiene 10, 15.01.1907, p. 29.

[75] Anonymous, Livingstone College, in: Journal of Tropical Medicine and Hygiene 11, 02.03.1908, p. 71–72.

anxious for him to adopt."[76] Scientists and colonial authorities recognised that the most effective way to promote hygienic knowledge overseas was through the training of missionaries since they had familiarised themselves with the climates and inhabitants of the colonies more thoroughly than any other group of Europeans.

Children in particular were considered important allies in disseminating hygienic knowledge, able to diffuse new behavioural norms into their wider communities. In 1903, the Colonial Office in London asked British administrators around the globe to write reports on the progress of the instruction of hygiene to colonial subjects. By 1911, these reports showed that education had shifted dramatically towards hygiene and sanitation.[77] Helen Tiffin has analysed how hygiene was conveyed in African and Australian textbooks from the late nineteenth century onwards, arguing that the teaching of hygiene featured technologies of literary learning rooted in religious instruction.[78] According to her, "learning by heart, the taking into the body of the (foreign) text, and the appending of questions to the text, were catechistical devices, which reinforced absorption of the material and its correct interpretation."[79]

Most texts used in the Basel Mission schools began with an explicit linkage between cleanliness and godliness. The "Catechism of Health," for example, had pupils recite: "I ought to take care of my body because my body is the house of God and ought to be well kept."[80] When the leaders in Basel mapped out hygienic training for African students, they recorded that the teaching of hygiene had to proceed from a solid grounding in Pietist principles of purity. At the same time, they valued the teaching of hygiene as a catechistical device, which had the capacity not only to prevent dirt and disease but also raise awareness for sin and penance. They believed that this type of bodily knowledge promoted

---

[76] Manson, Tropical Research in its Relation to the Missionary Enterprise, p. 11.

[77] Burke, Lifebuoy Men, Lux Women, p. 37.

[78] Helen Tiffin, The Mission of Hygiene: Race, Class and Cleanliness in African and Australian Textbooks 1885–1935, in: Gerhard Stilz (ed.), Colonies, Missions, Cultures in the English-Speaking World. General and Comparative Studies, Tübingen 2001, p. 41–54.

[79] Ibid., p. 42.

[80] Easy Lessons of Health, 1901, BMA, C.II.c.179; Friedrich Askani, Kurzer Leitfaden für den Unterricht in der Heidenmission mit einem Anhang von Missionsgeschichten, 1904, BMA, N.066; Friedrich Schütze, Leitfaden für den Unterricht in der Erziehungs- und Unterrichtslehre, 5th ed., Leipzig 1900, BMA, X.II.15.

social independence, private initiative and the creation of an autonomous self—attributes they considered to be the basis for a spiritual conversion. Scholars such as Peter van der Veer have argued that "both Catholic and Protestant missions" carried a "new conception of the self [...] to the rest of the world."[81] More specifically, some researchers have claimed that Pietists can be credited with inspiring both evangelicalism and modern individualism.[82] In recent years, however, there has been growing scepticism among historians about the longstanding assumption that missions acted as agents of individualisation.[83] The concept of individualism, with its close associations to ideas of the European Enlightenment and modernity, is certainly not without analytical pitfalls.[84]

The Pietist concept of a spiritual rebirth implied that becoming a born-again Christian was an individual's personal decision, regardless of race, gender or class. While the Basel Mission in West Africa operated with notions of individual conversion and had some individualising effects, the Committee in Basel was far from advocating self-determination and missionaries on the ground were driven by an unfaltering sense of cultural superiority. Both turned the missionary endeavour into a process characterised by marked asymmetries and conflicts. The communities targeted by the Basel missionaries were not only exposed to the pressures of colonialism but were also caught in an ideological quandary between the message of personal liberation and the reality of European domination. Furthermore, a number of conflicting social dynamics were constantly

[81] Peter van der Veer, Introduction, in: ibid. (ed.), Conversion to Modernities. The Globalization of Christianity, New York 1996, p. 9.

[82] See, for instance, Shantz, An Introduction to German Pietism.

[83] For a critical take on missionaries as agents of individualization, see Rebekka Habermas, Mission und Individualisierung – Togo um 1900. Über ein überraschendes Verhältnis, das *religion making* der Missionare und die Ursprünge der *microstoria*, in: Martin Fuchs/Antje Linkenbach/Wolfgang Reinhard (eds.), Individualisierung durch christliche Mission? Wiesbaden 2015, p. 536–554.

[84] On the historiography of individualism more generally, see Charles Taylor, Sources of the Self. The Making of the Modern Identity, Cambridge 1989; Richard van Dülmen (ed.), Entdeckung des Ich. Die Geschichte der Individualisierung vom Mittelalter bis zur Gegenwart, Köln/Weimar/Wien 2001; Magnus Schlette, Die Idee der Selbstverwirklichung. Zur Grammatik des modernen Individualismus, Frankfurt a. M. 2013.

competing in West African societies, which had their own individualising tendencies that further complicated the missionary dynamic.[85] The Basel Mission in West Africa displayed a sense of dialectic tension between the individual and the community, which is not abrogated by purely individualistic approaches. The whole purpose of isolating individual converts from their communities of origin was to integrate them into the Basel Mission's parishes. Community-building activities and the unity of the congregation played an important role since evangelical success meant more than merely growing tallies of converted individuals. True and lasting conversion was thought to be impossible outside of permanent Christian communities. Ultimately, the individual Christian could only be guarded from falling prey to the profane environment by the creation of safe havens. The Basel Mission thus not only engaged in preaching hygiene to individuals but also heavily focussed on creating pure spaces for the protection of their parishioners.

REFERENCES

Stephen Addae, The Evolution of Modern Medicine in a Developing Country: Ghana 1880–1960, Durham 1997.

Emmanuel Kwaku Akyeampong, Disease in West African History, in: ibid. (ed.), Themes in West Africa's History, Athens/Oxford/Accra 2006, p. 186–207.

Anonymous, Ein Wort zu Gunsten der Missionsschulen, in: Evangelisches Missionsmagazin 29 (1885), p. 234–240.

Anonymous, Livingstone College: Report for 1905–6, in: Journal of Tropical Medicine and Hygiene 10 (15.01.1907), p. 29.

Anonymous, Livingstone College, in: Journal of Tropical Medicine and Hygiene 11 (02.03.1908), p. 71–72.

Anonymous, Livingstone College Commemoration Day, in: Journal of Tropical Medicine and Hygiene 11 (15.07.1908), p. 218.

Basler Missionskomitee (ed.), An die Freunde des Ärztlichen Zweiges der Basler Mission, Basel 1891.

Judith Becker, Conversio im Wandel. Basler Missionare zwischen Europa und Südindien und die Ausbildung einer Kontaktreligiosität, 1834–1860, Göttingen 2015.

Iwan Bloch, Der Ursprung der Syphilis. Eine medizinische und kulturgeschichtliche Untersuchung, vol. 1, Jena 1901.

---

[85] Martin Fuchs/Antje Linkenbach/Wolfgang Reinhard (eds.), Individualisierung durch christliche Mission? Wiesbaden 2015.

236 L. M. RATSCHILLER NASIM

Walter Bruchhausen, Die "hygienische Eroberung" der Tropen. Gesundheitsschutz als europäischer Export in kolonialer und nachkolonialer Zeit, in: "Sei Sauber...!" Eine Geschichte der Hygiene und der öffentlichen Gesundheitsvorsorge in Europa, ed. by Musée d'Histoire de la Ville de Luxembourg, Köln 2004, p. 204–217.

Timothy Burke, Lifebuoy Men, Lux Women. Commodification, Consumption and Cleanliness in Modern Zimbabwe, Durham/London 1996.

Theodor Christlieb, Ärztliche Missionen, Gütersloh 1889.

John Comaroff/Jean Comaroff, Home-Made Hegemony: Modernity, Domesticity, and Colonialism in South Africa, in: Karen Tranberg Hansen (ed.), African Encounters with Domesticity, New Brunswick 1992, p. 37–74.

John Comaroff/Jean Comaroff, Of Revelation and Revolution, vol. 1: Christianity, Colonialism and Consciousness in South Africa, Chicago 1991.

Roger Davidson/Lesley A. Hall (eds.), Sex, Sin and Suffering. Venereal Disease and European Society since 1870, London/New York 2001.

Alfred Eckhardt, Ärztliche Missionsarbeit in Christiansborg, in: An die Freunde des Ärztlichen Zweiges der Basler Mission, Basel 1891, p. 8–19.

Alfred Eckhardt, Land, Leute und ärztliche Mission auf der Goldküste, Basel 1894.

Natasha Erlank, Missionary Views on Sexuality in Xhosaland in the Nineteenth Century, in: Le Fait Missionaire 11 (2001), p. 9–43.

Natasha Erlank, Strange Bedfellows. The International Missionary Council, the International African Institute, and Research into African Marriage and Family, in: Patrick Harries/David Maxwell (eds.), The Spiritual in the Secular. Missionaries and Knowledge about Africa, Grand Rapids 2012, p. 267–292.

Norman Etherington, Missionary Doctors and African Healers in Mid-Victorian South Africa, in: South African Historical Journal 19 (1987), p. 77–92.

Evangelische Missionsgesellschaft zu Basel (ed.), Neunundachtzigster Jahresbericht, Basel 1913.

Johannes Fabian, Time and the Work of Anthropology. Critical Essays 1971–1991, Chur et al. 1991.

Steven Feierman/John M. Janzen (eds.), The Social Basis of Health and Healing in Africa, Berkeley et al. 1992.

Rudolf Fisch, Die ärztliche Mission unter den Negern. Ansprache am Jahresfest der Basler Mission am 3. Juli 1895, in: Evangelisches Missionsmagazin 39 (1895), p. 371–377.

Rudolf Fisch, Über die Behandlung der Amöbendysenterie und einige andere tropenmedizinische Fragen, in: Archiv für Schiffs- und Tropenhygiene 8 (1904), p. 207–212.

Rudolf Fisch, Tropische Krankheiten. Anleitung zu ihrer Verhütung und Behandlung speziell für die Westküste von Afrika, für Missionare, Kaufleute, Pflanzer und Beamte, 1st ed., Basel 1891; 2nd ed., Basel 1894; 3rd ed., Basel 1903; 4th ed., Basel 1912.

Friedrich Hermann Fischer, Der Missionsarzt Rudolf Fisch und die Anfänge medizinischer Arbeit der Basler Mission an der Goldküste (Ghana), Herzogenrath 1991.

Ute Frevert, Professional Medicine and the Working Classes in Imperial Germany, in: Journal of Contemporary History 20 (1985) 4, p. 637–658.

Martin Fuchs/Antje Linkenbach/Wolfgang Reinhard (eds.), Individualisierung durch christliche Mission? Wiesbaden 2015.

Andreas Gestrich, Pietismus und ländliche Frömmigkeit in Württemberg im 18. und frühen 19. Jahrhundert, in: Norbert Haag/Sabine Holtz/Wolfgang Zimmermann/Dieter R. Bauer (eds.), Ländliche Frömmigkeit. Konfessionskulturen und Lebenswelten, Stuttgart 2002, p. 343–357.

Sander Gilman, Difference and Pathology: Stereotypes of Sexuality, Race and Madness, Ithaca 1985.

Gold Coast Colony Educational Department (ed.), Rules, London 1887.

Gold Coast Colony Educational Department (ed.), Code of Regulations with Schedules and Appendices, London 1894.

Gold Coast Colony Educational Department (ed.), Education Rules, Accra 1910.

Gold Coast Colony Educational Department (ed.), Imperial Education Conference Papers, London 1914.

Charles M. Good, The Steamer Parish. The Rise and Fall of Missionary Medicine on an African Frontier, Chicago/London 2004.

Patricia Grimshaw, Faith, Missionary Life, and the Family, in: Philippa Levine (ed.), Gender and Empire, Oxford 2004, p. 260–280.

Rebekka Habermas, Mission und Individualisierung – Togo um 1900. Über ein überraschendes Verhältnis, das *religion making* der Missionare und die Ursprünge der *microstoria*, in: Martin Fuchs/Antje Linkenbach/Wolfgang Reinhard (eds.), Individualisierung durch christliche Mission? Wiesbaden 2015, p. 536–554.

Julia Hauser, German Religious Women in Late Ottoman Beirut. Competing Missions, Leiden 2015.

Karl Hauss, Der Pionier der Balimission. Aus dem Leben von Ferdinand Ernst, Basel 1910.

Gottlob Haussleiter, Die Bedeutung der ärztlichen Mission in den deutschen Kolonien, in: Die ärztliche Mission 6 (1911), p. 5–16.

Erika Hebeisen, Leidenschaftlich fromm. Die pietistische Bewegung in Basel 1750–1830, Köln/Weimar/Wien 2005.

Friedrich Hey, Wegweiser für den Christen über Leiden, Krankheiten, Heilung, Offenbach 1905.

Friedrich Hey, Der Tropenarzt. Ausführlicher Ratgeber für Europäer in den Tropen, sowie für Besitzer von Plantagen und Handelshäusern, Kolonialbehörden und Missionsverwaltungen, 1st ed., Offenbach 1906.

Ludwig Külz, Die Abhängigkeit der geistigen und kulturellen Rückständigkeit der Naturvölker von ihren endemischen Krankheiten, in: Anthropos 14/15 (1919/1920) 1/3, p. 33–45.

Paul S. Landau, Explaining Surgical Evangelism in Colonial Southern Africa. Teeth, Pain and Faith, in: The Journal of African History 37 (1996) 2, p. 261–281.

Desiree Lewis, Representing African Sexualities, in: Sylvia Tamale (ed.), African Sexualities. A Reader, Cape Town et al. 2011, p. 199–216.

Sonja Malzner/Anne D. Peiter (eds.), Der Träger. Zu einer "tragenden" Figur der Kolonialgeschichte, Bielefeld 2018.

Emily J. Manktelow, Missionary Families: Race, Gender and Generation on the Spiritual Frontier, Manchester/New York 2013.

Patrick Manson, Tropical Research in its Relation to the Missionary Enterprise, Being an Address Delivered at Livingstone College on Commemoration Day, June 29th, 1908, London 1909.

David Maxwell, The Missionary Home as a Site for Mission: Perspectives from Belgian Congo, in: Studies in Church History 50 (2014), p. 428–455.

Carl Mense, Syphilis und venerische Krankheiten in den neu der Kultur erschlossenen Ländern besonders in Afrika, in: Archiv für Schiffs- und Tropenhygiene 4 (1900), p. 86–109.

Carl Mirbt, Die Missionsmethode der römisch-katholischen Kirche, in: Allgemeine Missionszeitschrift 28 (1901), p. 257–276.

Albert Neisser, Sind Syphilis und Frambösie verschiedene Krankheiten? in: Archiv für Schiffs-und Tropenhygiene 12 (1908), p. 173–179.

Theodor Oehler, An die Freunde des Ärztlichen Zweiges der Basler Mission, Basel 1892, p. 1–5.

Gottlieb Olpp, Die ärztliche Mission, ihre Begründung, Arbeitsmethode und Erfolge, 2nd ed., Barmen 1918.

Deborah Pellow, Sex, Disease, and Culture Change in Ghana, in: Philip W. Setel/Milton Lewis/Maryinez Lyons (eds.), Histories of Sexually Transmitted Diseases and HIV/AIDS in Sub-Saharan Africa, Westport/London 1999, p. 17–41.

Hermann Prätorius, Mittheilungen aus der afrikanischen Visitationsreise, in: Der Evangelische Heidenbote 56 (1883), p. 9–11, 17–19, 25–28, 33–35, 41–43.

Claude Quétel, Le mal de Naples. Histoire de la syphilis, Paris 1986.

Linda Ratschiller/Siegfried Weichlein (eds.), Der schwarze Körper als Missionsgebiet. Medizin, Ethnologie, Theologie in Afrika und Europa 1880–1960, Köln/Weimar/Wien 2016.

Lutz Sauerteig, Krankheit, Sexualität, Gesellschaft. Geschlechtskrankheiten und Gesundheitspolitik in Deutschland im 19. und frühen 20. Jahrhundert, Stuttgart 1999.

Heinrich Botho Scheube, Krankheiten der warmen Länder, 1st ed., Jena 1896; 2nd ed., Jena 1900; 3rd ed., Jena 1903; 4th ed., Jena 1910.

Magnus Schlette, Die Idee der Selbstverwirklichung. Zur Grammatik des modernen Individualismus, Frankfurt a. M. 2013.

Douglas H. Shantz, An Introduction to German Pietism: Protestant Renewal at the Dawn of Modern Europe, Baltimore 2013.

Ann Laura Stoler, Race and the Education of Desire. Foucault's History of Sexuality and the Colonial Order of Things, Durham/London 1995.

Charles Taylor, Sources of the Self. The Making of the Modern Identity, Cambridge 1989.

Helen Tiffin, The Mission of Hygiene: Race, Class and Cleanliness in African and Australian Textbooks 1885–1935, in: Gerhard Stilz (ed.), Colonies, Missions, Cultures in the English-Speaking World. General and Comparative Studies, Tübingen 2001, p. 41–54.

Peter van der Veer, Introduction, in: ibid. (ed.), Conversion to Modernities. The Globalization of Christianity, New York 1996.

Richard van Dülmen (ed.), Entdeckung des Ich. Die Geschichte der Individualisierung vom Mittelalter bis zur Gegenwart, Köln/Weimar/Wien 2001.

Megan Vaughan, Curing Their Ills. Colonial Power and African Illness, Cambridge 1991.

Megan Vaughan, Syphilis in Colonial East and Central Africa: The Social Construction of an Epidemic, in: Terence Ranger/Paul Slack (eds.), Epidemics and Ideas. Essays on the Historical Perception of Pestilence, Cambridge 1992, p. 269–302.

Hermann Vortisch, Der Arzt im Urwald, in: Der Feierabend, Nr. 19, Hannover 1905, p. 74–75.

Hermann Vortisch, Erfahrungen über einige spezifische Krankheiten an der Goldküste, in: Archiv für Schiffs- und Tropenhygiene 10 (1906), p. 537–539.

Hermann Vortisch, Die Nervosität als Störung zwischen Seele und Geist und ihre Überwindung, Hamburg 1921.

Daniel J. Walther, Sex and Control. Venereal Disease, Colonial Physicians, and Indigenous Agency in German Colonialism, 1884–1914, New York/Oxford 2005.

Daniel J. Walther, Sex and Control in Germany's Overseas Possessions: Venereal Disease and Indigenous Agency, in: Nina Berman/Klaus Mühlhahn/Patrice Nganang (eds.), German Colonialism Revisited: African, Asian, and Oceanic Experiences, Ann Arbor 2014, p. 71–84.

Gustav Warneck, Blicke in die römische Missionspraxis, in: Allgemeine Missionszeitschrift 10 (1885), p. 1–29, 49–66.

Gustav Warneck, Evangelische Missionslehre. Ein missionstheoretischer Versuch, ed. by Friedemann Knödler, Bonn 2015.
Karolin Wetjen, Gemeinde im Laboratorium. Aushandlungsprozesse des Christentums und Kirchenzucht in der Mission am Beginn des 20. Jahrhunderts, in: Linda Ratschiller/Karolin Wetjen (eds.), Verflochtene Mission. Perspektiven auf eine neue Missionsgeschichte, Köln/Weimer/Wien 2018, p. 89–116.
Endre Zsindely, Krankheit und Heilung im älteren Pietismus, Zürich/Stuttgart 1962.

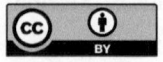

CHAPTER 6

Creating Pure Spaces: Edifices, Domesticity and the Temperance Movement

Missionaries at home and abroad identified and popularised corrupted spaces to emphasise the need for their interventions. They promised to protect and uplift people from these ostensibly detrimental surroundings by offering spaces where their ideal of purity held true in exemplary fashion. The very nature of the missionary endeavour assumed that a disorderly environment needed to be tidied up. From the point of view of the Basel missionaries in West Africa, Christians—Africans as well as Europeans—were constantly at risk of falling into heathen impurity in their profane surroundings. It was therefore particularly important to create pure spaces, in which the Christian community was shielded from undesirable influences and worldly distractions, or as the Basel missionary Johannes Müller expressed it, "one healthy apple should not lie under 100 rotten ones."[1]

---

[1] Johannes Müller, Report to the Committee, 1866, cited in: Schlatter, Geschichte der Basler Mission, vol. 3, p. 73.

© The Author(s) 2023
L. M. Ratschiller Nasim, *Medical Missionaries and Colonial Knowledge in West Africa and Europe, 1885–1914*,
Cambridge Imperial and Post-Colonial Studies,
https://doi.org/10.1007/978-3-031-27128-1_6

6.1   ARCHITECTURAL MEANS

The pursuit of creating pure spaces in West Africa materialised architec-
turally in the form of mission houses, hill stations, prayer halls, schools,
gardens and hospitals. The question of adequate housing for Europeans constituted a central theme in discussions on tropical hygiene
and frequently popped up in the Basel Mission doctors' publications.[2]
Since natural elements such as soil, water and air were believed to be
important factors that affected health, handbooks on tropical hygiene
declared that finding suitable locations and building proper houses were
preconditions for the survival of Europeans in the tropics. In 1895, the
Committee released a decree on building in Africa, recommending that
the best prophylaxis against tropical diseases was to elevate wood buildings on masonry piers and entirely surround dwellings with airy, spacious
verandas.[3] The mission doctors popularised this building design with
detailed floor plans in their handbooks on tropical hygiene.[4]

Missionaries, traders, explorers and colonial officials wrote extensively
about how important verandas were for survival in tropical colonies.
The veranda constituted a cornerstone of colonial imagery as a growing
number of readers in Great Britain, Germany and Switzerland familiarised themselves with colonial literature. The word "veranda" entered
the German language in the mid-nineteenth century when it was adopted
from the British, who, in turn, had appropriated it in India.[5] Popular
authors such as Rudyard Kipling exposed a broad audience to detailed
descriptions of life in the bungalows and verandas of British India. In
these colonial narratives, verandas appeared not only as part of health
provision but also as important public spaces with good views over the

---

[2] See selectively Alfred Eckhardt, Häuserbau in Westafrika und die Station Ho, in:
Deutsche Kolonialzeitung 4 (1891), p. 43–46; Ibid., Land, Leute und ärztliche Mission
auf der Goldküste, p. 15–18; Hey, Der Tropenarzt, 1st ed., p. 91–104; Fisch, Tropische
Krankheiten, 1st ed., p. 10–13; Ibid., Tropische Krankheiten, 4th ed., p. 29–44.

[3] Über afrikanisches Bauwesen, Basel 1895, BMA, D-10.4.18.

[4] See for example Hey, Der Tropenarzt, 1st ed., p. 101; Fisch, Tropische Krankheiten,
1st ed., p. 226–229; Fisch, Tropische Krankheiten, 3rd ed., p. 212–215.

[5] Itohan Osayimwese, Colonialism and Modern Architecture in Germany, Pittsburgh
2017, p. 205.

area, where Europeans could symbolically scan the horizon and plan further expansion.[6]

The Basel missionaries assumed much of the early construction work themselves but quickly proceeded to outsource the strenuous task to the West Indian Christians and later to African workers. Despite their invisibility in official accounts, African labourers did much of the arduous and perilous work of excavating, hauling and assembling materials. The Basel Mission established workshops in West Africa where missionaries, most of whom were skilled artisans, trained Africans to become specialised craftsmen such as bricklayers and carpenters. These craftsmen were much sought after by colonial governments because of their familiarity with European construction techniques and styles.[7]

The Basel Mission doctors' building advice not only comprised health considerations but also promulgated a specific aesthetic, including "half-timbered houses"—known as *Fachwerk* in their home towns—and edifices with "interlocking tiles" and "solid walls" made of sandstone.[8] They emphasised that buildings ought to have a "noble" structure, believing that European architecture and geometry fascinated and had a refining influence on African people. John MacKenzie has shown that missionaries in nineteenth-century Africa considered buildings "as books, which could convey lessons and messages as much as paper and print."[9] Edifices were therefore supposed to inspire respect and served as a clear indictor of what Christians could achieve. Although conditions often fell far below the ideal, much attention was paid to the appearance and arrangement of mission structures. By combining strong horizontal and vertical lines,

---

[6] On the meaning of architecture, and particularly verandas, in colonial and postcolonial African cities, see Garth Andrew Myers, Verandahs of Power: Colonialism and Space in Urban Africa, New York 2003.

[7] Osayimwese, Colonialism and Modern Architecture in Germany, p. 9; Wolfgang Lauber, Deutsche Architektur in Kamerun 1884–1914: Deutsche Architekten und Kameruner Wissenschaftler dokumentieren die Bauten der deutschen Epoche in Kamerun/Afrika, Stuttgart 1988, p. 49.

[8] Eckhardt, Häuserbau in Westafrika und die Station Ho; Peter A. Schweizer, Mission an der Goldküste: Geschichte und Fotografie der Basler Mission im kolonialen Ghana, Basel 2002, p. 108.

[9] MacKenzie, Missionaries, Science, and the Environment in Nineteenth-Century Africa, p. 120–121.

mission buildings were designed to protrude in the architectural and natural landscape of West Africa.[10]

The Basel Mission doctors repeatedly highlighted the key role of mission hospitals, which they assumed impressed values and behaviours of hygiene on African patients.[11] The hospital wards were designed to demonstrate order and cleanliness with beds in neat rows and clean white sheets while medical equipment and pharmaceuticals were thought to undermine what the medical missionaries saw as irrational healing practices. Mission hospitals were praised for their effectiveness in curative health care, their potential to gain the support of the wider population and their evangelising value. The Basel Mission's medical magazine stated that "hospitals are necessary not only for the sake of treatment but particularly to serve the main purpose of the medical mission, to win souls for the Lord."[12]

Rudolf Fisch referred to the mission hospital in Aburi as "the place where God had revealed Himself" to him.[13] In addition to providing "modern medical science," mission hospitals were also "imbued with a unique Christian spirit," as David Hardiman demonstrated.[14] Religious rituals were part of everyday life at the Basel Mission hospitals with frequent bedside prayers and daily services. Alfred Eckhardt highlighted the importance of establishing mission hospitals in West Africa in an article in 1892 by emphasising their value for evangelisation: "All mission doctors experience that spiritual success is far greater with people who are

---

[10] For descriptions of West African building styles, see Tarikhu Farrar, Building Technology and Settlement Planning in a West African Civilization: Precolonial Akan Cities and Towns, Lewiston 1996; Anthony King, The Bungalow: The Production of a Global Culture, London/Boston 1984.

[11] Hermann Vortisch, Wie kann man in Missionsspitälern evangelistisch tätig sein? in: Die ärztliche Mission 8 (1913), p. 13–17; Ibid., Ein barmherziger Samariter, in: Johannes Kammerer (ed.), Bilder aus dem Missionsspital, Basel 1912, p. 3–4; Theodor Müller, Bilder aus einem afrikanischen Missionsspital, in: Die ärztliche Mission 8 (1913), p. 35–37; Rudolf Fisch, Aus einer afrikanischen Poliklinik, in: Der Evangelische Heidenbote 79 (1906), p. 44.

[12] Basler Missionskomitee (ed.), Unsere ärztliche Mission. Bericht vom Jahr 1897, Basel 1898, p. 2. See further Bruchhausen, Medicine Between Religious Worlds; Hardiman, Introduction.

[13] Fisch, Vierzig Jahre ärztliche Mission auf der Goldküste, p. 22.

[14] Hardiman, The Mission Hospital 1880–1960, p. 198.

under daily spiritual influence for a longer period of time, who come to worship daily, who see Christian life daily, who experience mercy daily."[15]

The photograph of Friedrich Hey and his patients at the mission hospital in Odumase, however, puts the image of the mission hospital as a place of rigid Christian regime into perspective (Fig. 6.1).[16] It appeared in the journal for medical mission *Unsere ärztliche Mission* and in the popular monthly magazine *Der Evangelische Heidenbote* in 1898. The caption read: "Due to a lack of space, work takes place outdoors. Larger operations are also performed here on the veranda."[17] To generate donations, the visual message of the Basel Mission followed a binary pattern that highlighted both the urgent need for action and the achievements to date. The multitude of patients in the photograph thus provided evidence for both the success of the Basel medical mission and its constant lack of financial and human resources. Even though the picture is clearly staged and the production conditions remain fuzzy, photographs offer a glimpse into how African spaces might have been imagined by European readers.

Moreover, the ambivalent character of mission photographs revealed inconsistencies, allowing historians to question dominant narratives. The picture implied that medical treatment took place under open skies, although the Basel Mission had evidently built a hospital in Odumase. Rather than demonstrating exemplary hygiene and Christian orderliness, it suggested rudimentary medical care and improvisation. The image composition also contained mixed messages. The white, bearded mission doctor stands next to his sitting black patients and clearly stands out. He wears a white shirt, an apron and leather shoes while most Africans wear a piece of cloth. These contrasts, however, are softened by Hey's hand, resting on a patient's shoulder, and the people standing in the background. The intricacy of the photograph reflected the complex reality in West Africa, which was often unpredictable and required permanent adaptation.

A look back at the theological origins of the Basel Mission shows that Pietists had developed a particular approach to architecture and

---

[15] Eckhardt, Ein Arbeitsjahr in Odumase, here p. 9.

[16] Friedrich Hey, Hospital at Odumase. Dr. Hey with wounded, BMA, D-30.06.19.

[17] Basler Missionskomitee (ed.), Unsere ärztliche Mission. Bericht vom Jahr 1897, Basel 1898, p. 11; Anonymous, Blicke in die Thätigkeit unserer Missionsärzte, in: Der Evangelische Heidenbote 71 (1898), p. 46–47, here p. 46.

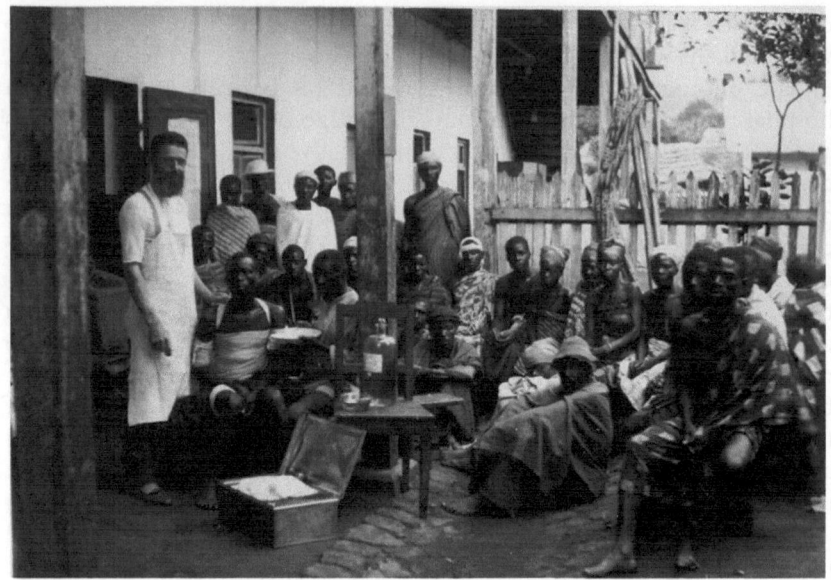

Fig. 6.1 Friedrich Hey, Hospital at Odumase. Dr. Hey with wounded, BMA, D-30.06.19

communal life. Members of the Unity of Moravian Brethren—*Herrnhuter Brüdergemeine*—founded the first autonomous Pietist settlement in 1722 at Herrnhut in eastern Germany. There, they implemented new ideas about religious organisation and spiritual life, for example by developing the concept of the *Betsaal*—prayer hall. In line with the Pietist reassessment of Christian practices, the prayer hall replaced the church as the site of religious worship, parish centre and administrative headquarters.[18] In the nineteenth century, Gottlieb Wilhelm Hoffmann, the father of the second Basel Mission Inspector Wilhelm Hoffmann, founded two prominent Pietist settlements in Wurttemberg.[19]

[18] Hartmut Beck, Die Herrnhuter Baukultur im pietistischen Zeitalter des 18. Jahrhunderts, in: Kunst und Kirche 50 (1987) 3, p. 186–189.

[19] Albrecht Rittmann, Vor 200 Jahren: Die Gründung der Brüdergemeinde Korntal, in: Schwäbische Heimat (2019) 1, p. 18–27; Renntisch, Mission und wirtschaftliche Entwicklung, p. 349–352; Jenkins, Württemberg als Hauptsäule der historischen Basler Mission, p. 32.

Korntal was established on the grounds of an existing town in 1819 to prevent the emigration of Pietists due to discrimination and economic hardship following years of famine. A conscious process of development guided the location, height and aesthetic of new buildings and maintained the centrality of the *Betsaal*. The entire town was surrounded by fields and orchards in which the residents pursued agriculture.[20] Wilhelmsdorf was established five years later in 1824. Unlike Korntal, it was built according to a predetermined plan. The settlement formed the outline of a cross, in the centre of which lay the prayer hall in a prominent position. Clear boundaries defined the towns of Korntal and Wilhemlsdorf and strict edicts maintained their isolation from broader society.[21]

In West Africa, the Basel missionaries implemented three spatial policies to come closer to their ideal of Pietist purity. The first one emphasised the primacy of rural over urban location and was framed in terms of protecting Africans from the colonial presence along the coast. The Basel missionaries frequently alluded to the administrative and commercial towns in West Africa as dirty, corrupted and sinful places, mirroring their aversion of industrialised cities in Europe. They advocated instead for a communal life close to the soil and dedicated to God, encouraging Christian converts to build their own houses and cultivate their own land on mission grounds. For the Basel missionaries, cultivation was practically synonymous with salvation. Johannes Zimmermann, who spent more than twenty years in Krobo on the Gold Coast, reflected upon his return to Basel:

> The original command to the whole of humanity is, 'Be fruitful and multiply, fill the earth and subdue it.' According to this ancient word of God, every human, by virtue of the fact that he is human, has the right to possess land, to settle on it, to build up a homestead and found a family.[22]

[20] Lothar Sigloch, Zur Geschichte von Korntal und Münchingen, vol. 1: Korntaler Ansichten – Siedlungsaspekte der Gemeinde Korntal, Korntal-Münchingen 1994, p. 32.

[21] Andreas Gestrich, Alltag im pietistischen Dorf: Bürgerliche Religiosität in ländlicher Lebenswelt, in: Die Alte Stadt 20 (1993) 1, p. 47–59.

[22] Johannes Zimmermann, Letztes Wort eines alten afrikanischen Missionars an sein deutsches Vaterland, in: Evangelisches Missionsmagazin 21 (1877), p. 225–245, here p. 226.

Zimmermann maintained that God had created and designed mankind to live in small rural communities, using simple agrarian technology and joining together to worship Him. The mobility of West Africans, their complex territorial arrangements and the transhumance of women during the agricultural cycle thwarted the Basel Mission's plans and offended their sense of order. The Basel missionaries thus encouraged converts to take possession of the land by investing themselves in it. They argued that the only way for parishioners to maintain a sustainable web of family, education and stable vocation, which they considered indispensable for a truly pious life, was through the creation of self-sustaining villages patterned on an idealised Alemannic agrarian model.[23]

Therefore, the Basel Mission's second policy consisted of establishing separate Christian settlements, referred to as "salems," for their missionaries and parishioners within rural contexts. In 1886, the Committee asked the missionaries in West Africa "whether the housing of Christians among heathens should be abolished entirely."[24] The veteran Gold Coast missionary Adolf Mohr replied that the separation of Christians from the non-Christian population was "desirable" since Christians who lived among "heathens and their heathen relatives often have a communal courtyard, where heathen nonsense spreads without shame."[25] He explained that the "Negro homesteads" were so close to each other that only a narrow path divided them and each room had direct access to the shared courtyard. Therefore, he concluded that "the constant noise makes quiet life or Christian devotion impossible" and that Christians were lonely and vulnerable in their communities of origin.[26]

Salems were established on mission land just outside existing African towns, clearly separated by fences, walls and roads.[27] They comprised the central mission house, a prayer hall, gardens, an outpatient clinic or hospital, schools and housing for European and African Christians.

---

[23] Paul Jenkins, Villagers as Missionaries: Wuerttemberg Pietism as a Nineteenth-Century Missionary Movement, in: Missiology. An International Review 8 (1980) 4, p. 425–432; Lehmann, Pietismus und weltliche Ordnung; Troeltsch, Die Soziallehren der christlichen Kirchen und Gruppen, ch. 2.

[24] Schlatter, Geschichte der Basler Mission, vol. 3, p. 72–74.

[25] Adolf Mohr, Annual report for 1886, 02.03.1887, BMA, D-01.45.IV.63.

[26] Ibid.

[27] Itohan Osayimwese, Pietism, Colonialism, and the Search for Utopia: Pietist Space in Germany and the Gold Coast, in: Thresholds 30 (2005), p. 74–79.

By physically separating converts from their communities of origin, the leaders in Basel expected that they would move away from the "dirt of their heathen environment."[28] The underlying assumption was that new converts would be easier to supervise and would develop a deeper sense of community once united in a settlement. Apart from an interest in retaining new converts, this policy of separation also reflected concern for the spiritual health of missionaries themselves since exposure to non-Christian practices was seen as a temptation for those in the field. By staying together, Christians were expected to be more likely to live according to Pietist purity ideals, outlined in the Basel Mission's congregational rules.

The situation of the mission house at the centre of the Christian village was a third way for the Basel Mission to live up to their concept of purity.[29] In the words of the missionary Eugen Schwarz in Cameroon, the mission house was a "green oasis in the middle of the barren, dark heathen land."[30] Built in an Alemannic style and surrounded by gardens, the mission house formed the symbolic core of the Pietist settlement.[31] Auxiliary buildings, including boys' and girls' schools, homes for European and African personnel, storerooms, workshops, houses for African converts and medical facilities were arranged orthogonally around the mission house. The mission house also provided space for religious worship until a prayer hall could be built. The quarters for African converts were often located on the periphery of the ensemble, implying a socio-spatial hierarchy between the mission house at the core of the village and the people on the margins.[32]

[28] Oettli, Gegenwärtige Missionsprobleme der Basler Mission in Kamerun, p. 39, BMA, E.28.

[29] Dagmar Konrad, Die Missionsstation, in: Museum der Kulturen Basel (ed.), Mission Possible? Die Sammlung der Basler Mission – Spiegel kultureller Begegnungen, Basel 2015, p. 69–75.

[30] Eugen Schwarz, Eine Reise zu zweien ins Innere Kameruns. Travel report recorded in 1917, Personal File Eugen Schwarz, BMA, BV 1681.

[31] On the garden as a metaphor in missionary and related contexts, see Sujit Sivasundaram, Natural History Spiritualized. Civilizing Islanders, Cultivating Breadfruit, and Collecting Souls, in: History of Science 39 (2001), p. 417–443.

[32] Sonia Abun-Nasr, Afrikaner und Missionar. Die Lebensgeschichte von David Asante, Basel 2013, p. 79–108; Jenkins, The Basel Mission in West Africa and the Idea of the Christian Village Community.

Pietist settlements in West Africa shared many elements with their European counterparts in Herrnhut, Korntal and Wilhelmsdorf, including an overall separatist predilection, choice of rural over urban contexts, emphasis on communal life and mutual supervision, and the reliance on the material environment to inculcate morality. A plan of the mission station at Kyebi on the Gold Coast dating from 1876 showed remarkable similarities to the layout of Wilhelmsdorf.[33] In both cases, the central location of the *Betsaal* represented the perceived or intended centrality of religious life. However, a closer look at the salems in West Africa reveals that they combined Pietist building styles with regional materials, designs and know-how. The Basel Mission schools best exemplify this new type of architecture emerging in West Africa.

The Basel Mission schools consisted of a series of buildings oriented to create a quadrangle. The primary structure was a two-storey building with wide verandas on both floors. Because elevation above ground level provided access to cooler, supposedly healthier air, upper levels were designated as living areas for Europeans. The ground floor was occupied by classrooms and other administrative functions. Single-storey wings on either side of the central structure housed dormitories, kitchens and workshops. The courtyard, comprising a well, school bell and work gardens, constituted the centrepiece of the Basel Mission schools, an element clearly inspired by architectural norms in West Africa. Itohan Osayimwese made the case that "the obsessive repetition of the courtyard form and bungalow type in Basel Mission building activity across the region constituted an appropriation of indigenous West African forms and building practices."[34]

The overt symbolism of Pietist settlements represented a new perception of space and time, where Christianity could be inscribed on the landscape in order to mould human society. It is no coincidence that Europe was "discovering new worlds" during the period in which utopian thought and practice flourished. Images of seemingly unspoiled natural landscapes and humans, provided by explorers and missionaries, and circulated through travel narratives and missionary journals, offered viable alternatives if conditions at home were too confining for the active pursuit of utopian goals. Johannes Müller, who was based at Abokobi on the

---

[33] Plan of the Mission Plot in Kyebi, 1876, BMA, D-31.4.9.10.

[34] Osayimwese, Pietism, Colonialism, and the Search for Utopia, p. 77.

Gold Coast, declared that Abokobi was a "shining example" of the benefits of separate Christian settlements:

> Here we have a proper, civil community of Christians. They negotiate the cleaning of the streets with neighbouring villages without the missionary, they settle disputes, they serve as local police, they fine those who fire guns or beat the drum 1 Schilling, and the pretty village with its tranquillity, order and security makes an impression, not least on the heathens.[35]

Salems in West Africa were frequently portrayed as role models in the Basel Mission's media. This type of account not only attested to the mission's success abroad but also held a mirror up to evangelicals at home by propagating an idealised portrayal of life in Christian settlements. To many supporters in Europe, these depictions of bucolic Pietist villages based on preindustrial economic and social conditions must have appeared as memories of a long gone past. By 1900, Basel and many other regional towns had undergone industrialisation and major social upheavals, exposing Pietists to mounting pressure from the society around them. The salems in West Africa, by contrast, were depicted as utopian spaces that promised to protect the Pietist community from corrupting influences.

Patrick Harries drew attention to the fact that "woven into the missionaries' representation of Africa was a call for clergy and church to play a leading role in the development of European society, a role that had only recently been suppressed in Switzerland by radical politicians and the forces of secularization."[36] Regardless of the fact that West African societies underwent similar developments to the ones in Europe, the image of African village life left a lasting impression on knowledge about the continent. The Basel Mission settlements in West Africa, ostensibly untouched by secular forces, "cold logic" and "dry materialism," served as discursive idols and safe havens to develop and debate conservative theological concepts. Firmly established on the evangelical mental map, their meaning reached far beyond the confinements of the mission area abroad and appealed to the utopian longings and political demands of devout Christians at home.

---

[35] Johannes Müller, Report to the Committee, 1866, cited in: Schlatter, Geschichte der Basler Mission, vol. 3, p. 73.

[36] Harries, Butterflies and Barbarians, p. 58.

Frederick Cooper and Ann Laura Stoler notably argued that colonies were "laboratories of modernity," places "where missionaries, educators, and doctors could carry out experiments in social engineering without confronting the popular resistances and bourgeois rigidness of European society at home."[37] To view the salems as laboratories of modernity, however, would be flawed as it assumes that the Basel missionaries had modernising intentions.[38] Most of them were highly critical of the changes in the world around them and advocated instead for a return to preindustrial modes of production and craftsmanship together with corresponding community and family models.[39] Their missionary endeavours in Africa were an expression of a search for pristine nature, community spirit and Pietist purity in a time of increasing uncertainty. These aspirations were not anti-modern per se, but the Basel Mission certainly did not conceive of their mission fields as laboratories of modernity.

Furthermore, the analogy presumes a uniformity of objectives and standardisation of practice among missionaries and other European protagonists in the colonies, which does not hold up to scrutiny. The Basel missionaries in West Africa undoubtedly promoted an ethnocentric agenda by creating Christian settlements modelled on Alemannic agrarian ideals, where African converts were to experience the same kind of lifestyle, marriage and household that they themselves had grown up in. Paradoxically, however, to the extent that the model they promoted for African Christians stressed economic independence from the dominant colonial economy, it very often put the missionaries directly at odds with European powers and their imperial interests.

Moreover, the concept implies that Europeans were completely free to implement their ideas of modernity in the colonies, "without confronting the popular resistances." The Basel Mission's villages in West Africa were never mere reproductions of Herrnhut, Korntal and Wilhelmsdorf. The total separation of Christian converts from their communities of origin

---

[37] Stoler/Cooper, Between Metropole and Colony, p. 5.

[38] For a critical view of missionaries as agents of modernisation, see Richard Hölzl, Aus der Zeit gefallen? Katholische Mission zwischen Modernitätsanspruch und Zivilisationskritik, in: Christoph Bultmann/Jörg Rüpke/Sabine Schmolinsky (eds.), Religionen in Nachbarschaft. Pluralismus als Markenzeichen der europäischen Religionsgeschichte, Münster 2012, p. 143–164.

[39] Jenkins, Land und Arbeit als vergessene Werte in der Mentalität von Baseler MissionarInnen um 1900.

simply proved unviable. Affiliation to the parish and life in the salem did not exclude other associations and bonds, to the dislike of the Basel missionaries.[40] The Christian settlements constituted places of exchange, where experiments and innovations were possible in a number of areas, from farming to medicine and religion, not in spite but rather because of negotiations between European missionaries and African people. It is questionable, therefore, whether modernisation is an adequate term for describing a process that was non-linear and often characterised by appropriation and reinterpretation.

Robert Peckham and David M. Pomfret warned that the idea of colonies as laboratories of modernity "continues to be reiterated within postcolonial studies, even though such allusions inadvertently reaffirm a colonial discourse that sought to legitimate colonial rule in pseudo-scientific terms as 'experiment'."[41] Scientists long likened colonial territories to laboratories and it was those involved in empire-building in the last third of the nineteenth century who first used this analogy.[42] The photograph of Friedrich Hey and his patients in Odumase illustrates that the Basel Mission very much participated in presenting the European presence in West Africa as an experiment. Hey appears as a physician in a white coat, who by means of his medical chest and medicine bottle brings scientific progress to the region. At the same time, the image indicates that the Basel Mission's aspirations to implement a specific Christian spatial order in West Africa were always confined by the realities on site.[43]

[40] Harris W. Mobley, The Ghanaian's Image of the Missionary: An Analysis of the Published Critiques of Christian Missionaries by Ghanaians 1897–1965, Leiden 1970, p. 73–80.

[41] Robert Peckham/David M. Pomfret, Introduction: Medicine, Hygiene, and the Reordering of Empire, in: ibid. (eds.), Imperial Contagions. Medicine, Hygiene, and Cultures of Planning in Asia, Hong Kong 2013, p. 1–14, here p. 13.

[42] Helen Tilley has argued that the concept had heterogeneous roots and that scientists, who thought of Africa as a living laboratory, helped to challenge the very foundations of colonialism with their social criticism, interdisciplinary and transnational methods, study of interrelated phenomena and codification of new areas of ethno-scientific and vernacular research. Tilley, Africa as a Living Laboratory.

[43] Friedrich Hey, Hospital at Odumase. Dr. Hey with Wounded, BMA, D-30.06.19.

6.2   DOMESTIC SAFE HAVENS

The Basel Mission's aspirations to create pure spaces in West Africa did not stop at the external appearance of mission houses. At least as much time and effort was spent on designing the interior of Christian homes and propagating domestic values. Rather atypical for Basel missionaries, who planned most of their constructions from scratch, Alfred Eckhardt moved into in an existing house in Christiansborg when he began to work there as a mission doctor in 1888. According to his account, the house had been built in the second half of the eighteenth century and served as a house of a "mulatto" slave trader before the Basel Mission acquired it in the 1840s. The Basel Mission first used the historic building as a missionary home, then converted it into a boys' school before it became a mission factory from 1867 to 1887. Eckhardt, who used the house as his home and medical practice, decided that the first room to be refurbished was the prayer hall, which he described in detail:

> The mission's workshop supplied a number of benches. Many colourful biblical pictures were hung on the previously bare walls. The mission factory in Accra donated a small harmonium and a few chairs for Europeans and black 'dignitaries'. A table, several hymnbooks and a chorale book were added, completing the prayer hall.[44]

This account illustrates that the Basel missionaries went to great lengths not only in establishing architectural structures for their evangelising ambitions but also in furnishing them. Missionaries believed, as Jean and John Comaroff have shown, that Christian homes figuratively constructed their inhabitants and that "their functionally specific spaces laid out the geometry of cleanliness and godliness."[45] The furniture, Bible pictures and music instrument in Eckhardt's description symbolised the elevating refinement of the missionary home, as did clocks, books and crockery in many other reports by Basel missionaries. They were emblems of European domesticity, which promised to materialise the ideal Christian home by imparting values of orderliness, cleanliness and civilisation.

The realisation of these Christian model homes in West Africa crucially depended on the support from women in Alemannic villages and towns,

---

[44] Eckhardt, Ärztliche Missionsarbeit in Christiansborg, p. 10.
[45] Comaroff/Comaroff, Ethnography and the Historical Imagination, p. 281.

who produced and supplied household items and clothes such as bed linen, towels, cleaning cloths, hats, socks, napkins, tablecloths, pillows, mirrors, tableware and irons.[46] The *Frauenverein zur Erziehung des weiblichen Geschlechts in den Heidenländern*—Society for the Education of the Female Gender in the Heathen Lands—which was founded as an aid organisation for the Basel Mission in 1841, served as a coordination office for all female support groups in Europe.[47] The society pooled resources for the furnishing of mission houses and schools abroad by compiling lists of the needed items and by giving exact manufacturing instructions for the required goods:

> We require fine and very uniform and tightly knit footwear. We ask the honoured associations not to get annoyed at this request because it is not based on weakness or luxury, but it is the hot, sweat-provoking climate of India and Africa that compels us to this request. Widely knitted stockings would expose the missionary to the torment of mosquito bites, which could make it impossible for him to walk.[48]

By producing specific goods, female supporters at home were given the impression that they could contribute directly to the success of the Basel Mission abroad. This gave them the opportunity to palpably trace the progress resulting from their generosity, creating a form of emotional attachment.[49]

---

[46] Prodolliet, Wider die Schamlosigkeit, p. 21–23.

[47] Initiated by the Basel Mission's second Inspector Wilhelm Hoffmann, the *Frauenverein* was made up of thirteen women, seven of which were wives of Committee members and six of their friends.

[48] Nachricht an die weiblichen Hilfsvereine der evangelischen Missionsgesellschaft zu Basel über die zweckmässigste Unterstützung derselben durch Naturalabgaben und Arbeiten, 14.03.1844, handwritten document, in: Prodolliet, Wider die Schamlosigkeit, p. 23.

[49] Patricia R. Hill, The World Their Household: The American Woman's Foreign Mission Movement and Cultural Transformation, 1870–1920, Ann Arbor 1985, p. 95; Altena, "Ein Häuflein Christen mitten in der Heidenwelt des dunklen Erdteils", p. 87; Ulrike Sill, Wie das Harmonium in die Hängematte kam: Ein Beispiel für den Wandel im Berichtswesen der Basler Mission im 19. Jahrhundert, in: Artur Bogner/ Bernd Holtwick/Hartmann Tyrell (eds.), Weltmission und religiöse Organisationen. Protestantische Missionsgesellschaften im 19. und 20. Jahrhundert, Würzburg 2004, p. 377–395.

The Committee outlined furniture regulations for both married and single missionaries, in which each item in the mission household was described precisely.[50] Even though the leaders in Basel maintained that missionaries should live modestly and surround themselves with basic amenities and unpretentious furniture, reflecting the ideal of Pietist asceticism, bourgeois living concepts clearly played an important role in the selection of home furnishings. A lot of the items in the furniture regulations such as a writing desk, a washbasin, curtains, children's beds, mirrors, carpets, wardrobes and book shelves can be attributed to a bourgeois lifestyle that would have been more comfortable than what most Basel missionaries were familiar with.[51]

In contrast to their staff, the Committee members were part of the Protestant bourgeoisie, who defined their class in terms of a family model based on the notion of separate spheres. Religiosity was gendered through an ideological division of men and women, the public and the private, which stipulated that men would communicate with the outside world while women would raise the young in the sheltered atmosphere of the home, inculcating in them basic moral and religious values.[52] People or families that did not follow this model were considered to fall out, or rather fall short, of this allegedly universal societal norm. Hence, the homes of the poor were besieged by benevolent visitors, pastors and city missionaries, all eager to judge and improve their apparently deviant private lives by the standard of the middle-class home.[53]

The core of the Basel Mission's project revolved around the Christian family, in which women and domesticity ultimately guaranteed the

---

[50] Mobiliarordnung, in: Verordnungen und Mitteilungen für die Missionare der Basler Mission, I.–XII. (1891–1900), 1901, BMA, ZS1.z.3004; Mobiliarordnung, in: Verordnungen und Mitteilungen für die Missionare der Basler Mission, XIII.–XX., Basel 1910; Mobiliarordnung für die Goldküste, 1902, BMA, D-9.1a.5.

[51] Andrea Hauser, Dinge des Alltags. Studien zur historischen Sachkultur eines schwäbischen Dorfes, Tübingen 1994, p. 154–157, 275–281; Konrad, Missionsbräute, p. 276–282.

[52] Hey emphasised that women were the "natural guardians of morals". Hey, Der Tropenarzt, 1st ed., p. 182.

[53] Frevert, "Fürsorgliche Belagerung"; Weisbrod, "Visiting" and "Social Control"; Friedrich/Jähnichen, Geschichte der sozialen Ideen im deutschen Protestantismus; Przyrembel, Verbote und Geheimnisse.

perpetuation of cleanliness and purity.[54] Evangelicals attributed the social question in the nineteenth century to an erosion of religious piety and family values in the lower classes. They diagnosed a lack of hygiene as both cause and symptom of social ills, which they addressed by propagating morals of hygiene and a Christian family model. Women were vested with responsibility for domestic upkeep, a task newly imbued with moral status, and their family's cleanliness, health and spiritual integrity.[55]

The regeneration of society through what appeared to evangelicals as the restoration of the family was embraced as a key concept in both home and foreign missions over the nineteenth century.[56] The domestic space was increasingly construed as a religious site residing within a feminine sphere of influence. In West Africa, the leaders of the Basel Mission recognised that the stability of the Christian family was crucial to the perpetuation of Christian villages and that women were simply indispensable for the creation and sustenance of such settlements.[57] Missionary wives not only worked as what was seen as their natural profession as spouse, housewife and mother, but also instructed African women and became teachers and principals at the girls' schools. Moreover, they assumed the management of the mission station, while their husbands were away on travel in remote areas to gain more parishioners.[58]

---

[54] On the role of marriage, family and children within Pietism, see Andreas Gestrich, Ehe, Familie, Kinder im Pietismus. Der "gezähmte Teufel", in: Hartmut Lehmann (ed.), Geschichte des Pietismus, vol 4: Glaubenswelt und Lebenswelten, Göttingen 2004, p. 499–521. On the early modern period in Basel, see Susanna Burghartz, Zeiten der Reinheit – Orte der Unzucht. Ehe und Sexualität in Basel während der Frühen Neuzeit, Paderborn 1999.

[55] Cleall, Missionary Discourses of Difference, p. 29–47; Hauser, German Religious Women in Late Ottoman Beirut, p. 114–118.

[56] Many researchers have shown that Protestant missionaries devoted considerable energy to writing about domesticity and constructing model homes. See selectively Comaroff/Comaroff, Home-Made Hegemony; Grimshaw, Faith, Missionary Life, and the Family; Dana L. Robert, The 'Christian Home' as a Cornerstone of Anglo-American Missionary Thought and Practice, in: ibid. (ed.), Converting Colonialism: Visions and Realities in Mission History, 1706–1914, Grand Rapids 2008, p. 134–165; Manktelow, Missionary Families; Maxwell, The Missionary Home as a Site for Mission.

[57] Predelli/Miller, Piety and Patriarchy, p. 78.

[58] The Christian home thus "provided a rationale for the participation of women in all aspects of mission work, including homemaking, evangelism, fund raising, teaching and even social reform", as Dana Robert and many others argued. Robert, The 'Christian Home' as a Cornerstone of Anglo-American Missionary Thought and Practice, p. 135.

With the arrival of more and more missionary wives, African males present within the private sphere of the home, such as chefs, servants and other staff, came to pose a threat to the gender-segregated order of Pietist life. The presumed sexual threat posed by male domestic workers, which was a recurrent colonial trope, led to the training of African women to replace them. Missionary wives taught African maids to prepare food, wash, sew and wipe the veranda. These domestic tasks, including cleaning, laundry, cooking and childcare, were increasingly seen as the sole and inherent province of women. Consequently, male domestics were more likely to be viewed as transgressive, though many of them continued to work in missionary households.[59]

The Committee gradually embraced the idea that missionary wives were better suited to reach African women than male missionaries, believing that they could break through the perceived seclusion of African women's lives and elevate them to promoters of Christianity. In 1900, the secretary of the Basel Mission, Friedrich Würz, recorded that a total of 150 missionary wives, 100 African and Indian female teachers and 30 Bible women contributed to propagating the gospel abroad.[60] In keeping with the gendered norms, by which Christian middle-class women were sheltered in the private sphere, non-European women were increasingly viewed as the key to their families' salvation, as Warneck expounded in his seminal study on evangelical mission:

> The female population is a very important factor in the Christianisation and civilisation of humanity; as housewife and mother she exerts a beneficial or pernicious influence, which cannot be appreciated highly enough, and the quality of women and mothers depends on the education of girls.[61]

Women were central to the conception of the civilising mission, for they were seen as vital allies in establishing new household norms, bodily practices and forms of piety. The Basel missionaries attached great importance to the specifics of women's education in West Africa because, in their view, it was their poor education and ignorance that made them adhere to heathenism. Christian women, by contrast, were believed to exercise

---

[59] Burke, Lifebuoy Men, Lux Women, p. 35–62; Cleall, Missionary Discourses of Difference, p. 48–73.

[60] Friedrich Würz, Aus der Basler Frauenmission, p. 3, BMA, N.181a.

[61] Warneck, Evangelische Missionslehre, p. 439.

a civilising influence on their children and thereby on future society. The Basel Mission's efforts in promoting knowledge of hygiene in West Africa, therefore, intersected with home economics and gendered forms of schooling.[62] These educational offers were aimed at generating new practices of domesticity and female behaviour in African communities, as this statement in the bulletin of the *Frauenverein* in 1891 illustrates:

> The girls must learn to wash, iron, sew, mend and keep the whole household orderly and clean. The heathen usually wears his clothes until it falls from his body, but a Christian has to become better herein. The girls need to be educated as guardians of manners and discipline.[63]

The goal of the Basel Mission's girls' schools, and female education more generally, was not to produce intellectual or academic women but to tend to the formation of a modest Christian character, very much in line with the concept of conservative Protestant girls' education in Europe at the time.[64] There was little ambiguity in the expressed norms governing the positions of women and men among Committee members, who continually defended the "divinely inspired patriarchy" of the organisation over which they presided.[65] Protestant mission leaders conceived of mission stations and schools as "surrogate domestic spaces where women could exert their beneficial influence protected from the outside world," as Julia Hauser argued for deaconesses in Late Ottoman Beirut.[66]

The Basel missionaries' urge to tidy up the perceived disorder around them clearly manifested itself in their efforts to introduce familiar housekeeping practices. The daily routine on the Basel Mission stations in

---

[62] The classes reserved for female pupils at the Basel Mission schools included sewing, cooking and home economics. There is a series of pictures of these classes in Aburi in the Basel Mission archives. Although undated, they have almost certainly been taken before 1914. See Hauswirtschafts-Unterricht mit Miss Charlotte Anoofo, Aburi, BMA, D-30.67.174; Handarbeits-Unterricht, Aburi, BMA, D-30.67.175; Koch-Unterricht Aburi, BMA, D-30.67.176.

[63] Basler Missionskomitee (ed.), Schreiben des Frauenvereins zu Basel für weibliche Erziehung in den Heidenländern. An die teuren Hilfsvereine in Deutschland und der Schweiz, Nr. 50, Basel 1891, p. 32.

[64] Hauser, German Religious Women in Late Ottoman Beirut, p. 207; Prodolliet, Wider die Schamlosigkeit, p. 52.

[65] Predelli/Miller, Piety and Patriarchy.

[66] Hauser, German Religious Women in Late Ottoman Beirut, p. 2.

West Africa resembled that of German boarding schools, partly that of the mission seminary in Basel, and included daily home and bodily care and a more thorough clean on Saturdays. The *württembergische Kehrwoche*—the structured cleaning of communal areas—with its roots in late fifteenth century Wurttemberg, aimed to improve household cleanliness. It continued to be practised by the Basel missionaries in West Africa, who insisted for the cleaning day to take place on Saturdays just as it did in their homeland. The weekly full bath recommended by proponents of the hygiene movement was scheduled twice a week in the Christian villages abroad.[67]

The Basel missionaries followed the Pietist principle of a "methodisation of life" in which every minute of every day was intended for a specific task. They attached great importance to "exploiting time," meaning for instance that awaking early amounted to a virtue while sleeping in was considered a disgraceful waste of time. The mission doctor Friedrich Hey called "modern idleness" a "disgrace" and considered work "the best life elixir and health remedy to stay exempt from many modern diseases."[68] Karl Huppenbauer, who started practising as a mission doctor in Aburi in 1914, praised the work of German missionary wives and contrasted their diligence with the ostensible idleness of English women:

> For women in the tropics, it is indeed no small matter to run the household as conscientiously as it has become second nature to every German missionary wife. Only if one compares this to the position and activity of most English women in the tropics, who spend their months of colonial boredom with getting up late, reading novels and drinking tea, one fully recognises the high-value work missionary wives provide.[69]

Huppenbauer's account shows that the Basel missionaries not only drew lines of differentiation between Europeans and Africans, or Christians and non-Christians, but also clearly tried to demarcate themselves from other European actors and lifestyles in the imperial arena. Because missionary designs of the Christian household were demonstrated by example, missionary wives were more likely than female colonial settlers

---

[67] Konrad, Missionsbräute, p. 292; Prodolliet, Wider die Schamlosigkeit, p. 57.

[68] Hey, Der Tropenarzt, 1st ed., p. 185.

[69] Karl Huppenbauer, Letter to Committee, 12.06.1914, Personal File Karl Huppenbauer, BMA, BV 2090.

to be considered essential personnel of the civilising mission. With their help, the Basel missionaries hoped to inculcate new models of hygiene, work and behaviour through the exemplary model of their own families, domestic arrangements and work ethic.

The struggle for what missionaries perceived as the reinvigoration of the Christian family among the poor at home and the heathens abroad was a transregional expression of Pietist purity efforts. Jean and John Comaroff notably referred to the dialectic of domesticity and suggested "that colonialism itself, and especially colonial evangelism, played a vital part in the formation of modern domesticity *both* in Britain and overseas; that each became a model for, a mirror image of, the other."[70] These findings, however, need to be differentiated to do justice to the protracted trials of purity and domesticity taking place in the Basel Mission's West African mission areas. Firstly, the Basel missionaries maintained that their Pietist approach to domesticity, work and behaviour were inherently superior to the worldly approach of colonial governments and settlers. Secondly, existing West African notions of domesticity not only persisted but also shaped the Basel Mission's agenda.

The Basel missionaries relied on an African workforce to practise hygiene as they intended. Only half of the male missionaries were accompanied by wives—most of whom were heavily engaged in teaching, nursing and evangelising—which made African domestic workers an indispensable component of missionary households. The functioning of the missionary family crucially depended on reliable nannies. Many children born to Basel missionaries in West Africa spoke little or no German at all, as Marie Wittwer-Lüthi's letter about her son Hans demonstrates: "He speaks like the Negro children, you wouldn't understand him."[71] The children's religious education took place in regional languages and many of them received West African names in addition to their European names.[72] Wittwer-Lüthi, a Bernese missionary wife in Cameroon from

---

[70] Comaroff/Comaroff, Ethnography and the Historical Imagination, p. 267.

[71] Marie Wittwer-Lüthi's biography and letters are found in: Marie Wittwer-Lüthi, Mutter und Missionarin, 27. September 1879 bis 7. Oktober 1955, BMA, QF-10.24.01. The letter containing this quote is not dated but classified under the period "Cameroon 1904–1914".

[72] Konrad, Schweizer Missionskinder des 19. Jahrhunderts, p. 172.

1904 to 1914, reported about her daughter: "Ndolo – Love – is Hanni's black name."[73]

African maids, teachers, medical assistants, porters and many others played a key role in keeping missionary spaces—schools, hospitals, homes—up to hygienic standards. African teachers taught the latest hygiene guidelines to their pupils in the Basel Mission schools, medical assistants kept hospitals clean and conveyed hygienic knowledge to their patients. Porters continued to carry missionaries in hammocks, particularly women, as this was considered to be the most hygienic means of transport, despite the arrival of the bicycle. Rather than merely executing the Basel Mission's plans, however, West Africans participated in creating new values and behaviours of hygiene by merging the Basel missionaries' views of purity with their own concepts of cleanliness, as this account published by the Basel Mission's Women's Society illustrates:

> On Saturday mornings, the school, veranda etc. are rigorously swept and the floor is coated with prepared cow dung, following the local method; this keeps the floor solid and prevents the white ants from digging it up. Thereupon, all Africans bathe in their bathroom by the well while rubbing themselves with a soapy mimosa fruit and then shower with water; the same also happens every Wednesday night; but on Saturdays the hair is washed as well, which is always a long business. [...] Lastly they receive fresh clothes for Sunday.[74]

This excerpt gives an impression of how regional ideas and practices of cleanliness in West Africa influenced the ways in which hygiene was implemented in the Basel Mission's salems. While the missionaries modelled schools, mission stations and Christian homes on their Pietist purity ideal, their aspirations had to be constantly adapted to the specific material environments and climatic conditions in West Africa, the disparity in

---

[73] Marie Wittwer-Lüthi, Mutter und Missionarin, 27. September 1879 bis 7. Oktober 1955, Cameroon 1904–1914, BMA, QF-10.24.01.

[74] Basler Missionskomitee (ed.), Schreiben des Frauenvereins zu Basel für weibliche Erziehung in den Heidenländern. An die teuren Hilfsvereine in Deutschland und der Schweiz, Nr. 13, Basel 1851, p. 12.

numbers between male and female missionaries and the persistence of African notions of domesticity.[75]

6.3 COMBATTING SPIRITS

The Blue Cross movement offers another example of how born-again Christians aspired to create safe havens, where the people they sought to protect would find shelter from the harmful consequences of modern life. Awakened laypeople founded the Blue Cross Society in Basel in 1882.[76] Twenty-five years later, the Basel Mission doctor Rudolf Fisch initiated the first Blue Cross Society in Aburi, thereby contributing to the formation of an abstinence network in West Africa.[77] He hoped to mobilise the African population against what he called the "schnapps flood" or "spirit plague" with organisations known as *Anidaho*—sobriety—in Twi. Spirits had been described as obstacles to the evangelisation of West Africa since the inception of missionary efforts in the area. However, complaints markedly increased from the 1880s, blaming alcoholism in the West African "gin belt"[78] on growing prosperity due to the cacao boom and the massive imports of cheap spirits from Europe.[79]

---

[75] Emily Lynn Osborn, Our New Husbands Are Here: Households, Gender, and Politics in a West African State from the Slave Trade to Colonial Rule, Athens 2011; Serena Owusua Dankwa, 'Shameless Maidens': Women's Agency and the Mission Project in Akuapem, in: Agenda. Empowering Women for Gender Equity 63 (2005) 2,2, p. 104–116.

[76] On the history of the abstinence movement in Basel, see Fabian Brändle/Hans Jakob Ritter, Zum Wohl! 100 Jahre Engagement für eine alkoholfreie Lebensweise, Basel 2010.

[77] Ghartey VI, who would later become King of the Winneba, established the first temperance society on the Gold Coast upon his return from England in 1862. See Emmanuel Kwaku Akyeampong, Drink, Power, and Cultural Change: A Social History of Alcohol in Ghana, c. 1800 to Recent Times, Oxford/Portsmouth 1996, p. 73.

[78] For a comprehensive history, see Dmitri van den Bersselaar, The King of Drinks: Schnapps Gin from Modernity to Tradition, Leiden/Boston 2007.

[79] The most influential German-speaking evangelical prohibitionists included Reinhold Grundemann, Zwei Bittschriften an den Reichskanzler betreffend die Beschränkung des Branntweinimports in Westafrika, in: Allgemeine Missionszeitschrift 12 (1885), p. 290–299, 348–350; Franz Michael Zahn, Der überseeische Branntweinhandel. Seine verderblichen Wirkungen und Vorschläge zur Beschränkung desselben, in: Allgemeine Missionszeitschrift 13 (1886), p. 9–39; Gustav Warneck, Der westafrikanische Branntwein-handel, in: Allgemeine Missionszeitschrift 13 (1886), p. 268–280.

In 1891, Alfred Eckhardt warned the readers of his popular account about the Gold Coast that the "century-long contact with 'Christian' whites has not only not bettered the blacks, but even made them worse. The bad example of the whites and their terrible gift, spirits, have added new vices to the old heathen ones."[80] Alcohol had been part of the earliest colonial expeditions to West Africa. Samuel Braun, the ship surgeon from Basel, already reported in 1624 that people on the Gold Coast "were eager" to exchange "a little firewater" with domestic goods.[81] It became increasingly customary for Europeans to gain the favour of Africans by offering or paying them with spirits. This approach was still popular with colonial officers and plantation owners in the twentieth century, drawing sharp criticism from members of the Basel Mission Committee.[82]

From the mid-nineteenth century, the flourishing European spirits industry discovered the West African market as a lucrative sales area.[83] Germany, most notably "synthetic wine producers" from Hamburg, became a hub for the production and export of trade spirits. The schnapps export from Hamburg to West Africa saw a fourfold increase between 1874 and 1884.[84] Within a few decades, the booming West African trade consisted mainly of an exchange of African natural products with European spirits, weapons and gunpowder. By the 1890s, about 30 to 40 million litres of high-proof alcohol were exported from Europe and America to the west coast of Africa yearly. Germany was by far the market leader, accounting for 75 per cent of spirits imports in its own colonial

---

[80] Alfred Eckhardt, Die Basler Mission auf der Goldküste, in: O. Frick (ed.), Geschichten und Bilder aus der Mission, vol. 10, Halle 1891, p. 3–19, here p. 12.

[81] Samuel Braun, Des Wundarztes und Burgers zu Basels Schiffarten, Basel 1624, p. 72.

[82] Hermann Christ, Über die Wirkung des Alkohols in den Gebieten der evangelischen Heidenmission, in: Evangelisches Missionsmagazin 39 (1895), p. 505–510; Ibid., Die Wirkungen des Alkohols in den Gebieten der evangelischen Mission, in: Bericht über den V. Internationalen Kongress zur Bekämpfung des Missbrauchs geistiger Getränke, Basel 1895, p. 156–161.

[83] Leonhard Harding, Hamburg's West Africa Trade in the Nineteenth Century, in: Gerhard Liesegang/Helma Pasch/Adam Jones (eds.), Figuring African Trade, Berlin 1986, p. 363–391.

[84] Norbert Schröder, Hamburgs Schnapsfabrikanten und der deutsche Kolonialismus in Westafrika, in: Zeitschrift des Vereins für Hamburgische Geschichte 76 (1990), p. 83–116, here p. 91–92.

territories and 57 per cent in British colonies in West Africa.[85] The rapid expansion of spirits imports into West Africa even troubled a number of colonial officials, who typically downplayed its impact.[86]

Most of the captains and traders refused to drink the spirits they were exporting to West Africa due to the poor quality of the product. They suspected that the costly process of removing the harmful fusel oils had been skipped to cut production costs. The Basel missionary Christian Graf, based in Cameroon, described the imported drink as follows: "Its dark brown appearance, its acrid smell and its corrosiveness do not bode well. It is so pungent that it was impossible for me to hold a few drops in the palm of my hand. Europeans use it instead of ethanol to preserve killed snakes."[87] He concluded that the "fire water" would purely benefit traders, governments and farm owners, eventually leading to the extinction of "the Negro" just like it had done with the "Indians of North America".[88] Comparisons between "native races" in different colonial settings was a common feature not only of missionary discourse but also of the emerging temperance movement, which emphasised the vulnerability of Africans and other "native peoples" to distilled spirits.[89]

Many prohibitionist organisations, such as the Blue Cross founded in Geneva in 1877, had common roots and maintained close links with evangelical groups.[90] The Blue Cross in Basel arose at the initiative of fervent Protestants, many of whom were involved with the Basel Mission. The Committee member Hermann Christ, most prominently, was an active

---

[85] Akin Olorunfemi, German Trade with British West African Colonies, 1895–1918, in: Journal of African Studies 8 (1981) 3, p. 111–120, here p. 115.

[86] Charles Ambler, The Drug Empire: The Control of Drugs in Africa. A Global Perspective, in: Gernot Klantschnig/Neil Carrier/Charles Ambler (eds.), Drugs in Africa: Histories and Ethnographies of Use, Trade, and Control, New York 2014, p. 25–47.

[87] Christian Graf, Palmwein oder Branntwein? in: Afrika 2 (1895), p. 234.

[88] Ibid.

[89] Charles Ambler, The Specter of Degeneration. Alcohol and Race in West Africa in the Early Twentieth Century, in: Jessica R. Pliley/Robert Kramm/Harald Fischer-Tiné (eds.), Global Anti-Vice Activism, 1890–1950. Fighting Drinks, Drugs, and "Immorality", Cambridge 2016, p. 103–123.

[90] The Christian organisation became a loosely organised International Federation in 1886. The society in Aburi was the first non-European Blue Cross Society to join the International Federation of the Blue Cross in 1907. See Francesco Spöring, Mission und Sozialhygiene. Schweizer Anti-Alkohol-Aktivismus im Kontext von Internationalismus und Kolonialismus, 1886–1939, Doctoral Thesis, ETH Zurich, 2014, p. 34.

founding member of the Blue Cross in Basel and member of the *Schweizerische Zentralstelle für die Bekämpfung des Alkoholismus*—Swiss Central Office for Combatting Alcoholism.[91] The Blue Cross Society is one of oldest and most radical anti-alcoholism societies in Switzerland to this day. While many other organisations focussed on information campaigns and education policies, the Blue Cross addressed the social question more broadly by engaging in poverty relief work.[92]

The *Gesellschaft für das Gute und Gemeinnützige (GGG)* became another vessel for the advancement of the prohibitionist cause. As president of the *GGG* and director of the Basel *Bürgerspital* between 1851 and 1867, the physician and popular writer Theodor Meyer-Merian led many of the early campaigns. He was a fierce advocate of the hygiene movement and argued that virtues such as cleanliness and order had a positive impact on health and prosperity.[93] Karl Sarasin, member of the *GGG* and the Basel Mission board, took on these efforts once Meyer-Merian had passed. During his tenure as the president of the Commission for the Conditions of Factory Workers in the *GGG* from 1878 to 1882, he launched a competition in which he called for the submission of an educational pamphlet on the subject of *"gegen das Wirtshaus"*—"against the pub." The winner of the competition, the Basel school inspector Traugott Siegfried, had submitted a piece on *"Das Wirtshaus,"* which was published as a book in 1881 and distributed in working-class areas.[94]

---

[91] For a critical history of Swiss alcohol policy, see Juri Auderset/Peter Moser, Rausch und Ordnung. Eine illustrierte Geschichte der Alkoholfrage, der schweizerischen Alkoholpolitik und der Eidgenössischen Alkoholverwaltung (1887–2015), Bern 2016.

[92] Markus Mattmüller, Basler Blaukreuzgeschichte – ein Kapitel Basler Sozial- und Kirchengeschichte, in: Blaues Kreuz Basel (ed.), Bleibender Auftrag. Vorbeugen – helfen – heilen: 100 Jahre Blaues Kreuz Basel 1882–1982, Basel 1982, p. 4–22.

[93] Regula Zürcher, Gegen den "Sumpf des selbstverschuldeten Elends". Antialkoholbewegung und Armutsbekämpfung im 19. Jahrhundert, in: Josef Mooser/Simon Wenger (eds.), Armut und Fürsorge in Basel. Armutspolitik vom 13. Jahrhundert bis heute, Basel 2011, p. 123–132, here p. 127.

[94] Traugott Siegfried, Das Wirtshaus. Von der Gemeinnützigen Gesellschaft der Stadt Basel ausgeschriebene und gekrönte Preisschrift, Basel 1881.

Basel's temperance movement, supported by a broad coalition of patricians, scientists and Pietists, proved quite successful.[95] From the mid-nineteenth century, the city saw the creation of eating houses, where no alcohol was served, and the first completely alcohol-free restaurant *Kaffeehalle zu Schmieden* opened in the early 1880s on the initiative of the *GGG*. With growing pressure from the sobriety lobby, politicians in Basel also drafted new restaurant laws, regulating the consumption of alcohol.[96] These efforts, however, did not go far enough for radical prohibitionists, who began to grow in number in the late 1880s. They demanded total abstinence and accused the temperance movement of not addressing the root of the problem because it merely fought schnapps and not fermented beverages such as wine, beer and ciders. The Basel Professor for Physiological Chemistry, Gustav von Bunge, was a leading exponent of this view in Switzerland and beyond.[97]

The concern for alcoholism of the lower classes in Basel was mirrored in the growing apprehension of alcoholism among the people in the colonies.[98] The Basel Mission came to play an active role in the political struggle for regulations on alcohol imports into the West African "gin belt" from 1885. Disappointed by the outcome of the Congo Conference in Berlin, the Basel Mission, together with its affiliated trading company, addressed a petition to the German chancellor Otto von Bismarck in April of 1885, asking him to take government action against the liquor trade

[95] In 1904, 1300 people formed a cantonal abstinence association in Basel. Approximately, 6 per cent of the city's population were members of the movement by 1913 compared to 2.5 per cent in Switzerland. Brändle/Ritter, Zum Wohl!, p. 102.

[96] Zürcher, Gegen den "Sumpf des selbstverschuldeten Elends", p. 128.

[97] Bunge's inaugural lecture at the University of Basel *Die Alkoholfrage* in 1886 was published in several editions and various languages. It gained wide international recognition in radical prohibitionist circles. Markus Mattmüller, Der Kampf gegen den Alkoholismus in der Schweiz. Ein unbekanntes Kapitel der Sozialgeschichte im 19. Jahrhundert, Bern 1979, p. 30.

[98] Historians have identified two schnapps waves sweeping through Switzerland: the first one following the Napoleonic wars in 1815 and the second one in the 1870s, when freedom of trade was anchored in the amended federal constitution of 1874, which led to a sharp increase in the number of alcohol distributors. See Jakob Tanner, Die "Alkoholfrage" in der Schweiz im 19. und 20. Jahrhundert, in: Hermann Fahrenkrug (ed.), Zur Sozialgeschichte des Alkohols in der Neuzeit Europas, Lausanne 1986, p. 147–168.

with Africa.[99] The *Norddeutsche Missionsgesellschaft* and other mission societies composed similar petitions a few months later and the Continental Conference of Evangelical Mission Societies in Bremen made a joint appeal to the German public in late October 1885.[100]

A range of Protestant missionary societies, including the Basel Mission, as well as the German Blue Cross and the German Society Against the Abuse of Spirituous Beverages, created the Commission for the Control of the African Spirits Trade, at the suggestion of the *Evangelischer Afrika-Verein*—Evangelical Africa Association—in 1896. The Commission reached out to like-minded groups in other European countries, such as the Native Races and the Liquor Traffic United Committee based in Great Britain, with the ultimate aim to completely ban the export of spirits to the colonies. Testimonials by missionaries about the implications of the spirits trade in different areas in West Africa were printed as a series in *Afrika*, the journal of the Evangelical Africa Association, and distributed to members of the German Colonial Council as an offprint.[101]

The Commission for the Control of the African Spirits Trade submitted several petitions to the Reich Chancellor and the Colonial Department of the Foreign Office, demanding for restrictions to be placed on the alcohol trade with the colonies.[102] The importance of the spirits trade for German commerce and agriculture meant that the members of the Colonial Council, among them spirits traders, initially dismissed these petitions. Over the years, however, the German government came to

---

[99] The petition was also printed in *Der Evangelische Heidenbote*. See Anonymous, Eine Eingabe, in: Der Evangelische Heidebote 58 (1885), p. 33–34.

[100] The appeal appeared in *Der Evangelische Heidenbote*. See Anonymous, Erklärung der Konferenz der deutschen evangelischen Missions-Gesellschaften in Sachen des Branntweinhandels mit den Kolonien, in: Der Evangelische Heidenbote 58 (1885), p. 90–91.

[101] Anonymous, Der Branntwein in Afrika. Berichte von deutschen evangelischen Missionaren, Offprint of Afrika 4 (1897).

[102] Anonymous, Die Eingabe an den Reichskanzler, 14.08.1896, in: Afrika 3 (1896), p. 169–173; Anonymous, Eingabe der Kommission zur Bekämpfung des afrikanischen Branntweinhandels an den deutschen Kolonialrat, 26.10.1897, in: Gustav Müller, Der Kampf gegen den afrikanischen Branntweinhandel, in: Afrika 5 (1898), p. 169–178; Gustav Müller, Bericht über die Thätigkeit der Kommission zur Bekämpfung des Afrikanischen Branntweinhandels, in: Afrika 8 (1901), p. 81–83; Anonymous, Eingabe der Kommission zur Bekämpfung des afrikanischen Branntweinhandels, in: Afrika 15 (1908), p. 14–15; Gustav Müller, Bericht über die Thätigkeit der Kommission zur Bekämpfung des Afrikanischen Branntweinhandels, in: Afrika 17 (1910), p. 1–4.

rethink the role of the spirits trade in its African "protectorates."[103] The Basel missionaries, who were well connected to various civil society organisations through their headquarters in Basel, constituted an important source of information about the alleged destitution caused by alcoholism in West Africa.[104]

Articles by Basel missionaries active in the temperance and abstinence movements found their way into widely circulated anti-alcohol periodicals. The Blue Cross published a wide range of magazines, including *Der Illustrierte Arbeiterfreund* and the *Arbeiterfreund-Kalender*, which were addressed to large sections of the population and enjoyed great approval, not just in Switzerland but also in Germany and Austria-Hungary.[105] Most articles dealing with the alcohol situation in Africa in the *Illustrierte Arbeiterfreund* originated from missionary magazines such as the Basel Mission's *Der Evangelische Heidenbote*. They included missionary reports and photographs, told success stories of converted African teetotallers and praised education methods used by Basel missionaries in their anti-alcohol struggle.[106]

In 1908, the German Chancellor Bernhard von Bülow presented a memorandum to the Reichstag on "*Alkohol und Eingeborenenpolitik,*" in which he adopted most of the positions of the Commission for the Control of the African Spirits Trade.[107] A pivotal argument in his reasoning was the economic concern that the spirits trade would destroy the labour force and purchasing power of the African population. The newly appointed Governor of Cameroon, Theodor Seitz, became a stout advocate of a total ban of the spirits trade in the colonies.[108] The

---

[103] Dietrich Döpp, Humanitäre Abstinenz oder Priorität des Geschäfts? Die Diskussion um die Legitimität des kolonialen Alkoholhandels in der deutschen Öffentlichkeit (1885–1914), in: Horst Gründer (ed.), Geschichte und Humanität, Münster/Hamburg 1994, p. 121–135.

[104] Spöring, Mission und Sozialhygiene, p. 72.

[105] Rolf Trechsel, Die Geschichte der Abstinenzbewegung in der Schweiz im 19. und frühen 20. Jahrhundert, Lausanne 1990, p. 31–45.

[106] Spöring, Mission und Sozialhygiene, p. 320.

[107] Bernhard von Bülow, Alkohol und Eingeborenenpolitik. Bekämpfung des Alkoholkonsums in den afrikanischen Kolonien: Denkschrift an den Reichstag (817), 1908, BMA, J.77.

[108] Susan Diduk, European Alcohol, History, and the State in Cameroon, in: African Studies Review 36 (1993) 1, p. 1–42.

Basel missionaries in Cameroon were now perceived as valuable allies in the struggle against alcoholism. They founded a soda water and lemonade factory, which according to the official German medical reports, contributed to the "reduction in consumption of alcoholic beverages" in Cameroon.[109]

Over the next years, some Basel missionaries markedly increased their anti-alcohol activism in West Africa. They toured villages, parishes and mission schools to campaign for alcohol abstention by giving lectures and displaying slideshows on their magic lanterns.[110] Rudolf Fisch wrote a series of pamphlets in Twi to propagate prohibitionist ideas and practices among the population in Aburi and founded the *Anidaho* society in January of 1907.[111] After the society's initial meeting, the mission doctor met with a group of 28 male parishioners, who had come to listen to his speech on the detriments of alcohol and the emergence of Blue Cross Societies in Europe. Fisch proposed that they make abstinence vows for an initial period of four months.[112] The mission doctor was the first to take the oath, followed by pastor Korang, catechist Ofei and the parish elder Obeng, reciting:

> I promise in front of my brothers that from today I will not drink any intoxicating drink for four months. So help me God. I will fight against the drinking of intoxicating drinks among my friends and brothers. The wine for Holy Communion is exempt. If I break my vows and drink intoxicating drink again, I will return my commitment card and any society badges to the board of this society.[113]

[109] Reichskolonialamt (ed.), Medizinal-Berichte über die Deutschen Schutzgebiete Deutsch-Ostafrika, Kamerun, Togo, Deutsch-Südwestafrika, Neu-Guinea, Karolinen, Marshall-Inseln und Samoa für das Jahr 1903/1904, Berlin 1905, p. 141.

[110] Veit Arlt, Christianity, Imperialism and Culture: The Expansion of the Two Krobo States in Ghana, c. 1830 to 1930, Basel 2005, p. 187.

[111] The first pamphlet on "Mmorosa ne n'adwuma" – "Schnapps and Its Effects" appeared in 5000 Twi copies: D-1.88.22b. More pamphlets followed, see BMA D-1.88.22h.

[112] Rudolf Fisch, First Annual Report on the Blue Cross Societies on the Gold Coast, 1908, BMA, D-1.88.22k.7.

[113] Rudolf Fisch, Zum Kampf gegen die Trunksucht, 1907, p. 4, BMA J.078c. The Basel Mission archives also hold a specimen of the certificate in Twi: BMA, D-1.88.22e.

The weekly meetings of the Blue Cross Society in Aburi had a litur-
gical character with church bells signalling the start, followed by an
opening hymn and prayer.[114] Fisch composed a hymnbook for abstainers
containing 32 *Anidaho* songs for this purpose.[115] The association's
members decided to introduce a 10-penny fine for unexcused absences
during assemblies and made regular donations. Despite this financial
burden, more and more Africans took an interest in the organisation,
among them an increasing number of women.[116] Concerned about the
mixing of men and women, Fisch convinced the Committee to establish
a separate society for women and girls, which was headed by the Swiss
teacher Hanna Brugger.[117] Alcoholism, however, was seen as a problem
affecting the male population by and large, in contrast to many other
hygiene issues.[118]

To campaign for the creation of additional Blue Cross Societies,
members of the Aburi association organised a range of *Anidaho* excur-
sions to Apasare, Dodowa, Asantema, Mampong, Akropong, Krobo,
Bama, Odumase und Akuse in the spring of 1907 (Fig. 6.2).[119]
According to Fisch, he and his fellow campaigners entered villages
with "powerful singing" and in "good order" before propagating their
message during a sermon.[120] At the end of 1907, Fisch reported that
a total of 20 Blue Cross Societies in 18 different towns, counting 958
members, had seen the light of day on the Gold Coast.[121]

Fisch attached special importance to the flag of the Blue Cross Society
in Aburi, bearing the imprint *"Gin ne mmorosa di owu dwuma"*—"Gin
and Rum are on Death's Payroll."[122] He urged the members not to use

---

[114] The statutes of the Blue Cross Society were recorded in Twi: Twi man mu anidaho
feku, Akropong 1907, BMA, D.II.g.7b.

[115] Rudolf Fisch, Anidaho-Nnwom Twi Kasa Mu – Hymn-Book for Abstainers in the
Tshi-Language, Basel 1907, BMA, D.II.b.20.

[116] Fisch, First Annual Report on the Blue Cross Societies on the Gold Coast, p. 5.

[117] Personal File Hanna Brugger, BMA, SV 32.

[118] Akyeampong, Drink, Power and Cultural Change, p. xxi.

[119] Rudolf Fisch, The Aburi Society visiting Apasare. The Blue Cross Society Aburi on
trek with Dr. Fisch, 1885/1911, BMA, QW-30.006.0010.

[120] Fisch, First annual report on the Blue Cross Societies on the Gold Coast, p. 6.

[121] Ibid., p. 18–19; Fischer, Der Missionsarzt Rudolf Fisch, S. 382–389.

[122] Fisch, First Annual Report on the Blue Cross Societies on the Gold Coast, p. 12.

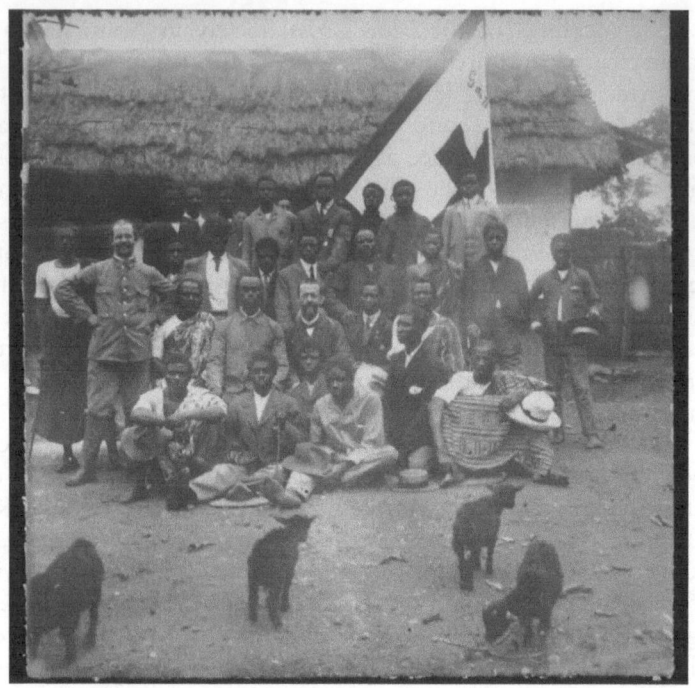

Fig. 6.2 Rudolf Fisch, The Aburi Society visiting Apasare. The Blue Cross Society Aburi on trek with Dr. Fisch, 1885/1911, BMA, QW-30.006.0010

the flag as a toy or load but to appreciate it as a representation of the society's honour. Objects such as the flag helped Fisch to combine adherence to the Blue Cross Society—a demarcated, ostensibly pure space—with social prestige. Members who had kept their vows for eight months were given a label pin in form of a blue cross. This "badge of honour," according to Fisch, had to be worn visibly and was highly coveted among the people in Aburi. It rewarded the compliant behaviour of a member and symbolised their perseverance and ideological affiliation.[123]

[123] Ibid., p. 6.

Fisch's fervent commitment earned him respect from eminent teetotallers such as his "highly venerated teacher" Gustav von Bunge.[124] However, his radical emphasis on abstinence rather than temperance placed him at odds with many of his missionary colleagues. Although a quarter of the Basel missionaries were members of the Blue Cross in 1913, they tolerated moderate consumption of beer, wine and palm wine, as well as African drinking practices during ceremonies such as obsequies.[125] Contrary to the dominant opinion among his fellow missionaries, Fisch argued that any type of alcohol caused grievous bodily harm, reduced fecundity, increased infant mortality and decimated the population in West Africa.[126]

The leadership in Basel merely recommended abstinence as an "evangelical advice" and for "health's sake" but did not make it an obligation.[127] Nonetheless, "without taking a stand on the question of abstinence at home or somehow impairing the moral freedom of the individual," they cautioned the missionaries that "even very small quantities of spirituous beverages" would have an "impact on the nervous system in the tropics, as only occurs with larger alcohol intake in our climate." Another aspect to consider, according to the Basel Mission's regulations, was "the influence of the missionaries' example on the native personnel, communities and heathens."[128] The consumption of spirits on the Basel Mission's premises in West Africa was therefore banned for both Africans and Europeans. The debate about alcoholism in the colonies was an arena in which competing values and visions of what it meant to be European and civilised played out.[129]

---

[124] Rudolf Fisch, Wirkungen des Schnapshandels in Westafrika, in: Internationale Monatsschrift 5 (1914), p. 145–155, here p. 150.

[125] In the early 1850s, the Basel missionaries had even planted vineyards in Akropong. See Spöring, Mission und Sozialhygiene, p. 73.

[126] Rudolf Fisch, Die bedrohte schwarze Rasse, in: Der Evangelische Heidenbote 86 (1913), p. 168–169.

[127] Verordnungen über die persönliche Stellung der Missionare, Basel 1914, p. 29, BMA, Q-09.26.

[128] Ibid.

[129] James H. Mills/Patricia Barton, Introduction, in: ibid. (eds.) Drugs and Empires. Essays in Modern Imperialism and Intoxication, c. 1500–c. 1930, Basingstoke 2007, p. 1–16.

With pressure intensifying from humanitarian and missionary lobbies, successive international agreements banned the production of spirits in West Africa, forbade their importation into the large zones where trade had not yet been extended, and imposed progressively higher duties in areas where the spirits trade already existed.[130] The Basel Mission introduced modules on the dangers of alcohol in their West African schools from 1907.[131] In a circular letter a few years later, the Committee urged all missionaries in Cameroon and on the Gold Coast to report on alcoholism in their areas and to propose appropriate countermeasures.[132]

The Basel missionaries tried to prevent the dilution of their Pietist beliefs and practices by punishing transgressions with exclusion from the Christian community. They expected that the strict enforcement of parish discipline would not only improve the individual sinner but also enhance the cohesion and integrity of their congregations. Parish exclusions constituted a key tool for upholding Pietist purity in West Africa between 1885 and 1914. The parishes in Cameroon, for example, counted a total of 8,882 members in 1910, of which 421 had been expelled by the end of the year. 260 of those excluded were re-admitted as parishioners after acknowledging their wrongdoing and promising to improve.[133] The ideal of purity could only be maintained in the long run if there were spaces where it was still visibly valid.[134] Therefore, the Basel missionaries aspired to create pure spaces in the form of Christian villages, domestic safe havens and sobriety societies.

---

[130] The Blue Cross Federation, the German Order of Good Templars and ten mission societies, including the Basel Mission, founded the *Deutsche Verband zur Bekämpfung des afrikanischen Branntweinhandels*—German Society for the Combat of the African Liquor Trade—in 1910, which replaced the Commission for the Control of the African Spirits Trade. Fischer, Der Missionsarzt Rudolf Fisch, p. 393–396.

[131] Wilhelm Rottmann, Über die Alkoholfrage in den Schulen, 13.05.1907, BMA, D-1.89.36; Committee report, 07.03.1907, BMA, Komitee-Protokoll 1907, §193; Committee report, 20.11.1907, BMA, Komitee-Protokoll 1907, § 1132.

[132] Circular letter to all stations on the Gold Coast and in Cameroon, 02.12.1913, BMA, D-9.2b.8a; Reports on the alcohol question, Cameroon, 1914, BMA, E-10.15.

[133] Walter Oettli, Gegenwärtige Missionsprobleme der Basler Mission in Kamerun, Basel 1911, p. 39–40, BMA, E. 28.

[134] Udo Simon, Why Purity? An Introduction, in: Petra Rösch/Udo Simon (eds.), How Purity is Made, Wiesbaden 2012, p. 1–37, here p. 4.

REFERENCES

Sonia Abun-Nasr, Afrikaner und Missionar. Die Lebensgeschichte von David Asante, Basel 2013.

Emmanuel Kwaku Akyeampong, Drink, Power, and Cultural Change: A Social History of Alcohol in Ghana, c. 1800 to Recent Times, Oxford/Portsmouth 1996.

Thorsten Altena, "Ein Häuflein Christen mitten in der Heidenwelt des dunklen Erdteils." Zum Selbst- und Fremdverständnis protestantischer Missionare im kolonialen Afrika 1884–1918, Münster 2003.

Charles Ambler, The Drug Empire: The Control of Drugs in Africa. A Global Perspective, in: Gernot Klantschnig/Neil Carrier/Charles Ambler (eds.), Drugs in Africa: Histories and Ethnographies of Use, Trade, and Control, New York 2014, p. 25–47.

Charles Ambler, The Specter of Degeneration. Alcohol and Race in West Africa in the Early Twentieth Century, in: Jessica R. Pliley/Robert Kramm/Harald Fischer-Tiné (eds.), Global Anti-Vice Activism, 1890–1950. Fighting Drinks, Drugs, and "Immorality", Cambridge 2016, p. 103–123.

Anonymous, Eine Eingabe, in: Der Evangelische Heidebote 58 (1885), p. 33–34.

Anonymous, Eingabe der Kommission zur Bekämpfung des afrikanischen Branntweinhandels an den deutschen Kolonialrat, 26.10.1897, in: Gustav Müller, Der Kampf gegen den afrikanischen Branntweinhandel, in: Afrika 5 (1898), p. 169–178.

Anonymous, Blicke in die Thätigkeit unserer Missionsärzte, in: Der Evangelische Heidenbote 71 (1898), p. 46–47.

Anonymous, Erklärung der Konferenz der deutschen evangelischen Missions-Gesellschaften in Sachen des Branntweinhandels mit den Kolonien, in: Der Evangelische Heidenbote 58 (1885), p. 90–91.

Anonymous, Die Eingabe an den Reichskanzler, 14.08.1896, in: Afrika 3 (1896), p. 169–173.

Anonymous, Der Branntwein in Afrika. Berichte von deutschen evangelischen Missionaren, Offprint of Afrika 4 (1897).

Anonymous, Eingabe der Kommission zur Bekämpfung des afrikanischen Branntweinhandels, in: Afrika 15 (1908), p. 14–15.

Veit Arlt, Christianity, Imperialism and Culture: The Expansion of the Two Krobo States in Ghana, c. 1830 to 1930, Basel 2005.

Juri Auderset/Peter Moser, Rausch und Ordnung. Eine illustrierte Geschichte der Alkoholfrage, der schweizerischen Alkoholpolitik und der Eidgenössischen Alkoholverwaltung (1887–2015), Bern 2016.

Basler Missionskomitee (ed.), Schreiben des Frauenvereins zu Basel für weibliche Erziehung in den Heidenländern. An die teuren Hilfsvereine in Deutschland und der Schweiz, Nr. 13, Basel 1851.

Basler Missionskomitee (ed.), Schreiben des Frauenvereins zu Basel für weibliche Erziehung in den Heidenländern. An die teuren Hilfsvereine in Deutschland und der Schweiz, Nr. 50, Basel 1891.

Basler Missionskomitee (ed.), Unsere ärztliche Mission. Bericht vom Jahr 1897, Basel 1898.

Hartmut Beck, Die Herrnhuter Baukultur im pietistischen Zeitalter des 18. Jahrhunderts, in: Kunst und Kirche 50 (1987) 3, p. 186–189.

Fabian Brändle/Hans Jakob Ritter, Zum Wohl! 100 Jahre Engagement für eine alkoholfreie Lebensweise, Basel 2010.

Samuel Braun, Des Wundarztes und Burgers zu Basels Schiffarten, Basel 1624.

Walter Bruchhausen, Medicine Between Religious Worlds: The Mission Hospitals of South-East Tanzania During the Twentieth Century, in: Mark Harrison/ Margaret Jones/Helen Sweet (eds.), From Western Medicine to Global Medicine. The Hospital Beyond the West, Hyderabad 2009, p. 172–192.

Susanna Burghartz, Zeiten der Reinheit – Orte der Unzucht. Ehe und Sexualität in Basel während der Frühen Neuzeit, Paderborn 1999.

Timothy Burke, Lifebuoy Men, Lux Women. Commodification, Consumption and Cleanliness in Modern Zimbabwe, Durham/London 1996.

Hermann Christ, Die Wirkungen des Alkohols in den Gebieten der evangelischen Mission, in: Bericht über den V. Internationalen Kongress zur Bekämpfung des Missbrauchs geistiger Getränke, Basel 1895, p. 156–161.

Hermann Christ, Über die Wirkung des Alkohols in den Gebieten der evangelischen Heidenmission, in: Evangelisches Missionsmagazin 39 (1895), p. 505–510.

Esme Cleall, Missionary Discourses of Difference. Negotiating Otherness in the British Empire, Basingstoke 2012.

John Comaroff/Jean Comaroff, Ethnography and the Historical Imagination, Boulder 1992.

John Comaroff/Jean Comaroff, Home-Made Hegemony: Modernity, Domesticity, and Colonialism in South Africa, in: Karen Tranberg Hansen (ed.), African Encounters with Domesticity, New Brunswick 1992, p. 37–74.

Serena Owusua Dankwa, 'Shameless Maidens': Women's Agency and the Mission Project in Akuapem, in: Agenda. Empowering Women for Gender Equity 63 (2005) 2, p. 104–116.

Susan Diduk, European Alcohol, History, and the State in Cameroon, in: African Studies Review 36 (1993) 1, p. 1–42.

Dietrich Döpp, Humanitäre Abstinenz oder Priorität des Geschäfts? Die Diskussion um die Legitimität des kolonialen Alkoholhandels in der deutschen Öffentlichkeit (1885–1914), in: Horst Gründer (ed.), Geschichte und Humanität, Münster/Hamburg 1994, p. 121–135.

Alfred Eckhardt, Ärztliche Missionsarbeit in Christiansborg, in: An die Freunde des Ärztlichen Zweiges der Basler Mission, Basel 1891, p. 8–19.

Alfred Eckhardt, Die Basler Mission auf der Goldküste, in: O. Frick (ed.), Geschichten und Bilder aus der Mission, vol. 10, Halle 1891, p. 3–19.

Alfred Eckhardt, Häuserbau in Westafrika und die Station Ho, in: Deutsche Kolonialzeitung 4 (1891), p. 43–46.

Alfred Eckhardt, Ein Arbeitsjahr in Odumase (Goldküste), in: An die Freunde des Ärztlichen Zweiges der Basler Mission, Basel 1893, p. 5–11.

Alfred Eckhardt, Land, Leute und ärztliche Mission auf der Goldküste, Basel 1894.

Tarikhu Farrar, Building Technology and Settlement Planning in a West African Civilization: Precolonial Akan Cities and Towns, Lewiston 1996.

Rudolf Fisch, Tropische Krankheiten. Anleitung zu ihrer Verhütung und Behandlung speziell für die Westküste von Afrika, für Missionare, Kaufleute, Pflanzer und Beamte, 1st ed., Basel 1891; 2nd ed., Basel 1894; 3rd ed., Basel 1903; 4th ed., Basel 1912.

Rudolf Fisch, Meine erste Motorradfahrt, in: Der Evangelische Heidenbote 78 (1905), p. 79–80.

Rudolf Fisch, Aus einer afrikanischen Poliklinik, in: Der Evangelische Heidenbote 79 (1906), p. 44.

Rudolf Fisch, Die bedrohte schwarze Rasse in: Der Evangelische Heidenbote 86 (1913), p. 168–169.

Rudolf Fisch, Wirkungen des Schnapshandels in Westafrika, in: Internationale Monatsschrift 5 (1914), p. 145–155.

Rudolf Fisch, Vierzig Jahre ärztliche Mission auf der Goldküste, in: Deutsches Institut für ärztliche Mission Tübingen (ed.), Die deutsche evangelische ärztliche Mission nach dem Stand des Jahres 1928, Stuttgart 1928, p. 16–27.

Friedrich Hermann Fischer, Der Missionsarzt Rudolf Fisch und die Anfänge medizinischer Arbeit der Basler Mission an der Goldküste (Ghana), Herzogenrath 1991.

Ute Frevert, "Fürsorgliche Belagerung": Hygienebewegung und Arbeiterfrauen im 19. und frühen 20. Jahrhundert, in: Geschichte und Gesellschaft 11 (1985) 4, p. 420–446.

Norbert Friedrich/Traugott Jähnichen, Geschichte der sozialen Ideen im deutschen Protestantismus, in: Helga Grebing (ed.), Geschichte der sozialen Ideen in Deutschland. Sozialismus – katholische Soziallehre – protestantische Sozialethik. Ein Handbuch, 2nd ed., Wiesbaden 2005, p. 867–1102.

Andreas Gestrich, Alltag im pietistischen Dorf: Bürgerliche Religiosität in ländlicher Lebenswelt, in: Die Alte Stadt 20 (1993) 1, p. 47–59.

Andreas Gestrich, Ehe, Familie, Kinder im Pietismus. Der "gezähmte Teufel", in: Hartmut Lehmann (ed.), Geschichte des Pietismus, vol 4: Glaubenswelt und Lebenswelten, Göttingen 2004, p. 499–521.

Christian Graf, Palmwein oder Branntwein? in: Afrika 2 (1895), p. 234.

Patricia Grimshaw, Faith, Missionary Life, and the Family, in: Philippa Levine (ed.), Gender and Empire, Oxford 2004, p. 260–280.

Reinhold Grundemann, Zwei Bittschriften an den Reichskanzler betreffend die Beschränkung des Branntweinimports in Westafrika, in: Allgemeine Missionszeitschrift 12 (1885), p. 290–299, 348–350.

David Hardiman, Introduction, in: ibid. (ed.), Healing Bodies, Saving Souls. Medical Missions in Asia and Africa, Amsterdam/New York 2006, p. 5–57.

David Hardiman, The Mission Hospital 1880–1960, in: Mark Harrison/ Margaret Jones/Helen Sweet (eds.), From Western Medicine to Global Medicine. The Hospital Beyond the West, Hyderabad 2009, p. 198–220.

Leonhard Harding, Hamburg's West Africa Trade in the Nineteenth Century, in: Gerhard Liesegang/Helma Pasch/Adam Jones (eds.), Figuring African Trade, Berlin 1986, p. 363–391.

Patrick Harries, Butterflies and Barbarians. Swiss Missionaries and Systems of Knowledge in South-East Africa, Oxford 2007.

Andrea Hauser, Dinge des Alltags. Studien zur historischen Sachkultur eines schwäbischen Dorfes, Tübingen 1994.

Julia Hauser, German Religious Women in Late Ottoman Beirut. Competing Missions, Leiden 2015.

Friedrich Hey, Der Tropenarzt. Ausführlicher Ratgeber für Europäer in den Tropen, sowie für Besitzer von Plantagen und Handelshäusern, Kolonialbehörden und Missionsverwaltungen, 1st ed., Offenbach 1906.

Patricia R. Hill, The World Their Household: The American Woman's Foreign Mission Movement and Cultural Transformation, 1870–1920, Ann Arbor 1985.

Richard Hölzl, Aus der Zeit gefallen? Katholische Mission zwischen Modernitätsanspruch und Zivilisationskritik, in: Christoph Bultmann/Jörg Rüpke/Sabine Schmolinsky (eds.), Religionen in Nachbarschaft. Pluralismus als Markenzeichen der europäischen Religionsgeschichte, Münster 2012, p. 143–164.

Paul Jenkins, Villagers as Missionaries: Wuerttemberg Pietism as a Nineteenth-Century Missionary Movement, in: Missiology. An International Review 8 (1980) 4, p. 425–432.

Paul Jenkins, The Basel Mission in West Africa and the Idea of the Christian Village Community, in: Godwin Shiri (ed.), Wholeness in Christ. The Legacy of the Basel Mission in India, Mangalore 1985, p. 13–25.

Paul Jenkins, Land und Arbeit als vergessene Werte in der Mentalität von Baseler MissionarInnen um 1900. Ein Essay mit Bildquellen, in: Inge Mager (ed.), Christentum und Kirche vor der Moderne. Industrialisierung, Historismus und die Deutsche Evangelische Kirche. Zweites Symposium der deutschen Territorialgeschichtsvereine, 9. bis 11. Juni 1995, Hannover 1995, p. 137–147.

Paul Jenkins, Württemberg als Hauptsäule der historischen Basler Mission – transregionale Erwägungen über Entwicklungen bis 1914, in: Blätter für württembergische Kirchengeschichte 116 (2016), p. 29–54.
Anthony King, The Bungalow: The Production of a Global Culture, London/ Boston 1984.
Dagmar Konrad, Missionsbräute. Pietistinnen des 19. Jahrhunderts in der Basler Mission, Münster 2001.
Dagmar Konrad, Die Missionsstation, in: Museum der Kulturen Basel (ed.), Mission Possible? Die Sammlung der Basler Mission – Spiegel kultureller Begegnungen, Basel 2015, p. 69–75.
Dagmar Konrad, Schweizer Missionskinder des 19. Jahrhunderts, in: Schweizerische Gesellschaft für Wirtschafts- und Sozialgeschichte 29 (2015), p. 163–185.
Wolfgang Lauber, Deutsche Architektur in Kamerun 1884–1914: Deutsche Architekten und Kameruner Wissenschaftler dokumentieren die Bauten der deutschen Epoche in Kamerun/Afrika, Stuttgart 1988.
Hartmut Lehmann, Pietismus und weltliche Ordnung in Württemberg vom 17. bis zum 20. Jahrhundert, Stuttgart 1969.
John MacKenzie, Missionaries, Science and the Environment in Nineteenth-Century Africa, in: Andrew Porter (ed.), The Imperial Horizons of British Protestant Missions, 1880–1914, Grand Rapids/Cambridge 2003, p. 106–130.
Emily J. Manktelow, Missionary Families: Race, Gender and Generation on the Spiritual Frontier, Manchester/New York 2013.
Markus Mattmüller, Der Kampf gegen den Alkoholismus in der Schweiz. Ein unbekanntes Kapitel der Sozialgeschichte im 19. Jahrhundert, Bern 1979.
Markus Mattmüller, Basler Blaukreuzgeschichte – ein Kapitel Basler Sozial- und Kirchengeschichte, in: Blaues Kreuz Basel (ed.), Bleibender Auftrag. Vorbeugen – helfen – heilen: 100 Jahre Blaues Kreuz Basel 1882–1982, Basel 1982, p. 4–22.
David Maxwell, The Missionary Home as a Site for Mission: Perspectives from Belgian Congo, in: Studies in Church History 50 (2014), p. 428–455.
James H. Mills/Patricia Barton, Introduction, in: ibid. (eds.) Drugs and Empires. Essays in Modern Imperialism and Intoxication, c. 1500–c. 1930, Basingstoke 2007, p. 1–16.
Harris W. Mobley, The Ghanaian's Image of the Missionary: An Analysis of the Published Critiques of Christian Missionaries by Ghanaians 1897–1965, Leiden 1970.
Gustav Müller, Der Kampf gegen den afrikanischen Branntweinhandel, in: Afrika 5 (1898), p. 169–178.
Gustav Müller, Bericht über die Thätigkeit der Kommission zur Bekämpfung des Afrikanischen Branntweinhandels, in: Afrika 8 (1901), p. 81–83.

Gustav Müller, Bericht über die Thätigkeit der Kommission zur Bekämpfung des Afrikanischen Branntweinhandels, in: Afrika 17 (1910), p. 1–4.

Theodor Müller, Bilder aus einem afrikanischen Missionsspital, in: Die ärztliche Mission 8 (1913), p. 35–37.

Garth Andrew Myers, Verandahs of Power: Colonialism and Space in Urban Africa, New York 2003.

Akin Olorunfemi, German Trade with British West African Colonies, 1895–1918, in: Journal of African Studies 8 (1981) 3, p. 111–120.

Itohan Osayimwese, Pietism, Colonialism, and the Search for Utopia: Pietist Space in Germany and the Gold Coast, in: Thresholds 30 (2005), p. 74–79.

Itohan Osayimwese, Colonialism and Modern Architecture in Germany, Pittsburgh 2017.

Emily Lynn Osborn, Our New Husbands Are Here: Households, Gender, and Politics in a West African State from the Slave Trade to Colonial Rule, Athens 2011.

Robert Peckham/David M. Pomfret, Introduction: Medicine, Hygiene, and the Re-ordering of Empire, in: ibid. (eds.), Imperial Contagions. Medicine, Hygiene, and Cultures of Planning in Asia, Hong Kong 2013, p. 1–14.

Line Nyhagen Predelli/Jon Miller, Piety and Patriarchy: Contested Gender Regimes in Nineteenth-Century Evangelical Missions, in: Mary Taylor Huber/Nancy C. Lutkehaus (eds.), Gendered Missions. Women and Men in Missionary Discourse and Practice, Ann Arbor 1999, p. 67–112.

Simone Prodolliet, Wider die Schamlosigkeit und das Elend der heidnischen Weiber. Die Basler Frauenmission und der Export des europäischen Frauenideals in die Kolonien, Zürich 1987.

Alexandra Przyrembel, Verbote und Geheimnisse. Das Tabu und die Genese der europäischen Moderne, Frankfurt a. M. 2011.

Reichskolonialamt (ed.), Medizinal-Berichte über die Deutschen Schutzgebiete Deutsch-Ostafrika, Kamerun, Togo, Deutsch-Südwestafrika, Neu-Guinea, Karolinen, Marshall-Inseln und Samoa für das Jahr 1903/1904, Berlin 1905.

Karl Renntisch, Mission und wirtschaftliche Entwicklung, Basel 1975.

Albrecht Rittmann, Vor 200 Jahren: Die Gründung der Brüdergemeinde Korntal, in: Schwäbische Heimat (2019) 1, p. 18–27.

Dana L. Robert, The 'Christian Home' as a Cornerstone of Anglo-American Missionary Thought and Practice, in: ibid. (ed.), Converting Colonialism: Visions and Realities in Mission History, 1706–1914, Grand Rapids 2008, p. 134–165.

Wilhelm Schlatter, Geschichte der Basler Mission 1815–1915, 3 vol., Basel 1916.

Norbert Schröder, Hamburgs Schnapsfabrikanten und der deutsche Kolonialismus in Westafrika, in: Zeitschrift des Vereins für Hamburgische Geschichte 76 (1990), p. 83–116.

Peter A. Schweizer, Mission an der Goldküste: Geschichte und Fotografie der Basler Mission im kolonialen Ghana, Basel 2002.

Traugott Siegfried, Das Wirtshaus. Von der Gemeinnützigen Gesellschaft der Stadt Basel ausgeschriebene und gekrönte Preisschrift, Basel 1881.

Lothar Sigloch, Zur Geschichte von Korntal und Münchingen, vol. 1: Korntaler Ansichten – Siedlungsaspekte der Gemeinde Korntal, Korntal-Münchingen 1994.

Ulrike Sill, Wie das Harmonium in die Hängematte kam: Ein Beispiel für den Wandel im Berichtswesen der Basler Mission im 19. Jahrhundert, in: Artur Bogner/Bernd Holtwick/Hartmann Tyrell (eds.), Weltmission und religiöse Organisationen. Protestantische Missionsgesellschaften im 19. und 20. Jahrhundert, Würzburg 2004, p. 377–395.

Udo Simon, Why Purity? An Introduction, in: Petra Rösch/Udo Simon (eds.), How Purity is Made, Wiesbaden 2012, p. 1–37.

Sujit Sivasundaram, Natural History Spiritualized. Civilizing Islanders, Cultivating Breadfruit, and Collecting Souls, in: History of Science 39 (2001), p. 417–443.

Francesco Spöring, Mission und Sozialhygiene. Schweizer Anti-Alkohol-Aktivismus im Kontext von Internationalismus und Kolonialismus, 1886–1939, Doctoral Thesis, ETH Zurich, 2014.

Ann Laura Stoler/Frederick Cooper, Beetween Metropole and Colony: Rethinking a Research Agenda, in: ibid. (eds.), Tensions of Empire. Colonial Cultures in the Bourgeois World, Berkeley et al. 1997, p. 1–56.

Jakob Tanner, Die "Alkoholfrage" in der Schweiz im 19. und 20. Jahrhundert, in: Hermann Fahrenkrug (ed.), Zur Sozialgeschichte des Alkohols in der Neuzeit Europas, Lausanne 1986, p. 147–168.

Helen Tilley, Africa as a Living Laboratory. Empire, Development, and the Problem of Scientific Knowledge, 1870–1950, Chicago 2011.

Rolf Trechsel, Die Geschichte der Abstinenzbewegung in der Schweiz im 19. und frühen 20. Jahrhundert, Lausanne 1990.

Ernst Troeltsch, Die Soziallehren der christlichen Kirchen und Gruppen. Gesammelte Schriften, vol. 1, Tübingen 1912.

Dmitri van den Bersselaar, The King of Drinks: Schnapps Gin from Modernity to Tradition, Leiden/Boston 2007.

Hermann Vortisch, Ein barmherziger Samariter, in: Johannes Kammerer (ed.), Bilder aus dem Missionsspital, Basel 1912, p. 3–4.

Hermann Vortisch, Wie kann man in Missionsspitälern evangelistisch tätig sein? in: Die ärztliche Mission 8 (1913), p. 13–17.

Gustav Warneck, Der westafrikanische Branntweinhandel, in: Allgemeine Missionszeitschrift 13 (1886), p. 268–280.

Gustav Warneck, Evangelische Missionslehre. Ein missionstheoretischer Versuch, ed. by Friedemann Knödler, Bonn 2015.

Bernd Weisbrod, "Visiting" and "Social Control". Statistische Gesellschaften und Stadtmissionen im Viktorianischen England, in: Christoph Sachsse/Florian Tennstedt (eds.), Sozial Sicherheit und soziale Disziplinierung. Beiträge zu einer historischen Theorie der Sozialpolitik, Frankfurt a. M. 1986, p. 181–208.

Franz Michael Zahn, Der überseeische Branntweinhandel. Seine verderblichen Wirkungen und Vorschläge zur Beschränkung desselben, in: Allgemeine Missionszeitschrift 13 (1886), p. 9–39.

Johannes Zimmermann, Letztes Wort eines alten afrikanischen Missionars an sein deutsches Vaterland, in: Evangelisches Missionsmagazin 21 (1877), p. 225–245.

Regula Zürcher, Gegen den " Sumpf des selbstverschuldeten Elends." Antialkoholbewegung und Armutsbekämpfung im 19. Jahrhundert, in: Josef Mooser/Simon Wenger (eds.), Armut und Fürsorge in Basel. Armutspolitik vom 13. Jahrhundert bis heute, Basel 2011, p. 123–132.

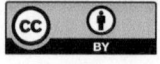

CHAPTER 7

Subverting Purity: Magic, Medical Pluralism and Tenacious Syncretism

The Basel Mission doctors proclaimed that they possessed a magic bullet that convincingly demonstrated the superiority of their medical knowledge and Christian faith over African medicine and beliefs. Despite their hegemonic assertions, however, they faced constant competition from other influential medical practitioners and spiritual leaders, eventually forcing them to revise their course of action. At the same time, the Basel Mission doctors constituted a permanent source of hazard for their own organisation by disregarding and shifting existing boundaries of purity. Their arrival in West Africa had far-reaching repercussions, transforming the existing relationship between the Basel missionaries and African healers, questioning key tenets of Pietist purity and exposing the fragility and inconsistencies within the missionary project.

7.1 Of Healers and Doctors

Before the dawn of High Imperialism and scientific medicine, Europeans on the west coast of Africa often consulted resident medical men and considered African medical texts and practices as bodies of knowledge to learn from.[1] The Basel missionaries, who had lived on the

---

[1] Gordon, Some Observations on Medicine and Surgery as Practised by the Natives.

© The Author(s) 2023
L. M. Ratschiller Nasim, *Medical Missionaries and Colonial Knowledge in West Africa and Europe, 1885–1914,*
Cambridge Imperial and Post-Colonial Studies,
https://doi.org/10.1007/978-3-031-27128-1_7

Gold Coast since 1828, did not adopt a uniformly negative approach to African healers, despite the fact that they often saw themselves as battling with "heathen humbug" and "quackery." After all, like naturopaths back home, African healers made use of herbs, heat and water. The anthropologist Adam Mohr demonstrated that before the arrival of the Basel Mission doctors in West Africa in 1885, European missionaries and African Christians on the Gold Coast "followed local patterns of therapeutic inclusion" by consulting a variety of African healers when they attempted to procure relief from illness and misfortune.[2]

Archival sources show that up to the 1880s the Basel missionaries mainly relied on African remedies based on plants, roots and barks as well as hydrotherapies, ablutions and baths. They reported, for example, that in the case of amoeba dysentery, which they called the "scourge of the tropics," they resorted to African herbal medicine since their own remedies proved ineffective.[3] They also consulted African medical men when dealing with ailments such as obstipation, headaches, skin diseases and fever.[4] Their laxative salts, in turn, found wide distribution among the population in West Africa since bowel cleansing constituted a significant aspect of health provision there, as it did in Europe.[5]

Healing and medical care created a relationship of trust between the Basel missionaries and the people on the Gold Coast, as numerous early sources indicate. Andreas Riis, for example, who struggled with what he identified as "severe jaundice" in 1832, turned his back on the Danish government physician as his condition continually deteriorated. He subsequently sought the help of a "Negro doctor," who performed six to eight cold ablutions on him daily: "Each time he washed my whole body with soap and lemon first, before rinsing me with cold water."[6] Riis reported

---

[2] Mohr, Missionary Medicine and Akan Therapeutics, p. 432.

[3] Johannes Zimmermann, Letter to Committee, Ussu, 01.04.1851, BMA, D-1.3.7; Gottlieb Schmid, Letter to Committee, 15.11.1882, BMA, D-1.35.40; Ibid., Letter to Committee, 22.01.1883, BMA, D-1.35.47; Adolf Mohr, Letter to Committee, 21.07.1905, BMA, D-1.84.15.

[4] Johannes Binder, Letter to Committee, Christiansborg, 27.11.1871, BMA, D-1.23.43b; Ibid., Letter to Committee, 12.09.1875, BMA, D-1.27.161; Ibid., Letter to Committee, 18.09.1875, BMA, D-1.27.163.

[5] Fisch, Über die Darmparasiten der Goldküstenneger; Vortisch, Statistik und Bericht über das 1. Halbjahr 1904 der ärztlichen Mission auf der Goldküste, p. 352.

[6] Andreas Riis, Letter to Committee, Christiansborg, 02.12.1832, BMA, D-1.1.15.

that he recovered from his illness within four days. Henceforth, he relied on the African medical man entirely and discredited the Danish government physician as a "fifth wheel," who had failed to prevent deaths and lost the Europeans' trust.[7] Fifteen years later, the Basel missionary Johannes Stanger described cold ablutions as the most effective "African fever therapy."[8]

The Basel missionaries' testimonies indicate that water and ablutions were essential parts of West African bodily practices, long before they took root in European societies and symbolised the epitome of European superiority. Christian missionaries studied African concepts of sickness and healing in considerable depth, in contrast to government doctors and colonial authorities.[9] They had some understanding of the complexities of African medicine and often made distinctions between medicine men, herbalists and the people they characterised as "witch doctors." Their extensive studies were indispensable for both their own health and a better understanding of the Africans' conceptual world. Considering the scarcity of knowledge on African medicine in Europe, they also attracted the interest of early anthropologists.[10]

For most of the nineteenth century, the Basel Mission stations were sites where a wide range of healthcare providers, including African medicine men, herbalists, bonesetters, cauterisers, village midwives and diviners, as well as European missionaries and government physicians, worked alongside each other. They promoted a large variety of bodily practices and therapeutic techniques until the 1880s, when the arrival of scientifically trained physicians triggered a shift in attitudes towards

---

[7] Andreas Riis, Letter to Committee, Christiansborg, 10.06.1834, BMA, D-1.1.35.6a.

[8] Johannes Stanger, Letter to Committee, Christiansborg, 25.08.1847, BMA, D-1.2.17.

[9] Bruchhausen/Roelcke, Categorising 'African Medicine', p. 78–83.

[10] Patrick Harries, Anthropology, in: Norman Etherington (ed.), Missions and Empire, Oxford 2005, p. 238–260; Ibid., From the Alps to Africa: Swiss Missionaries and the Rise of Anthropology, in: Helen L. Tilley/Robert J. Gordon (eds.), Ordering Africa. Anthropology, European Imperialism and the Politics of Knowledge, Manchester 2007, p. 201–224; David Maxwell, The Soul of the Luba. W.F.P. Burton, Missionary Ethnography and Belgian Colonial Science, in: History and Anthropology 19 (2008) 4, p. 325–351; Alexandra Przyrembel, Wissen auf Wanderschaft. Britische Missionare, ethologisches Wissen und die Thematisierung religiöser Selbstgefühle um 1830, in: Historische Anthropologie 19 (2011) 1, p. 31–53.

African healers within the Basel Mission.[11] The Basel Mission doctors saw themselves as academically approved experts on questions of hygiene, the body and healing. Their medical mission in West Africa, however, represented an intrusion into an existing system of healing, which constituted an essential part of people's lives in the face of frequent disease and physical suffering. The Basel missionary Otto Lädrach reported in 1904:

> In the field of illness and death, the fetish priests still assert themselves persistently in certain places. [...] From chicken & sheep entrails, they deduce whether a patient will die or recover, they ask the advice & answers of ghosts at night in the jungle – nobody is able to control their answers! Their therapy is nothing but a mix of medical advice & crude ceremonies, pungent herbs & smeary salves, all sorts of potions & baths, fetish strings & amulets.[12]

The Basel Mission doctors staged a campaign against African healers, trying to devalue them by making three main allegations. Firstly, the medical missionaries portrayed them as inherently brutal by claiming, for example, that they scarified their patients "to grasp the disease"[13] and exposed new born children to smoke, rubbing their eyes with "'indigenous pepper."[14] By accentuating scientific thinking and the use of empirical methods, the medical missionaries tried to delineate themselves from other forms of knowledge, thereby negating their value. Nonetheless, they were constantly confronted with established medical practitioners that offered an alternative way of treating the body and mind. African medicine men constituted a rival source of medical and spiritual authority, which the Basel Mission doctors tried to undermine.

Secondly, they condemned "the greed of fetish priests," who purportedly staged collusive ceremonies and issued "outrageous treatment bills."[15] Although patients who could afford it were expected to pay

---

[11] Kwasi Konadu, Medicine and Anthropology in Twentieth Century Africa: Akan Medicine and Encounters with (Medical) Anthropology, in: African Studies Quarterly 10 (2008) 2, p. 45–69.

[12] Otto Lädrach, Insert to the annual account for 1904, 31.01.1905, BMA, D-1.81.85.

[13] Rudolf Fisch, Annual report for 1908, 13.01.1909, BMA, D-1.90.20.

[14] Hermann Vortisch, Bilder aus der ärztlichen Mission auf der Goldküste, in: Die ärztliche Mission 1 (1906), p. 3–10, here p. 6.

[15] Fisch, Die ärztliche Mission unter den Negern, p. 375.

for their drugs and consultations with the Basel Mission doctors, greed served as a powerful image by which to degrade African healers as morally corrupt. The medical mission on the Gold Coast broke even in 1895, with African patients paying 8066.95 Swiss francs for consultations and 5500.20 Swiss francs for drugs, making yearly profits from then on.[16] Nevertheless, African medical men were presented as avaricious quacks, who deceived and exploited their own people.[17] This image was consolidated by Paulo Mohenu, a former "witch doctor" who became a member of the Basel Mission on the Gold Coast. He testified that "fetish priests" formed secret societies to cover their fraudulent practices and deceptive conduct in a widely circulated book published by the Basel missionary Heinrich Bohner.[18]

Thirdly, the Basel Mission doctors argued that African medicine was irrational, lumping it together with witchcraft, magic and superstition. In contrast to earlier missionaries, they usually referred to African medical men as "witch doctors" and "fetish priests" without specifying and distinguishing between the different types of healers in West Africa. Due to this undifferentiated approach and hostile attitude, African healers were increasingly reluctant to disclose their expert knowledge, contributing to the image of African medicine as something mysterious. Consequently, reliable information on African healing was hard to come by and informants, often the Basel Mission doctors' assistants, were reluctant to offend healers and acquaintances. Once information, however reliable, had been gained, the medical missionaries applied the criteria of scientific medicine to assess its validity within their own supposedly rational framework.[19]

[16] In 1895, the expenses amounted to 13,737.65 Swiss francs while the earnings came to 13,567.15 Swiss francs. See Basler Missionskomitee (ed.), Unsere ärztliche Mission. Bericht vom Jahr 1896, Basel 1897.

[17] Rudolf Fisch, Annual report for 1886, 08.01.1887, BMA, D-1.45.9; Alfred Eckhardt, Annual report for 1887, 04.02.1888, BMA, D-1.47.14; Friedrich Hey, Annual report for 1896, 05.02.1897, BMA, D-1.64.167.

[18] Heinrich Bohner, Im Lande des Fetischs, Basel 1890.

[19] Eckhardt, Die Basler Mission auf der Goldküste; Hermann Vortisch, Die Neger der Goldküste, in: Globus 89 (1906), p. 277–283, 293–297; Ibid., Aus der Arbeit eines Missionsarztes, in: Schweizerische Rundschau für Medizin 38 (1912), p. 1025–1036; Theodor Müller, Krankheitsbilder von der Goldküste, in: Die ärztliche Mission 7 (1912), p. 131–136; Rudolf Fisch, Die Dagbamba. Eine ethnographische Skizze, in: Baessler-Archiv 3 (1912) 2/3, p. 132–164.

The arrival of the Basel Mission doctors in West Africa promised greater evangelisation success, not only by attenuating suffering and lowering death rates among the missionary community and the wider population, but also by creating a close link between scientific medicine and Christianity.[20] Committee members now viewed mission medicine based on scientific grounds as a practical manifestation of the gospel, undertaken in obedience to Christ's commands. The medical missionaries asserted that effective medical care undermined superstitious beliefs upon which supposedly irrational healing practices depended.[21] Healing, however, remained a particularly contested realm, where missionaries had a hard time asserting the superiority of European knowledge and Christian religion, as an article in the Basel Mission's medical journal in 1892 exemplifies:

> All views of the people, as long as they were heathens, were permeated by superstition, but particularly their notions of disease and healing. Often it proves difficult for converts to leave behind not only idolatry but also superstition. When a disease appears again, they are easily tempted to resort to old remedies or at least their heathen relatives urge them to.[22]

By offering an all-encompassing cosmology of healing that addressed the needs of body, mind and soul, the Basel Mission doctors hoped to break the spell of Christian converts consulting African healers in times of unease and hardship. They believed that scientific thought and treatment successes would embolden their patients to renounce the charms of healers and free themselves from their faith in intrusive social and spiritual forces. Their campaign against African medical men was not just an expression of the increasing support for scientific medicine within evangelical circles but also an attempt to undermine the healers' moral status

---

[20] Ranger, Godly Medicine, p. 259. Also see Terence O. Ranger, Medical Science and Pentecost: The Dilemma of Anglicanism in Africa, in: W. J. Shiels (ed.), The Church and Healing, Oxford 1982, p. 333–365.

[21] Alfred Eckhardt, Annual report for 1887, 04.02.1888, BMA, D-1.47.14.

[22] An die Freunde des Ärztlichen Zweiges der Basler Mission, Basel 1892, p. 2.

and political authority. Steven Feierman demonstrated that medical practices in African societies were deeply connected with political power and control over resources.[23]

The British and German colonial governments in West Africa tried to diminish the influence of African healers by instituting laws that banned certain treatments from the early 1890s.[24] They branded many African healing practices as barbaric and superstitious rituals, forcing people on the Gold Coast and in Cameroon to act in covert and subversive ways. In 1893, Fisch deplored that he had to give up his consultation days in Odumase after rumours of foul play in the death of the Basel Mission nurse Klara Finckh:

> During the illness of Miss Finckh, and especially after her death, people circulated in Krobo that I had poisoned Miss F., and many other absurd allegations. I have reason to believe that the fetish people used this trick to regain their old practice. It looks like they succeeded quite well. On two consecutive consultation days, no sick person came to see me.[25]

Fisch's report shows that African medicine men and the Basel medical missionaries continually competed with each other for the favour of their patients. The Basel Mission doctors recognised that one of their advantages in this competition, which clearly distinguished mission medicine from African medical practice, was medical equipment and surgical procedures, such as the removal of cataracts, limbs and tumours. Medical devices and physical interventions were compelling arguments for resorting to mission medicine, as Alfred Eckhardt's account about a consultation in Christiansborg illustrates: "Sometimes I don't examine a person more precisely because I have already seen what condition it is; upon which he protests and says: 'You haven't tapped on my chest yet and used your small tube (he means the stethoscope)!'".[26]

---

[23] Steven Feierman, Struggles for Control: The Social Roots of Health and Healing in Modern Africa, in: African Studies Review 28 (1985) 2/3, p. 73–147.

[24] Akeyampong, Disease in West African History; Mohr, Missionary Medicine and Akan Therapeutics.

[25] Rudolf Fisch, Jahresbericht für 1893, in: An die Freunde des Ärztlichen Zweiges der Basler Mission, Basel 1894, p. 10–13, here p. 11.

[26] Eckhardt, Ärztliche Missionsarbeit in Christiansborg, p. 15.

The Basel medical men used different medical instruments, procedures and remedies from their African peers but they shared a common source of authority. Both sets of experts combined their healing methods with belief in a higher power. African healers and medical missionaries both offered a metaphysical healing cosmos with a specific view of the human body in its social and spiritual dimension. Megan Vaughan pointed to this analogy by showing that "mission medicine demanded belief in both the scientific and the supernatural."[27] While the Basel Mission doctors condemned West Africans for their belief in miracles, their medical interventions were based on the same rationale.

Upon completion of a cataract surgery, Hermann Vortisch asserted: "People notice after all that the mission doctor has a stronger, greater God behind him than the quacks."[28] The apparent ability to make the blind see must have resonated with West African concepts of magic around 1900, but the Basel medical missionaries were keen to evoke biblical references, likening their cures to Jesus' miracles.[29] The missionary Paul Steiner wrote a popular tractate on *How a Blind Negro Came to See Again! A True Incident from the West African Mission* in 1894, which was sold for 5 Swiss cents or 4 German pfennig to the Basel Mission's supporters at home. The booklet emphasised that regaining eyesight was not merely a medical intervention but a spiritual process, reassuring the readers in its opening sentence that "God still does miracles today."[30]

The apparently magical effectiveness of anaesthesia was also held up by the Basel medical missionaries as a miraculous intervention in line with Jesus' story. They used chloroform to anaesthetise their patients in West Africa during procedures such as amputations, reporting that the performance in which "the European doctor killed the sick, then cut him open and brought him back to life" evoked "deep admiration" among the

---

[27] Vaughan, Curing Their Ills, p. 60.

[28] Vortisch, Bilder aus der ärztlichen Mission auf der Goldküste, p. 5.

[29] Worboys has argued that this held true for many medical missions. Worboys, Colonial and Imperial Medicine, p. 234.

[30] Paul Steiner, Wie ein blinder Neger wieder sehend wurde! Eine wahre Begebenheit aus der westafrikanischen Mission, Basel 1894, p. 3.

resident population.[31] An anecdote by Hermann Vortisch, dating from 1906, further illustrates how the Basel Mission doctors used their medical performances to allude to the supernatural element of their trade:

> When I was performing my operation here in a small room of the mission house, a large number of people stood in front of the door and the window, trying to catch a glimpse of the wonder. 'Eh', they exclaimed, 'first he kills the sick person, so that he can cut him without pain, and then he will reawaken him.' And how excited they were, when I carried the successfully operated man outside, to see whether he would really reawaken from apparent death. Soon he opened his eyes, and the people told each other: 'Now the doctor has brought him back to life.'[32]

Although no faith was particularly successful at dealing with the most intractable illnesses in West Africa, they all claimed to offer healing and tried to persuade the public that their apparent accomplishments were due to their privileged relations with the divine.[33] The Basel medical missionaries attempted to stage their procedures as biblical miracles, dramatising the wonders of chloroform or cataract removal, but they did not attempt to perform spiritual healing and deliverance practices. While prayer accompanied scientifically understood treatments, suggestions of spiritual cures for physical ailments that had permeated Pietist healing at home were not part of the Basel medical mission in West Africa. Yet in calling upon their own magic, the Basel Mission doctors operated within a paradox.

The criticism of African superstition and the simultaneous exploitation of seemingly supernatural powers point to contentious production processes of religious and secular knowledge at the time. The very notions of religion and secularism were products of negotiations conducted with a newfound intensity in the late nineteenth and early twentieth centuries.[34] In his book, *The Invention of World Religion*, Tomoko

[31] Friedrich Hey, Bericht aus Odumase, in: Unsere ärztliche Mission. Bericht vom Jahr 1897, Basel 1898, p. 7–10; Friedrich Hey, Annual report for 1897, 16.04.1898, BMA, D.1.66.198; Rudolf Fisch, Annual report for 1905, 02.02.1906, BMA, D.1.84a.19.

[32] Vortisch, Bilder aus der ärztlichen Mission auf der Goldküste, p. 6.

[33] Peel, Religious Encounter and the Making of the Yoruba, p. 221.

[34] Asad (ed.), Formations of the Secular; Dressler/Mandair (eds.), Secularism and Religion-Making; Rebekka Habermas, Introduction: Negotiating the Religious and the Secular in Modern German History, in: ibid. (ed.), Negotiating the Secular and the

Masuzawa argued that categories such as religion, magic and fetishism emerged at the end of nineteenth century as a result of colonial encounters.[35] Missionaries played a key role in these developments by producing and circulating knowledge on the religious and the secular with case studies and interpretations from their mission fields around the globe.[36]

Until the beginnings of the medical mission, the displacement of African healers was not necessarily the Basel Mission's intention, as their bodies of knowledge were interpreted as cultural customs rather than religious beliefs and practices. From 1885, however, the Basel Mission's activities in West Africa not only engendered conflicts between different belief systems but also between competing healing systems. The mission doctors were exponents of an increasingly assertive and exclusionary type of medicine, which defined itself as scientific and European in sharp opposition to what they perceived as quackery. Scientific medicine was not conceived of as one medical system among many; it was the standard to which all other medical systems had to aspire, and which they inevitably failed to meet.[37]

The Basel Mission doctors mapped the disjuncture between science and superstition onto metropolitan and colonial spaces respectively. According to their narrative, the decline of magic in Europe was the direct and inevitable consequence of advances in medicine, which rendered belief in occult principles obsolete. They invariably viewed themselves as scientists, whose rational, empirical and experimental approach was what

Religious in the German Empire: Transnational Approaches, New York/Oxford 2019, p. 1–29.

[35] Tomoko Masuzawa, The Invention of World Religions, or, How European Universalism Was Preserved in the Language of Pluralism, Chicago 2005. See further Arie L. Molendijk/Peter Pels (eds.), Religion in the Making: The Emergence of the Sciences of Religion, Leiden/Boston/Köln 1998.

[36] Wetjen, Mission als theologisches Labor; Richard Hölzl/Karolin Wetjen, Negotiating the Fundamentals? German Missions and the Experience of the Contact Zone, 1850–1918, in: Rebekka Habermas (ed.), Negotiating the Secular and the Religious in the German Empire. Transnational Approaches, New York/Oxford 2019, p. 196–234; Karolin Wetjen. Religionspädagogische Resonanzen und die Mission: "Christianity Making" im missionarischen Bildungsraum am Ende des 19. Jahrhunderts, in: David Käbisch/Michael Wermke (eds.), Transnationale Grenzgänge und Kulturkontakte. Historische Fallbeispiele in religionspädagogischer Perspektive, Leipzig 2017, p. 23–38.

[37] Andrew Cunningham/Birdie Andrews, Introduction, in: ibid. (eds.), Western Medicine as Contested Knowledge, Manchester 1997, p. 1–23, here p. 12.

distinguished them from African healers.[38] Imagining European medicine as scientific, however, required considerable discursive work. In his publication on the "fundamentals of colonial indigenous hygiene," Ludwig Külz noted about Europeans: "The idea that supernatural forces are the cause for diseases sits deep in our blood for many of us still today, and to this day medicine has not completely emancipated itself from priesthood and belief in miracles."[39]

Scientific, technological and medical novelties were the subjects of controversial debates around 1900. Scientific medicine still used century-old techniques such as bloodletting, later considered harmful, and vast gaps in medical understanding remained. The notion of scientific medicine with its suggestion of internal coherence obscures the complex and often conflicting interpretations of disease that persisted well into the twentieth century.[40] Scientific medicine was not consistently accepted, far less practised, anywhere in the world. The gradual breakthrough of scientific medicine did not mean that all other existing forms of healing vanished. Beliefs in witchcraft, magic and the occult continued to be widespread in European societies.[41]

Healing and the body remained contested territories at home and abroad. While 1885 marked the beginning of a transitional period in West Africa, evidence shows that some Basel missionaries continued consulting African healers into the twentieth century. Private diaries and family letters demonstrate that the non-medical missionaries widely resorted to African remedies and practitioners but these accounts are generally missing from official reports and publications. It seems likely, therefore, that the missionaries no longer reported their use of African medicine to the board in Basel once their medically qualified colleagues began to

---

[38] Martin Lengwiler/Nigel Penn, Science between Africa and Europe. Creating Knowledge and Connecting Worlds (Introduction), in: ibid./Patrick Harries (eds.), Science, Africa and Europe. Processing Information and Creating Knowledge, London/New York 2019, p. 1–12.

[39] Külz, Grundzüge der kolonialen Eingeborenenhygiene, p. 389.

[40] Porter, What is Disease; Jacyna, Localization of Disease.

[41] Marijke Gijswijt-Hofstra/Brian P. Levack/Roy Porter, Witchcraft and Magic in Europe, vol. 5: The Eighteenth and Nineteenth Centuries, London 1999; Diethard Sawicki, Leben mit den Toten: Geisterglauben und die Entstehung des Spiritismus in Deutschland 1770–1900, Paderborn 2002; Christoph Ribbat, Religiöse Erregung: Protestantische Schwärmer im Kaiserreich, Frankfurt a. M. 1996; Ulrich Linse, Geisterseher und Wunderwirker: Heilssuche im Industriezeitalter, Frankfurt a. M. 1996.

work in West Africa. Missionary Otto Lädrach, for instance, admitted to the Committee that he had successfully taken African herbal medicine in 1898, nine years after the fact, to argue for the administering of African remedies to a missionary wife in 1907:

> At home in Europe, in the canton of Berne, one would say: 'Ah, what's the use of calling a quack now! [...] But when you are days away from any medical help and must see your neighbour, co-worker and station companion suffer and endure for days, you try everything and you stop philosophising about the dangers of quackery.[42]

Many Basel missionaries continued to consult African healers after 1885 out of necessity due to a lack of medical help but also because they quietly accepted their efficacy. They had grown up with folk medicine practised in Swabian and Swiss villages that was much closer to African forms of medicine than that of the academically trained medical missionaries. They followed a therapeutic pattern that was inclusive, unlike the exclusive claims of scientific treatment. This complex medical pluralism, however, was concealed by an elite, scientific discourse. In West Africa, scientific medicine was represented as a cohesive European body of knowledge framed in opposition to other, less civilised, forms of thinking. African medicine thus appeared as a threat to the secularity and singularity of European medical and scientific modernity.[43]

Through their copious writings, the Basel Mission doctors shaped notions of magic, fetishism and heathenism about West Africa while presenting themselves as promoters of scientific medicine, individualism and reason. They pointed out that knowledge of hygiene, in particular, was an effective method of demarcating and replacing faith in intrusive social and spiritual forces with causal, rational thinking and individual responsibility. Beatrice Mesmer has argued for nineteenth-century Switzerland that "hygiene rituals" became the "exorcism, which was expected to expel social poisons."[44] While social reformers saw

---

[42] Otto Lädrach, Letter to Committee, 23.09.1907, p. 9–10, BMA, D-1.87.196.

[43] Walter Bruchhausen, Magie und Besessenheit in Übersee. Der Diskurs über das fremde Okkulte um 1900, in: Barbara Wolf-Braun (ed.), Medizin, Okkultismus und Parapsychologie im 19. und frühen 20. Jahrhundert, Wetzlar 2009, p. 45–68; Harries/Dreier, Medizin und Magie in Afrika.

[44] Mesmer, Reinheit und Reinlichkeit, p. 491.

hygiene as a means of cleansing society of undesirable social and political elements, the Basel Mission doctors made use of hygiene as a way of purifying Christianity of medical knowledge they considered unscientific and irrational.

7.2 THE MISSION DOCTORS AS PURITY HAZARDS

The arrival of scientifically qualified mission doctors in West Africa introduced a new dynamic into the stable social structure and knowledge system of the Basel Mission. As academically trained physicians, they presented a challenge to the tight-knit missionary community and embodied a threat to the perpetuation of Pietist purity ideals. An essential dimension of Pietist purity consisted in complying with the social hierarchy, mirroring the individual's devotion to God. Patriarchal supervision within the family and the larger parish was thought to prevent the transgression of boundaries and therefore uphold the divine order. What's more, their scientific views risked subverting certain established religious bodily practices and were repeatedly met with incomprehension, even hostility at times, by their missionary colleagues. These pious physicians thus posed a threat to the cohesion of the Basel Mission by challenging long-standing organisational and conceptual tenets.[45]

The medical missionaries trained at the Basel Mission seminary for five years, like ordinary missionaries, but unlike them, they completed subsequent medical studies at university, thereby eluding the control and gaze of the mission leadership. Worried about this worldly influence, the Committee encouraged medical pupils to stay in the mission house during their period of study. Josef Haller, a pastor in Tuttlingen who worked as a teacher at the Basel Mission seminary for five years, specified: "To counterbalance the naturalistic and materialistic enterprise of medical studies, it is desirable for the students to stay in the mission house. Still, this does not guarantee that our young doctors will not deviate from Christianity."[46] The perceived danger in allowing missionaries to attend medical faculties is illustrated by a letter that Rudolf Fisch obtained from his mother during his university studies:

---

[45] Gottlob Haussleiter, Die Stellung des Missionsarztes im Organismus der Mission, in: Die ärztliche Mission 4 (1909), p. 73–79.

[46] Josef Haller, Die Vorbildung unserer Missionare, Basel 1904, p. 38.

May your faith at university not suffer any damages. Oh since it is generally said: 'There are no religious physicians, faith does not get along with science.' I know that there are exceptions but there are few. What matters is to be constantly equipped with vigil and prayer. [...] Above all, what matters is to request strength from the Lord so that arrogance does not take possession of the poor heart. [...] You still lack a lot to be selfless, that's why many temptations arise when you socialise with the different minds that are to be found at university. Rather be the humble missionary with a merry, faithful heart than losing your faith through science.[47]

This letter is a vivid expression of Pietists' concerns and fears towards academia and science. By integrating physicians into their agenda, the Committee jeopardised the social hierarchy within the Basel Mission, which was considered a key element of the purity process. The homogenous and relatively modest social makeup of the Basel missionaries was thought to guarantee practical harmony and divine order. Although some of the Basel Mission doctors had a background in agriculture and craftwork like the majority of the ordinary missionaries, their subsequent medical studies clearly set them apart from their brothers and sisters. This social gap certainly contributed to the numerous conflicts that erupted between them. The medical missionaries struggled to justify their work to their non-medical colleagues, who oftentimes felt that the medical mission was a superficial method of attracting converts.[48]

The Basel Mission doctors were experts in health, outclassing their colleagues in this regard, but at the same time, they remained in a subordinate position in relation to the Committee. They were born-again Christians and self-confessed members of their mission society, who had sworn obedience to their superiors and subscribed to uphold their programme and goals.[49] In West Africa, however, they enjoyed relative autonomy from Basel and acquired a degree of authority over non-medical missionaries. The Committee expected the mission doctors to be proactive, resourceful and innovative in order to save lives and advance the evangelising cause, but they also clearly feared a loss of cohesion. When

---

[47] Rudolf Fisch, Self-composed CV until 1911, p. 9, Personal File Rudolf Fisch, BMA, BV 985.

[48] Fisch, Die ärztliche Mission unter den Negern, p. 371–372.

[49] Basler Missionskomitee (ed.), Bedingungen für den Eintritt in die ärztliche Mission, in: Unsere ärztliche Mission. Bericht vom Jahr 1896, Basel 1897, p. 31.

discussing the posting of a second mission doctor to West Africa in 1885, some Committee members warned against this plan by pointing out "that brother Fisch is not a very compatible character."[50]

The Basel Mission board allowed the mission doctors to prescribe certain measures such as home leaves without their consent but their autonomy represented a threatening element of uncertainty to their superiors' hegemony. Before their employment, the Committee had been the decisive authority in granting or denying permissions for home leave. Shortly after Fisch's arrival on the Gold Coast, the Committee reported: "Brother Schopf wants to return home – 'at the instigation of the physician' – on this occasion the concern is raised that we need to keep our eyes open with regards to the mission doctor to make sure he does not overreach with his instructions."[51]

By outranking Committee instructions that were to be followed by all missionaries, the mission doctors disrupted entrenched organisational procedures and social hierarchies. Their position within the organisation remained a constant source of disruption. Ordinary missionaries in West Africa relied on their medical assistance but continued to be highly sceptical of their scientific approach.[52] While they approved of surgical procedures such as the removal of tumours and cataracts, they distrusted the medical missionaries' treatment of internal diseases and often disregarded their hygiene guidelines and prophylactic measures, including the regular use of quinine to prevent malarial fevers. Rudolf Fisch continually condemned the missionaries' insufficient quinine intake and demanded that the Committee issue a binding directive.[53]

In 1907, Inspector Theodor Oehler sent a circular letter to the mission members in Cameroon and on the Gold Coast in which he stated: "If you notice that brothers or sisters are putting their health and lives at risk through refusing to take quinine, an unreasonable lifestyle or improper overexertion, you have the duty to inform the Committee and

---

[50] Committee report, 22.01.1885, BMA, Komitee-Protokoll 1885, §71.

[51] Committee report, 11.09.1885, BMA, Komitee-Protokoll 1885, §588.

[52] Fischer, Der Missionsarzt Rudolf Fisch, p. 356–357.

[53] Rudolf Fisch, Circular letter about malaria and black water fever, 18.09.1902, BMA, D-11.77.8; Ibid., Letter to Committee, 24.09.1902, BMA, D-11.77.9; Ibid., Letter to Committee, 05.10.1906, BMA, D-1.86.6.

potentially file an application for dismissal."[54] Oehler's circular not only stressed the importance of health and hygiene but also consolidated the mission doctors' authority on these questions. Henceforth, missionaries who wished to submit a request for approval to marry had to be vetted by a medical missionary.[55] The leadership issued several instructions concerning the "hygienic behaviour" of missionaries, refusing, however, to make quinine prophylaxis a mandatory requirement despite the firm support of the doctor in the seminary, Adolf Hägler-Gutzwiller.[56]

Hägler-Gutzwiller was a sought-after medical practitioner and social reformer who had initiated the founding of the Basel sanatorium in 1896. Supported and financed by the *GGG*, and located in Davos, this charitable institution hosted patients suffering from tuberculosis and became a model for benevolent pulmonary sanatoriums across Europe.[57] The fact that the Committee members did not follow Hägler-Gutzwiller's generally appreciated advice when it came to issuing a binding directive on quinine intake highlights that they feared the resistance of the missionaries in West Africa. Hygiene and health remained contentious topics among the Basel missionaries.

In February 1907, Fisch asked the Committee to be dispensed from providing medical care to his missionary colleagues.[58] One of them had suffered from severe malaria a couple of months earlier because, according to Fisch, he had only taken "minuscule homeopathic doses" of quinine. The patient, however, remained intransigent and Fisch made him sign a liability form for the "adequate" intake of quinine.[59] The mission doctor took a hard line with his fellow missionaries, whom he

---

[54] Theodor Oehler, Circular letter to the mission members in Cameroon and the Gold Coast concerning the duty to follow the mission doctor's instructions, 20.04.1907, BMA, D-9.2b.6a/b.

[55] Ibid.

[56] Hägler-Gutzwiler gave medical classes in the Basel Mission seminary and served as doctor in the Basel Mission house from 1875 to 1905. Adolf Hägler-Gutzwiler, Statement on quinine prophylaxis, 13.11.1906, BMA, D-1.86.7.

[57] Archiv der Basler Höhenklinik Davos, 1896–1992, StABS, PA 878. On the history of sanatoriums in Switzerland see Iris Ritzmann, Sanatorien, in: Historisches Lexikon der Schweiz, http://www.hls-dhs-dss.ch/textes/d/D14073.php, version 04.05.2017 (last access: 22.07.2022).

[58] Rudolf Fisch, Letter to Committee, 25.02.1907, BMA, D-1.87.156.

[59] Rudolf Fisch, Letter to Committee, 05.10.1906, BMA, D-1.86.6.

dismissed as laypeople, making him increasingly unpopular.[60] In March 1907, a group of missionaries filed a motion to reappoint Friedrich Hey as mission doctor to the Gold Coast. Hey had become a staunch advocate of homeopathy and naturopathy in the meantime, which matched the missionaries' therapeutic preferences.[61] Although the Committee decided against this proposition, Fisch felt that the basis of trust with his fellow missionaries had been irrevocably destroyed.[62]

The Basel Mission doctors produced and circulated divisive knowledge on hygiene and health beyond evangelical circles, generating considerable potential for discord within their own organisation. Their extensive publications, including medical monographs and contributions to scientific and colonial journals, jeopardised the Committee's well-monitored information policy. The Committee tried to tighten their control of the mission doctors' prolific writing, as a 1904 letter by Hermann Vortisch to Inspector Oehler illustrates: "Henceforth I will submit all manuscripts intended for publication to the inspectorate in compliance with your request."[63]

Financial matters created another source of conflict since the leaders in Basel tried to keep the doctors' expenses in West Africa under their control and accused them of undermining their authority by acting too autonomously. The purchase of often expensive medical instruments was subject to the Committee's approval.[64] When Friedrich Hey commissioned construction work on the mission hospital in Douala in 1902 without asking for permission, the Committee members issued a clear warning:

No brother, no physician either, has the right to change plans approved by the Committee; if he does it anyway, the general treasurer is simply

---

[60] Rudolf Fisch, Letter to Committee with statements by Wilhelm Jacob Rottmann and Philipp Johannes Rösler, 05.10.1906, BMA, D-1.87.156/157; Fisch, Die ärztliche Mission unter den Negern, p. 372.

[61] Committee report, 13.03.1907, BMA, Komitee-Protokoll 1907, §250; Committee report, 17.04.1907, BMA, Komitee-Protokoll 1907, §373.

[62] Theodor Oehler, Letter to Rudolf Fisch, 08.05.1907, copy book, p. 288–292, BMA, D-2.22.

[63] Hermann Vortisch, Letter to Theodor Oehler, 21.08.1904, Personal File Hermann Vortisch, BMA, BV 1674.

[64] Committee report, 17.03.1885, BMA, Komitee-Protokoll 1885, §271.

instructed to deny the relevant payments and to direct the person in question and their requests to the Committee.[65]

The medical missionaries challenged the social hierarchy within the Basel Mission, making them highly suspicious in the leadership's eyes. Moreover, their dedication to scientific medicine questioned religious approaches to healing and the body. They were divisive figures and potential troublemakers, whose medical notions of hygiene contradicted Pietist views on purity in many ways. Theodor Müller's disclosure that the syphilis epidemic on the Gold Coast had been misdiagnosed for over twenty-five years illustrates that the mission doctors embodied a potential threat to approved knowledge and the established order. By promoting new ideas and practices of hygiene, they transgressed and pushed the boundaries of purity. They acted as taboo breakers who aroused the resentment and mistrust of the larger missionary community.

7.3   Tenacious Syncretism

"Why" asked Hermann Vortisch in 1906 about the population on the Gold Coast "do they send me wounded people straight after an accident? Why did a father bring his son, who had fallen from a house and broken his spine, to me, a 3–4 days' journey away?"[66] By formulating these rhetorical questions, the mission doctor purported that the patients who came to see him had taken an ultimate decision for mission medicine exclusively. Yet his reasoning neglected that for most West Africans, the consultation of a mission doctor was just one aspect of a multifaceted cosmos of healing. African Christians did not simply give up their existing medical concepts und bodily practices, even though the Basel Mission doctors insisted that those who made use of their medical facilities had to distance themselves from African medicine. They often found themselves waging a losing battle in this respect.

By 1914, the Basel Mission parishes counted 25,042 members on the Gold Coast and 15,112 in Cameroon. These West African parishioners had developed a healing system in which they merged Christian faith and

---

[65] Committee report, 03.12.1885, BMA, Komitee-Protokoll 1885, §1007.

[66] Vortisch, Bilder aus der ärztlichen Mission auf der Goldküste, p. 5.

scientific medicine with African beliefs and medicine.[67] The missionary Adolf Mohr, who worked on the Gold Coast for over 30 years, wrote an unpublished letter to the Basel Mission board in 1905 in which he stated:

> Despite our physicians and their European drugs, ointments and powders, the indigenous are still tied to their boiled herbs and cortices. Even our pastors and catechists mainly use local medicine. In case of injuries, ulcers and where surgical interventions are needed, European medicine is being bought or the help of the physician is sought; but overall the indigenous remain with local medicine.[68]

This quote illustrates that West African Christians incorporated the consultation of European doctors and the use of European drugs into their existing cosmos of healing. If one became sick in West Africa, there were a variety of therapeutic practitioners one could choose from to alleviate one's illness. There was the prophet, the amulet maker, the herbalist and the medicine maker, all of whom had the capacity to heal. All these healers made different sorts of medicine: some were material and consumed, like pharmacopeia, some were material and not consumed, like amulets, and others were purely spiritual, like prayers. All four practitioners incorporated some form of spiritual ritual into their healing techniques.[69]

In a letter to the Committee, Alfred Eckhardt admitted that Africans saw the mission doctor as a "last resort" after they had tried "all sorts of hocus-pocus and nearly succumbed to their agony."[70] A closer look at the type of medical care that African patients sought from the Basel Mission doctors shows that the dressing of wounds, treatment of bone fractures and surgical interventions proved most popular. European drugs, too, found wide approval among the African population since they were often plant and mineral based in the same vein as their own remedies. The mission doctors' treatment of internal diseases, by contrast, proved far less convincing. Fisch deplored that his patients on the Gold Coast

---

[67] Evangelische Missionsgesellschaft zu Basel (ed.), Neunundneunzigster Jahresbericht, Basel 1914, p. 8.

[68] Adolf Mohr, Remarks to a letter from R. Fisch, 21.07.1905, BMA, D-1.84.15.

[69] Patterson, Health in Colonial Ghana, p. 11–31; Mohr, Missionary Medicine and Akan Therapeutics, p. 444–447.

[70] Alfred Eckhardt, Letter to Committee, 02.10.1887, BMA, D-1.47.10.

turned to African medical men if they could not see a speedy recovery or remarkable improvement, especially when facing internal illnesses.[71]

There were numerous ailments for which the medical missionaries did not have a cure, causing many parishioners to look elsewhere for treatment. While they resorted to the mission doctors in the case of certain diseases, such as yaws, which scientific medicine was fairly effective against, they generally viewed them as one alternative among others. Some diseases came to be seen as treatable by drugs but beliefs in social and spiritual forces persisted. The Basel Mission doctors did not revolutionise West Africans' understanding of disease causation nor did they replace African healers. Mission medicine, therefore, did not necessarily serve as a conversion tool, as had been hoped by advocates of the medical mission. Disillusioned, Fisch came to a sobering conclusion in this regard in his speech at the annual Basel Mission festival on 3 July 1895:

> Indeed, most people that we invite to reconcile themselves with God, reply: 'What you say is good, but heal my disease first and then I shall become a Christian', and when people are cured from their disease, then they do not become Christians after all.[72]

The Basel medical missionaries gradually came to realise that growing patient numbers did not directly translate to the demise of African forms of healing either. The clearer they drew boundaries between themselves and African healers, the more often and evidently these boundaries were transgressed. Steven Feierman observed that "the problem is not that therapeutic efficacy is lacking in African medicine; it is that diverse healing traditions, each with legitimate claims to efficacy, co-exist with little capacity to exclude one another from the range of practical options."[73] Mission medicine thus became another possibility within the existing range of therapeutic options for both European and African Christians in West Africa.

At the same time, African medicine underwent substantial transformation during the colonial period. Many African healers incorporated scientific approaches into their ancestral practices and thus became serious

---

[71] Rudolf Fisch, Annual report for 1886, 08.01.1887, BMA, D-1.45.9.

[72] Fisch, Die ärztliche Mission unter den Negern, p. 376.

[73] Feierman, Struggles for Control, p. 80.

competitors for European physicians.[74] Scientific medicine gained global significance not simply because European men exported it to the colonies but because of its protracted trials, encounters and appropriations overseas.[75] Megan Vaughan, Nancy Hunt, Luise White, Julie Livingston and others have demonstrated how Africans, particularly intermediaries such as medical assistants, hospital clerks and midwives, appropriated concepts and tools of scientific medicine to suit their own purposes.[76] In most regions of the world, navigating between multiple systems of medical knowledge was part of the everyday experience.[77]

Hospitals provide interesting insights into mediated histories of medicine, incorporating a range of actors from different backgrounds that worked alongside each other, sharing knowledge and experiences. Walima T. Kalusa examined the role of lower class medical workers such as ward attendants, orderlies and nurses at the hospitals run by the Christian Missions in Many Lands in Zambia, challenging their depiction as mere agents of missionary endeavours and scientific medicine.[78] His study shows that these medical brokers used African languages and supposedly heathen concepts to interpret medical terms and technologies, and thereby "drained Christian medicine of its scientific connotations and simultaneously invested in it 'pagan' meanings."[79]

Pluralism was a characteristic of medical practices in most societies.[80] Frequently, plurality in medicine was accompanied by the development of stereotypical images of the competing practitioners and their therapeutic

[74] Karen Flint, Healing Traditions: African Medicine, Cultural Exchange, and Competition in South Africa, 1820–1948, Ohio 2008; Cunningham/Andrews, Introduction.

[75] Mark Harrison, A Global Perspective: Reframing the History of Health, Medicine, and Disease, in: Bulletin of the History of Medicine 89 (2015) 4, p. 639–689; Mark Jackson (ed.), A Global History of Medicine, Oxford 2018.

[76] Vaughan, Curing Their Ills; Hunt, A Colonial Lexicon of Birth Ritual; White, Speaking with Vampires; Livingston, Debility and the Modern Imagination in Botswana.

[77] Good, The Steamer Parish; Hokkanen, Medicine and Scottish Missionaries in the Northern Malawi Region; Kalusa, Christian Medical Discourse and Praxis on the Imperial Frontier.

[78] Walima T. Kalusa, Language, Medical Auxiliaries, and the Re-interpretation of Missionary Medicine in Colonial Mwinilunga, Zambia, 1922–1951, in: Journal of Eastern African Studies 1 (2007) 1, p. 57–78.

[79] Ibid., p. 74.

[80] Bruchhausen, Medical Pluralism as a Historical Phenomenon; Ibid., Medizin zwischen den Welten.

methods. These images were part of public discourse and oftentimes constitutive for the self-image of medical men and their clientele.[81] Walter Bruchhausen and Volker Roelcke have shown that many of the categories and paradigms that were used to explain African medicine were in fact European. They were the result of political and scientific developments, ethnographic and psychological approaches, administrative activities and controversies about orthodox and heterodox medicine in Europe itself. This re-definition of African healing practices through a colonial lens came to full blossom during the age of High Imperialism from the Berlin Conference in 1884–1885 up to World War I.[82]

The Basel medical missionaries who practised in West Africa in this time period declared that African medicine was incompatible with scientific medicine and attempted to create Christian communities in which mission medicine, based on rational foundations, would prevail. Their agenda meant that the population in West Africa had to be converted not only to Christ but also to their scientific doctrine. Despite their efforts to establish a medical hegemony, however, African Christians exercised a great deal of autonomy with respect to medicine, and other cultural practices, within the Basel Mission parishes. Fisch lamented that his "proclamation of the only great doctor and the only remedy" referring to Christianity and mission medicine "is either not understood or entirely misunderstood"[83] and that even the African pastor of the Basel Mission in Aburi had a high opinion of "indigenous quacks."[84]

The refusal of Africans to give up their medical practices and dismiss their cosmos of healing caused considerable frustration among the Basel Mission doctors, most evident in violent disputes. Fisch described a series of physical altercations in his personal diary: he hit a villager who did not get out of his way on a narrow path,[85] he beat one of his medical assistants after seeing him "patting with a girl in the courtyard"[86] and he intervened in a mass brawl and "properly beat up a few guys."[87] Fisch's

---

[81] Chakrabarti, Medicine and Empire, p. 182–199.

[82] Bruchhausen/Roelcke, Categorising 'African Medicine', p. 76–77.

[83] Rudolf Fisch, Report for the 2nd half-year 1888, 26.02.1889, BMA, D-1.49.11.

[84] Rudolf Fisch, Annual report for 1898, 27.01.1899, BMA, D-1.69.36.

[85] Fisch, Diary Entry on 31.03.1908, BMA, D-10-24.

[86] Fisch, Diary Entry on 22.10.1908, BMA, D-10-24.

[87] Fisch, Diary Entry on 27.12.1908, BMA, D-10-24.

propensity for violence, which fundamentally contradicted the Pietist code of conduct, indicates a sense of impotence in the face of constant challenges from African protagonists and his fellow missionaries. The mission doctors desperately attempted to introduce an all-encompassing system of knowledge, including an exclusive claim to the truth, by combining Christianity with scientific medicine. They did not succeed, however, in suppressing the medical and religious syncretism in the areas in which they operated.

Confronted with this tenacious syncretism, the Basel medical missionaries had no choice but to accommodate African ways of thinking and acting if they wanted to gain them for their cause. They refashioned their medical discourse and praxis to popularise their system of healing among the population in West Africa. They integrated, for example, allusions to magical powers and the use of medicinal plants into their medical explanations and practices, which, ironically, they had promised to dislodge. Therefore, the popularity of mission medicine was not so much the result of its supposed superior effectiveness but rather the result of deliberate adaptations. The Basel Mission doctors continually had to negotiate and adjust their concepts of purity, health and cleanliness.

West Africans did not adopt Christianity and scientific medicine in terms of a fixed set of meanings and practices. They chose to reconcile their old and new faiths, blending Christian tenets and mission medicine with African beliefs and medical treatments without seeing this as a problem. They incorporated new norms of hygiene into existing African concepts of purity and cleanliness. While it remains difficult to establish the exact nature of this syncretism given the lack of sources by African protagonists and the complex and creative nature of this process of selection, appropriation and reinterpretation, it is clear that the Basel Mission doctors' knowledge of hygiene emerged from these protracted and contentious exchange processes in West Africa. These trials and tribulations of hygiene on the supposed margins of civilisation reverberated across the globe, transforming religious tenets of purity, scientific assumptions of health and hygiene, and colonial views of cleanliness and civilisation.

REFERENCES

Emmanuel Kwaku Akyeampong, Disease in West African History, in: ibid. (ed.), Themes in West Africa's History, Athens/Oxford/Accra 2006, p. 186–207.

Talal Asad (ed.), Formations of the Secular: Christianity, Islam, Modernity, Stanford 2003.

Basler Missionskomitee (ed.), Unsere ärztliche Mission. Bericht vom Jahr 1896, Basel 1897.

Basler Missionskomitee (ed.), Bedingungen für den Eintritt in die ärztliche Mission, in: Unsere ärztliche Mission. Bericht vom Jahr 1896, Basel 1897, p. 31.

Heinrich Bohner, Im Lande des Fetischs, Basel 1890.

Walter Bruchhausen/Volker Roelcke, Categorising 'African Medicine': The German Discourse on East African Healing Practices, 1885–1918, in: Waltraud Ernst (ed.), Plural Medicine, Tradition and Modernity, 1800–2000, London/New York 2002, p. 76–94.

Walter Bruchhausen, Medizin zwischen den Welten. Geschichte und Gegenwart des medizinischen Pluralismus im südöstlichen Tansania, Göttingen 2006.

Walter Bruchhausen, Magie und Besessenheit in Übersee. Der Diskurs über das fremde Okkulte um 1900, in: Barbara Wolf-Braun (ed.), Medizin, Okkultismus und Parapsychologie im 19. und frühen 20. Jahrhundert, Wetzlar 2009, p. 45–68.

Walter Bruchhausen, Medical Pluralism as a Historical Phenomenon: A Regional and Multi-Level Approach to Health Care in German, British and Independent East Africa, in: Anne Digby/Waltraud Ernst/Projit B. Mukharji (eds.), Crossing Colonial Historiographies. Histories of Colonial and Indigenous Medicines in Transnational Perspective, Newcastle 2010, p. 99–113.

Pratik Chakrabarti, Medicine and Empire, 1600–1960, Basingstoke 2014.

Andrew Cunningham/Birdie Andrews, Introduction, in: ibid. (eds.), Western Medicine as Contested Knowledge, Manchester 1997, p. 1–23

Markus Dressler/Arvind-Pal S. Mandair (eds.), Secularism and Religion-Making, Oxford 2011.

Alfred Eckhardt, Die Basler Mission auf der Goldküste, in: O. Frick (ed.), Geschichten und Bilder aus der Mission, vol. 10, Halle 1891, p. 3–19.

Alfred Eckhardt, Ärztliche Missionsarbeit in Christiansborg, in: An die Freunde des Ärztlichen Zweiges der Basler Mission, Basel 1891, p. 8–19.

Evangelische Missionsgesellschaft zu Basel (ed.), Neunundneunzigster Jahresbericht, Basel 1914.

Steven Feierman, Struggles for Control: The Social Roots of Health and Healing in Modern Africa, in: African Studies Review 28 (1985) 2/3, p. 73–147.

Rudolf Fisch, Jahresbericht für 1893, in: An die Freunde des Ärztlichen Zweiges der Basler Mission, Basel 1894, p. 10–13.

Rudolf Fisch, Die ärztliche Mission unter den Negern. Ansprache am Jahresfest der Basler Mission am 3. Juli 1895, in: Evangelisches Missionsmagazin 39 (1895), p. 371–377.

Rudolf Fisch, Über die Darmparasiten der Goldküstenneger, in: Archiv für Schiffs- und Tropenhygiene 12 (1908), p. 711–718.

Rudolf Fisch, Die Dagbamba. Eine ethnographische Skizze, in: Baessler-Archiv 3 (1912) 2/3, p. 132–164.

Friedrich Hermann Fischer, Der Missionsarzt Rudolf Fisch und die Anfänge medizinischer Arbeit der Basler Mission an der Goldküste (Ghana), Herzogenrath 1991.

Karen Flint, Healing Traditions: African Medicine, Cultural Exchange, and Competition in South Africa, 1820–1948, Ohio 2008.

Marijke Gijswijt-Hofstra/Brian P. Levack/Roy Porter, Witchcraft and Magic in Europe, vol. 5: The Eighteenth and Nineteenth Centuries, London 1999.

Charles M. Good, The Steamer Parish. The Rise and Fall of Missionary Medicine on an African Frontier, Chicago/London 2004.

Charles Alexander Gordon, Some Observations on Medicine and Surgery as Practised by the Natives of the Portion of the West Coast of Africa, in: Edinburgh Medical Journal 2 (1856/1857), p. 529–537.

Rebekka Habermas, Introduction: Negotiating the Religious and the Secular in Modern German History, in: ibid. (ed.), Negotiating the Secular and the Religious in the German Empire. Transnational Approaches, New York/Oxford 2019, p. 1–29.

Josef Haller, Die Vorbildung unserer Missionare, Basel 1904.

Patrick Harries, Anthropology, in: Norman Etherington (ed.), Missions and Empire, Oxford 2005, p. 238–260.

Patrick Harries, From the Alps to Africa: Swiss Missionaries and the Rise of Anthropology, in: Helen L. Tilley/Robert J. Gordon (eds.), Ordering Africa. Anthropology, European Imperialism and the Politics of Knowledge, Manchester 2007, p. 201–224.

Patrick Harries/Marcel Dreier, Medizin und Magie in Afrika. Eine Sozialgeschichte des Wissens, in: David Guggerli et al. (eds.), Nach Feierabend. Zürcher Jahrbuch für Wissensgeschichte, vol. 8: Gesundheit, Zürich 2012, p. 85–104.

Mark Harrison, A Global Perspective: Reframing the History of Health, Medicine, and Disease, in: Bulletin of the History of Medicine 89 (2015) 4, p. 639–689.

Gottlob Haussleiter, Die Stellung des Missionsarztes im Organismus der Mission, in: Die ärztliche Mission 4 (1909), p. 73–79.

Friedrich Hey, Bericht aus Odumase, in: Unsere ärztliche Mission. Bericht vom Jahr 1897, Basel 1898, p. 7–10.

Markku Hokkanen, Medicine and Scottish Missionaries in the Northern Malawi Region 1875–1930. Quests for Health in a Colonial Society, Lewiston 2007.

Richard Hölzl/Karolin Wetjen, Negotiating the Fundamentals? German Missions and the Experience of the Contact Zone, 1850–1918, in: Rebekka Habermas (ed.), Negotiating the Secular and the Religious in the German Empire. Transnational Approaches, New York/Oxford 2019, p. 196–234.

Nancy Rose Hunt, A Colonial Lexicon of Birth Ritual, Medicalization and Mobility in the Congo, Durham 1999.

Mark Jackson (ed.), A Global History of Medicine, Oxford 2018.

L. S. Jacyna, Localization of Disease, in: Deborah Brunton (ed.), Medicine Transformed. Health, Disease and Society in Europe, 1800–1930, Manchester/New York 2004, p. 1–30.

Walima T. Kalusa, Language, Medical Auxiliaries, and the Re-interpretation of Missionary Medicine in Colonial Mwinilunga, Zambia, 1922–1951, in: Journal of Eastern African Studies 1 (2007) 1, p. 57–78.

Walima T. Kalusa, Christian Medical Discourse and Praxis on the Imperial Frontier. Explaining the Popularity of Missionary Medicine in Mwinilunga District, Zambia, 1906–1935, in: Patrick Harries/David Maxwell (eds.), The Spiritual in the Secular. Missionaries and Knowledge about Africa, Grand Rapids 2012, p. 245–266.

Kwasi Konadu, Medicine and Anthropology in Twentieth Century Africa: Akan Medicine and Encounters with (Medical) Anthropology, in: African Studies Quarterly, 10 (2008) 2, p. 45–69.

Ludwig Külz, Grundzüge der kolonialen Eingeborenenhygiene, in: Beihefte zum Archiv für Schiffs- und Tropenhygiene 15 (1911), p. 386–475.

Martin Lengwiler/Nigel Penn, Science between Africa and Europe. Creating Knowledge and Connecting Worlds (Introduction), in: ibid./Patrick Harries (eds.), Science, Africa and Europe. Processing Information and Creating Knowledge, London/New York 2019, p. 1–12.

Ulrich Linse, Geisterseher und Wunderwirker: Heilssuche im Industriezeitalter, Frankfurt a. M. 1996.

Julie Livingston, Debility and the Modern Imagination in Botswana, Bloomington 2005.

Tomoko Masuzawa, The Invention of World Religions, or, How European Universalism Was Preserved in the Language of Pluralism, Chicago 2005.

David Maxwell, The Soul of the Luba. W.F.P. Burton, Missionary Ethnography and Belgian Colonial Science, in: History and Anthropology 19 (2008) 4, p. 325–351.

Beatrix Mesmer, Reinheit und Reinlichkeit. Bemerkungen zur Durchsetzung der häuslichen Hygiene in der Schweiz, in: Nicolai Bernard/Quirinus Reichen (eds.), Gesellschaft und Gesellschaften. Festschrift zum 65. Geburtstag von Professor Dr. Ulrich Im Hof, Bern 1982, p. 470–494.

Adam Mohr, Missionary Medicine and Akan Therapeutics: Illness, Health and Healing in Southern Ghana's Basel Mission, 1828–1918, in: Journal of Religion in Africa 39 (2009) 4, p. 429–461.

Arie L. Molendijk/Peter Pels (eds.), Religion in the Making: The Emergence of the Sciences of Religion, Leiden/Boston/Köln 1998.

Theodor Müller, Krankheitsbilder von der Goldküste, in: Die ärztliche Mission 7 (1912), p. 131–136.

Karl David Patterson, Health in Colonial Ghana. Disease, Medicine, and Socio-Economic Change, 1900–1955, Waltham 1981.

John D. Y. Peel, Religious Encounter and the Making of the Yoruba, Bloomington 2003.

Roy Porter, What is Disease? in: ibid (ed.), The Cambridge History of Medicine, Cambridge 2006, p. 71–102.

Alexandra Przyrembel, Wissen auf Wanderschaft. Britische Missionare, ethologisches Wissen und die Thematisierung religiöser Selbstgefühle um 1830, in: Historische Anthropologie 19 (2011) 1, p. 31–53.

Terence O. Ranger, Medical Science and Pentecost: The Dilemma of Anglicanism in Africa, in: W. J. Shiels (ed.), The Church and Healing, Oxford 1982, p. 333–365.

Terence O. Ranger, Godly Medicine. The Ambiguities of Medical Mission in Southeastern Tanzania 1900–1945, in: Steven Feierman/John M. Janzen (eds.), The Social Basis of Health and Healing in Africa, Berkley/Los Angeles/Oxford 1992, p. 256–282.

Christoph Ribbat, Religiöse Erregung: Protestantische Schwärmer im Kaiserreich, Frankfurt a. M. 1996.

Iris Ritzmann, Sanatorien, in: Historisches Lexikon der Schweiz, http://www.hls-dhs-dss.ch/textes/d/D14073.php, version 04.05.2017 (last access: 22.07.2022).

Diethard Sawicki, Leben mit den Toten: Geisterglauben und die Entstehung des Spiritismus in Deutschland 1770–1900, Paderborn 2002.

Paul Steiner, Wie ein blinder Neger wieder sehend wurde! Eine wahre Begebenheit aus der westafrikanischen Mission, Basel 1894.

Megan Vaughan, Curing Their Ills. Colonial Power and African Illness, Cambridge 1991.

Hermann Vortisch, Statistik und Bericht über das erste Halbjahr 1904 der ärztlichen Mission auf der Goldküste, in: Archiv für Schiffs- und Tropenhygiene 9 (1905), p. 346–354.

Hermann Vortisch, Bilder aus der ärztlichen Mission auf der Goldküste, in: Die ärztliche Mission 1 (1906), p. 3–10.

Hermann Vortisch, Die Neger der Goldküste, in: Globus 89 (1906), p. 277–283, 293–297.

Hermann Vortisch, Aus der Arbeit eines Missionsarztes, in: Schweizerische Rundschau für Medizin 38 (1912), p. 1025–1036.

Karolin Wetjen, Religionspädagogische Resonanzen und die Mission: "Christianity Making" im missionarischen Bildungsraum am Ende des 19. Jahrhunderts, in: David Käbisch/Michael Wermke (eds.), Transnationale Grenzgänge und Kulturkontakte. Historische Fallbeispiele in religionspädagogischer Perspektive, Leipzig 2017, p. 23–38.

Karolin Wetjen, Mission als theologisches Labor: Koloniale Aushandlungen des Religiösen in Ostafrika um 1900, Stuttgart 2020.

Luise White, Speaking with Vampires. Rumor and History in Colonial Africa, Berkley 2000.

Michael Worboys, Colonial and Imperial Medicine, in: Deborah Brunton (ed.), Medicine Transformed. Health, Disease and Society in Europe 1880–1930, Manchester/New York 2004, p. 211–238.

PART III

Reverberations of Hygiene 1885–1914

Part II

Reverberations of Hygiene 1882-1914

Shaping Colonial Science: Missionary Challenges, Racial Segregation and the Locality of Science

The imperial expansion in Africa both required and promoted scientific explanations and medical strategies, such as the ones developed in the field of tropical medicine and hygiene around 1900. As missionaries, explorers, traders, military personnel, scientists, settlers and colonial officials travelled to different parts of the world and encountered different people, knowledge of purity, health and cleanliness changed. How did the Basel Mission doctors participate in scientific controversies, political discussions and popular debates on hygiene from 1885 to 1914? By shaping ideas about tropical diseases and their prevention, the Basel medical missionaries introduced a wide audience of scientists, politicians and colonial enthusiasts to distinctive arguments and specific methods formed through their missionary vocation and experience in West Africa. Crucially, their negotiations of hygiene not only had cognitive reverberations but also practical and material implications both abroad and at home.

8.1 Trials from the Periphery

In 1891, Alfred Eckhardt made a clear statement about a misconception that was still widely held among tropical doctors and colonial officials at the time: "The indigenous also suffer from tertian fever (climate fever)

© The Author(s) 2023   313
L. M. Ratschiller Nasim, *Medical Missionaries and Colonial Knowledge in West Africa and Europe, 1885–1914*,
Cambridge Imperial and Post-Colonial Studies,
https://doi.org/10.1007/978-3-031-27128-1_8

frequently; it is a mistake to think that it only occurs with whites."[1] Myths about the innate resistance of Africans to tropical diseases go back to the earliest explorations of Africa. Europeans, who reached the west coast of Africa, labelling it as the "white man's grave," reported that Africans were significantly less affected by tropical fevers than themselves. This was partly due to the fact that early explorers and ship surgeons had little knowledge of African societies and the diseases they suffered from. However, European observers continued to view people living in the tropical world to be generally healthier due to their seemingly more natural way of life into the twentieth century. The "noble savage" stood as the epitome of health in contrast to the "modern civilised man."[2]

The suspected disease resistance of the "natives" in the colonies was one of the scientific arguments brought forward to pay less attention to, or not engage at all in, the subject of their health care.[3] Colonial governments showed very limited interest in the well-being of their African subjects until the turn of the twentieth century. The Basel missionaries, by contrast, depicted disease, suffering and death as an inherent part of Africans' lives since the onset of their mission on the Gold Coast in 1828.[4] While to many European visitors it seemed that Africans enjoyed good health compared to themselves, increasing missionary activity in the nineteenth century made it abundantly clear that Africans experienced poor health at least as much as Europeans.

---

[1] Eckhardt, Ärztliche Missionsarbeit in Christiansborg, p. 16.

[2] The idea that many aspects of European civilisation were harmful to health, as advocated by the French philosopher Jean-Jacques Rousseau in the eighteenth century, for instance, found wide recognition in medical circles. Bruchhausen, Die "hygienische Eroberung" der Tropen; Birthe Kundrus, Moderne Imperialisten. Das Kaiserreich im Spiegel seiner Kolonien, Köln et al. 2003, p. 162–173.

[3] Walter Bruchhausen, Sind die "Primitiven" gesünder? Völkerkundliche Perspektiven um 1900, in: Céline Kaiser/Marie-Luise Wünsche (eds.), Die "Nervosität der Juden" und andere Leiden an der Zivilisation. Konstruktionen des Kollektiven und Konzepte individueller Krankheit im psychiatrischen Diskurs um 1900, Paderborn et al. 2003, p. 41–56.

[4] Their letters describe for example how Africans struggled with bouts of fever, smallpox epidemics and the Guinea worm. Johannes Stanger, Letter to Committee, Christiansborg, 25.08.1847, BMA, D-1.2.17; Johannes Zimmermann, Letter to Committee, Ussu, 07.10.1850, BMA, D-1.3.16; Johann Georg Widman, Letter to Committee, Akropong, 18.01.1850, BMA, D-1.3.3; Johannes Stanger, Letter to Committee, Ussu, 02.07.1851, BMA, D-1.3.9.

Due to their prolonged stays in tropical regions, the Basel missionaries were able to study the specific disease environments thoroughly. During his medical research expedition in 1882–1883, Mähly observed that numerous African children succumbed to malaria, suggesting that it affected them as much as it did European adults. Therefore, he argued that African adults, who had survived malaria as children, had developed "a kind of tolerance" to the disease agent making them more resistant.[5] It was not until Robert Koch popularised his immunity theory in the early twentieth century, however, that tropical doctors generally accepted this view.[6] Upon his return from Oceania in 1900, Koch argued that "native" children in New Guinea represented the biggest reservoir of malaria infection, while adults had developed a relative immunity.[7]

Instead of examining climatic and environmental conditions exclusively, medical scientists in tropical colonies started searching for and identifying new germs in water, soil and in the bodies of both animals and humans. They became "microbe hunters," who isolated and cultivated pathogenic bacteria.[8] In the tropics, the notion of "hunting for microbes" developed in relation to colonial hunting sports. Koch was a passionate game hunter. During his 1906–1907 sleeping sickness expedition to East Africa, he shot and autopsied several animals, including herons, eagles, crocodiles and hippopotami, ostensibly to identify the animal hosts of trypanosomiasis.[9]

Colonies provided fertile ground for medical research and the development of new ideas that gained currency through formal and informal networks of physicians and researchers across the world. The acclaim for Fisch's first edition of *Tropische Krankheiten* in 1891, both in the scientific press and in the wider market, led to the publication of a second

[5] Ernst Mähly, Akklimatisation und Klimafieber, in: Deutsche Kolonialzeitung 3 (1886), p. 72–83, here p. 78.

[6] Thomas D. Brock, Robert Koch. A Life in Medicine and Bacteriology, New York 1988; Worboys, Germs, Malaria and the Invention of Mansonian Tropical Medicine, p. 192–193.

[7] Robert Koch, Ergebnisse der vom Deutschen Reich ausgesandten Malariaexpeditionen. Vortrag vom 05.11.1900, in: Julius Schwalbe (ed.), Gesammelte Werke von Robert Koch, Leipzig 1912, vol. 2, p. 435–447.

[8] Wolfgang U. Eckart, Robert Koch. Ein Bakteriologe für die Kolonien, in: Ulrich van der Heyden/Joachim Zeller (eds.) Kolonialmetropole Berlin. Eine Spurensuche, Berlin 2002, p. 102–106.

[9] Gradmann, Laboratory Disease, p. 222–224.

edition merely three years later. In the foreword of the 1894 version, Fisch assured that his "very abundant experiences" had produced "new insights," which he hoped, would act as a "faithful and reliable adviser" to Europeans in the tropics.[10] By emphasising the importance of first-hand experience and long-time practice in tropical climates, in contrast to armchair research in Europe, the Basel Mission doctors positioned themselves as experts in the field of tropical medicine and hygiene.

Fisch specified that the diagnosis of "bilious fever" in particular required revisions following "advances in recent research" and "our increasing experience."[11] By the 1870s, over 150 Basel missionaries had lost their lives in West Africa, with most deaths attributed to this specific condition. The Committee thus instructed Fisch to conduct a "medical-scientific study of bilious fever" to find out by what means it might be reduced or checked.[12] While the condition was fairly well-known as "black water fever" in French and English medical texts, German publications were limited to a few case studies. The disease started gaining more attention in the German medical press once the German Empire formalised its influence in Africa. Friedrich Plehn, who was a government physician in Cameroon from 1893 to 1894 before moving to German East-Africa, first used the term "*Schwarzwasserfieber*"—adopted from the English designation "black water fever"—instead of "*Gallenfieber*"—"bilious fever"—in an article in 1895, stating that he had adopted it in Cameroon.[13]

Mähly had described "bilious fever" as a misleading term for the prevalent condition as early as 1885 in the *Correspondenz-Blatt für Schweizer Ärzte*.[14] His observations, however, went unnoticed in German medical circles. Building on Mähly's findings, Fisch did not refer to the condition as "*Gallenfieber*" anymore from 1893, using the term "*Schwarzwasserfieber*" instead in his reports to the Committee.[15] After attributing Klara Finckh's death that same year to black water fever, he

---

[10] Fisch, Tropische Krankheiten, 2nd ed., foreword.

[11] Ibid.

[12] Committee report, 04.02.1885, BMA, Komitee-Protokoll 1885, §71.

[13] Friedrich Plehn, Über das Schwarzwasserfieber an der afrikanischen Westküste, in: Deutsche medizinische Wochenschrift 21 (1895), p. 397–400, 416–418, 434–437.

[14] Mähly, Über das sogenannte "Gallenfieber" an der Goldküste.

[15] Rudolf Fisch, Letter to Committee, 10.10.1893, BMA, D-1.59.36.

wrote a circular letter to the Basel missionaries in West Africa informing them of his reassessment and new insights into the disease.[16] It seems likely, therefore, that it was Fisch who first coined the term in the German language and that Friedrich Plehn adopted it shortly thereafter when he met the Basel missionaries in Cameroon.

The German-speaking scientific community entertained a ferocious debate about the cause and treatment of black water fever in the 1890s. The use and effect of quinine—the only anti-malarial remedy in those days—occupied centre stage in this dispute. Tropical doctors made contrasting observations about the effects of quinine on black water fever. While some of them thought that the intake of quinine for malaria prevention or treatment caused black water fever, others argued it proved effective against the latter condition too. Most physicians warned of the possible side effects of high quinine doses, including temporary deafness and permanent blindness, and therefore only recommended it in small quantities of one-tenth of a gram per day or on specific occasions such as expeditions.[17]

Rudolf Fisch, by contrast, questioned the prophylactic use of small quinine doses, assuming that it accumulated undesirable side effects while building up resistance of the malaria agent against the drug.[18] He started to experiment with higher and regular quinine doses for the Gold Coast missionaries in the early 1890s. While the mortality rate of black water fever was believed to be around 50 per cent at that time, Fisch's approach markedly reduced this figure among the missionaries, from 42.7 per cent in 1890 to 9.3 per cent in 1895.[19] Only the German colonial doctors Friedrich and Albert Plehn reached a comparable mortality rate dealing with back water fever.[20] In 1896, Fisch published the results of his long-term experiment in several medical and colonial journals in Switzerland

---

[16] Rudolf Fisch, Circular letter about black water fever, 08.02.1894, BMA, D-1.61.56.

[17] Grant, West African Hygiene, p. 11–12.

[18] Fisch, Tropische Krankheiten, 1st ed., p. 47.

[19] Rudolf Fisch, Über Schwarzwasserfieber, in: Correspondenz-Blatt für Schweizer Ärzte 26 (1896), p. 271–276, here p. 273; Ibid., Das Schwarzwasserfieber nach den Beobachtungen und Erfahrungen auf der Goldküste Westafrikas, in: Deutsche Medizinal-Zeitung 17 (1896), p. 223–225, 235–236, 247–249, here p. 236, 248.

[20] Albert Plehn, Beitrag zur Kenntnis von Verlauf und Behandlung der tropischen Malaria in Kamerun, Berlin 1896, p. 54.

and Germany, advancing the theory that an "adequate and consequent quinine prophylaxis" prevented both malaria and black water fever.[21]

Robert Koch joined this debate a couple of years later by stating that black water fever was caused by "pure quinine poisoning."[22] His speech to the German Colonial Society in June 1898 caused considerable turmoil among tropical doctors, who had been prescribing quinine extensively as an anti-malarial drug.[23] Koch, whose reflections were based on short research expeditions to Africa and Asia, merely recommended it as an occasional malaria prophylaxis.[24] His theory on quinine as the cause for black water fever appeared in a paper widely published in medical journals in 1899. Fisch, who read Koch's thesis in the *Afrika-Post* available on the Gold Coast, feared that it would cause Europeans to reject quinine therapy and thus increase the occurrence of malarial fevers. He replied with an article, explaining that most black water fever cases affected people who only rarely took quinine.[25]

Missionary texts such as Fisch's studies on quinine served as trials from the periphery in a period when sciences were adopting their present form.[26] Fisch arrived at the conclusion that quinine must be amply used during fever intervals, applying what is accepted as the most effective method today. During his 26-year tenure on the Gold Coast, he was able to reduce the overall mortality among missionaries from 36 per

---

[21] Rudolf Fisch, Das Schwarzwasserfieber nach den Beobachtungen und Erfahrungen auf der Goldküste Westafrikas, in: Deutsche Medizinal-Zeitung 17 (1896) p. 223–225, 235–236, 247–249; Ibid., Das Schwarzwasserfieber, in: Deutsche Kolonialzeitung 9 (1896), p. 139–141; Ibid., Über Schwarzwasserfieber, in: Correspondenz-Blatt für Schweizer Ärzte 26 (1896), p. 271–276.

[22] Robert Koch, Über Schwarzwasserfieber (Hämoglobinurie), in: Julius Schwalbe (ed.), Gesammelte Werke von Robert Koch, Leipzig 1912, vol. 2, p. 348–370.

[23] Stephan Besser, Die hygienische Eroberung Afrikas. 9. Juni 1898: Robert Koch hält seinen Vortrag *Ärztliche Beobachtungen in den Tropen*, in: Alexander Honold/Klaus R. Scherpe (eds.), Mit Deutschland um die Welt. Eine Kulturgeschichte des Fremden in der Kolonialzeit, Stuttgart/Weimar 2004, p. 217–225.

[24] Koch, Über Schwarzwasserfieber (Hämoglobinurie); Ibid., Ergebnisse der vom Deutschen Reich ausgesandten Malariaexpeditionen.

[25] In their case, he argued, a small dose of only 0.25 grams of quinine could potentially trigger black water fever. Rudolf Fisch, Ist Schwarzwasserfieber Chininvergiftung? in: Afrika-Post 2 (1899), p. 277–278.

[26] Livingstone, Scientific Inquiry and the Missionary Enterprise; Johnston, Missionary Writing and Empire.

cent in 1885 to 6 per cent in 1911.[27] Albert Plehn, Friedrich's brother, who worked as a German government doctor in Cameroon from 1894 to 1903, wrote an enthusiastic review of Fisch's research in the *Archiv für Schiffs- und Tropenhygiene* in 1900.[28] He drew on Fisch's results to introduce a large-scale "consequent quinine prophylaxis" for Europeans in Cameroon.[29] Physicians working in tropical colonies had to be dedicated to long-term field observation and open to experimentation in challenging environments—the "stuff of missionary medicine," as Maryinez Lyons put it.[30]

The effectiveness of quinine prophylaxis created the impression among scientists, and Europeans more generally, that Africa had become accessible to them. Although the application of quinine remained highly controversial throughout the nineteenth century, the drug combatted the pessimism that pervaded the colonial public about the health and survival of Europeans in the tropics.[31] This optimism did not entirely abolish the image of the "white man's grave" but it helped to introduce a new hope and impulse in the colonisation of the continent.[32]

The four editions of Fisch's *Tropische Krankheiten* show how new findings in bacteriology and parasitology were gradually incorporated into existing knowledge on tropical diseases. The rapid changes in medical knowledge were particularly visible in Fisch's observations on malaria. The first edition in 1891 presented and discussed studies conducted in Italy, where malaria was endemic and resurgent around Rome. In 1885–1886, Camillo Golgi, Angelo Celli and Ettore Marchiafava were able to link the life cycle of the protozoan parasite causing malaria to the clinical

---

[27] Fischer, Der Missionsarzt Rudolf Fisch, p. 516.

[28] Albert Plehn, Besprechung des Artikels von R. Fisch: Ist Schwarzwasserfieber Chininvergiftung? in: Archiv für Schiffs- und Tropenhygiene 4 (1900), p. 63–65, here p. 64.

[29] Ibid., Zur Chininprophylaxe der Malaria nebst Bemerkungen zur Schwarzwasserfieberfrage, in: Archiv für Schiffs- und Tropenhygiene 5 (1901), p. 380–393.

[30] Lyons, The Colonial Disease, p. 67.

[31] Philip D. Curtin, The Image of Africa: British Ideas and Action, 1780–1850, vol. 1, London 1964, p. 361–362; Headrick, The Tools of Empire, p. 231–237.

[32] Although medical factors, such as quinine prophylaxis, did not directly contribute to the Scramble for Africa, the decline in European morality in Africa from the mid-nineteenth century certainly facilitated imperial expansion. Philip D. Curtin, Death by Migration. Europe's Encounter with the Tropical World in the Nineteenth Century, Cambridge 1989, p. 132–137; Chakrabarti, Medicine and Empire, p. 126–129.

syndrome.[33] Despite this discovery, scientists still needed to explain how it spread from one human to another. Patrick Manson had provided an earlier clue in 1877, when he demonstrated in his research on lymphatic filariasis that mosquitoes transmitted filarial worms.[34]

Significantly, while the first three editions of *Tropische Krankheiten* were structured around what Fisch identified as the most pressing conditions in West Africa, the fourth edition in 1912 listed diseases according to their vectors, such as mosquitoes, flies and worms. Twenty years after Manson's vector theory, Ronald Ross, an officer of the Indian Medical Services for twenty-five years, created the formal link between the malaria parasite and the mosquito vector. In 1897, he was able to demonstrate that the protozoan parasite causing malaria was spread by mosquitoes, which set the agenda for the formation of metropolitan institutions devoted to tropical medicine and hygiene at the turn of the twentieth century. Ross' discovery of the anopheles mosquito as both intermediate host and vector of malaria implied that environment, albeit very differently constituted from that of the miasma theories, was of vital importance after all.[35]

The discoveries of microbes, parasites and vectors of particular diseases gave rise to new optimism for their eradication. Yet while scientists were well equipped to identify many agents of tropical diseases under the microscope, there were far fewer definitive cures. Prevention, therefore, remained a major focus in tropical medicine, as Fisch's continuously revised advice on tropical hygiene in the four editions of *Tropische Krankheiten* illustrates.

Precisely when bacteriology was making significant strides, several epidemic outbreaks of cholera and plague afflicted different parts of the colonies, killing millions of people and often threatening European interests. These epidemics in the 1880s and 1890s established the link between germs and the tropics, imprinting in popular and scientific discourse the need for bacteriological intervention to protect primarily European lives and commercial interests.[36] Mark Harrison has shown

---

[33] Worboys, Germs, Malaria and the Invention of Mansonian Tropical Medicine, p. 189–190.

[34] Haynes, Imperial Medicine, p. 29–56.

[35] Worboys, Germs, Malaria and the Invention of Mansonian Tropical Medicine, p. 194.

[36] Olaf Briese, Angst in den Zeiten der Cholera. Über kulturelle Ursprünge des Bakteriums, Berlin 2003; Rod Edmond, Returning Fears: Tropical Disease and the

that, in India, an earlier respect for Indian medical knowledge, not least when cholera began to ravage Europe in the 1830s, gave way to an unfavourable recasting of the environment as "intrinsically pathogenic and its indigenous inhabitants as reservoirs of dirt and disease."[37]

Medical research at the end of the nineteenth century increasingly focussed on the human body as the site of germs, particularly after Koch argued that Africans were carriers of trypanosomiasis, also known as sleeping sickness.[38] Now human bodies—some more than others— were prone to host germs and needed to be vaccinated or isolated. This allowed for more intrusive public health measures whereby the state could order medical officers to inject antigens into the bodies of subjects or take brutal sanitary measures.[39] Colonial administrations started to introduce a range of measures in West Africa from garbage collection, water purification and "mosquito brigades" to the restriction of Africans' movements and their confinement in camps, where they were treated under force and often subjected to painful and risky drug tests.[40] But the easiest and most effective measure, they argued, was racial segregation, especially in urban centres, where most Europeans in the colonies lived.

8.2   The Question of Segregation

The turn of the twentieth century marked the beginning of a new phase in public health and hygiene both at home and abroad. The theory of human germ carriers, which suggested that even healthy individuals could carry microbes in their bodies and infect others without themselves showing symptoms of the disease, reinstated medical segregation based

Metropolis, in: Felix Driver/Luciana Martins (eds.), Tropical Visions in the Age of Empire, Chicago 2005, p. 175–194; Valesca Huber, The Unification of the Globe by Disease? The International Sanitary Conferences on Cholera, 1851–1894, in: The Historical Journal 49 (2006) 2, p. 453–476.

[37] Harrison, Tropical Medicine in Nineteenth-Century India, p. 301.

[38] Christoph Gradmann, Robert Koch and the Invention of the Carrier State: Tropical Medicine, Veterinary Infections and Epidemiology around 1900, in: Studies in History and Philosophy of Biological and Biomedical Sciences 41 (2010) 3, p. 232–240.

[39] Paul Weindling, Epidemics and Genocide in Eastern Europe, 1890–1945, Oxford 2000; Thomas Rütten/Martina King (eds.), Contagionism and Contagious Diseases. Medicine and Literature 1880–1933, Berlin/Boston 2013.

[40] Helen Tilley, Medicine, Empires, and Ethics in Colonial Africa, in: AMA Journal of Ethics 18 (2016) 7, p. 743–753.

on race and class.[41] Segregation policies stemmed from a new scientific understanding of the body as an anatomical container of disease.[42] The localisation of pathogens in the individual body led to the problematisation of the boundary between the inside and outside of the body. David Armstrong argued that states used hygiene to oversee the passage between the two: "The focus of late nineteenth century public health became the zone which separated anatomical space from environmental space, and its regime of hygiene developed as the monitoring of matter which crossed between these two great spaces."[43]

Social and racial segregation, especially the segregation of urban space, was frequently justified by reference to images of disease and dirt. Proponents of the hygiene movement, public health officers and bacteriologists fought the eradication of disease in the tropics, or among the poor in European cities, not just through vaccines and immunisation but also by enacting social and cultural reforms. Ambitious medical projects such as the segregation of whole cities were rarely viable in Europe, in contrast to the colonies. Professional planners revelled in the relative freedom that colonial contexts seemed to offer for the realisation of what they considered to be modern, hygienically informed city planning. Although these freedoms proved to be chimeric in practice, scores of experts drew inspiration from the notion of the colony as a laboratory, comparing and contrasting ameliorative interventions across empires.[44]

By the early twentieth century, many Europeans in West Africa lived in settlements, segregated from the African population, which was seen

---

[41] On the effect of the theory of human germ carriers in the colonies, see Warwick Anderson, "Where Every Prospect Pleases and Only Man is Vile". Laboratory Medicine as Colonial Discourse, in: Critical Inquiry 18 (1992) 3, p. 506–529; Stephan Besser, Tropische Infektionsphantasmen. Zur kulturellen Typologie der Malaria um die Jahrhundertwende, in: Alexander Honold/Klaus R. Scherpe (eds.), Das Fremde. Reiseerfahrung, Schreibformen und kulturelles Wissen, Bern et al. 1999, p. 175–195; Bauche, Medizin und Herrschaft, p. 310–333.

[42] Alexander Butchart, The Anatomy of Power. European Constructions of the African Body, London/New York 1998, esp. p. 74–91; Philipp Sarasin/Silvia Berger/Marianne Hänseler/Myriam Spörri (eds.), Bakteriologie und Moderne. Studien zur Biopolitik des Unsichtbaren 1870–1920, Frankfurt a. M. 2007.

[43] Armstrong, Public Health Spaces and the Fabrication of Identity, p. 396.

[44] Carl Nightingale, Segregation: A Global History of Divided Cities, Chicago 2012.

to be a source of infection.[45] Whereas the hitherto assumed immunity of Africans towards a range of tropical diseases was used as an argument to prove medical differences and not engage in their health care, the contrary point of view now legitimised racial segregation. Anxieties over Africans as containers of disease and dirt grew.[46] Experts in tropical medicine declared segregation to be "the first law of hygiene in the tropics" and the justification for the preferential treatment of Europeans was framed against the supposed ignorance of the "native" population.[47]

The British Colonial Secretary Joseph Chamberlain recommended the segregation of European and African housing as early as 1900 to prevent the spread of malaria. Knowledge produced in the field of tropical hygiene was instrumental in instituting residential segregation along racial lines. The Governor of the Gold Coast Colony, Matthew Nathan thought that African towns and villages were "native reservoirs" of infection and relocated the capital from Accra to Christiansborg in 1902. He further expedited racial segregation by demanding the implementation of a 44 feet protection zone separating European and African neighbourhoods. Nathan's plans, however, did not materialise since they were met with considerable resistance from the African population as well as European traders and missionaries, who simply refused to move their trading and mission posts for fear that spatial separation would damage their respective purposes.[48]

The Basel missionaries in the town of Akropong on the Gold Coast had seen a wave of heavy fevers in 1901, which Fisch accredited to "the proximity of Negro houses with their gruesome mosquito hotbeds" to the missionary compound and the presence of "Negro children," who he saw as a "constant source of infection." He thus filed for the relocation of the

---

[45] Philip D. Curtin, Medical Knowledge and Urban Planning in Tropical Africa, in: American Historical Review 90 (1985) 3, p. 594–613; John Cell, Anglo-Indian Medical Theory and the Origins of Segregation in West Africa, in: American Historical Review 91 (1989) 2, p. 307–335.

[46] This tendency to regard the proximity of Africans as a primary source of contagion has been referred to by Maynard Swanson as the "sanitation syndrome". Maynard Swanson, The Sanitation Syndrome: Bubonic Plague and Urban Native Policy in the Cape Colony, 1900–1909, in: The Journal of African History 18 (1977) 3, p. 387–410.

[47] Walter Myers, Seventy Second Annual Meeting of the British Medical Association, in: British Medical Journal, 1904, p. 631.

[48] Thomas S. Gale, Segregation in British West Africa, in: Cahiers d'Études Africaines 20 (1980) 80, p. 495–507; Patterson, Health in Colonial Ghana, p. 35–40.

mission station at greater distance from the neighbouring African town.[49] The Committee initially agreed to this costly measure but the plan failed to materialise due to the resolute objection of the other missionaries.[50] Most of them still questioned the validity of the mosquito theory and, more importantly, argued that segregation would undermine an essential tenet of missionary work: the necessary proximity to the people they sought to convert.[51]

The Basel Mission doctors, in contrast, insisted on the hygienic imperative of segregation measures in line with the majority of their medical colleagues.[52] Following the fever outbreak in Akropong, Fisch was assigned to design the plans for the reconstruction of the secondary school in Krobo. He recommended that the school should be situated at least one kilometre away from the houses of Africans and that the residence of the European school principal ought to be in the opposite direction to the wind on a slightly elevated site, as far as possible from the rooms of the African pupils but still close enough to exercise the necessary discipline. Upon completion of the secondary school in Krobo, however, the actual distance between the principal's home and the pupils' dorms amounted to only 30 meters, which shows that medical segregation was hardly reconcilable with missionary work.[53]

German scientists closely followed urban segregation projects developed by British and French doctors and administrators in the tropical world. Friedrich Plehn noted approvingly after a visit to India that the British kept European and "indigenous" neighbourhoods apart in most colonial cities in an article in the *Archiv für Schiffs- und Tropenhygiene* in 1899: "The European district is, without exception, and in full contrast to the native district, laid out in an irreproachably hygienic way, from the capital to the medium-sized and smaller provincial cities."[54] Ludwig Külz turned to French Guinea, arguing that although the French were

[49] Rudolf Fisch, Annual report for 1901, 12.02.1902, p. 3–4, BMA, D-1.75.19.

[50] Deliberation on new building plans in Akropong with several statements, 27.08.–20.09.1902, BMA, D-1.77.30–34; Committee report, 09.11.1902, BMA, Komitee-Protokoll 1902, §650.

[51] Letter from the station conference in Akropong, 27.08.1902, BMA, D-1.77.30.

[52] Arthur Häberlin, Letter to Inspector Oehler, Duala, 25.03.1908, BMA, E-2.27.123.

[53] Rudolf Fisch, Letter to Committee, 14.03.1902, BMA, D-1.76.191.

[54] Friedrich Plehn, Bericht über eine Informationsreise nach Ceylon und Indien, in: Archiv für Schiffs- und Tropenhygiene 3 (1899), p. 273–311.

"not by any means superior to us in areas of tropical scientific research," they had "in many ways a huge lead over us in our West African protectorates" regarding the organisation of colonial cities. He commented on Conakry's segregated cityscape, observing that "everything that has been created in Conakry since 1890 is according to plan, and equally hygienic and comfortable."[55]

At the International Medical Congress in Paris in 1900, the German government doctor Hans Ziemann declared that "native settlements" in West Africa should be "transferred approximately one kilometre away from the European districts, according to the flying range of the Anopheline," to prevent the spread of malaria among the European population.[56] He repeatedly submitted this proposal to the German colonial government in Cameroon in the following years, citing hygienic reasons for the segregation of the capital, Douala. From 1910, the colonial administration officially pursued the ambitious plan to completely remove the African population and landowners of Douala from their ancestral homes on the left bank of the Wouri River. The Duala people were to be relocated outside of the townscape, separated by a one-kilometre wide undeveloped cordon sanitaire, to make Cameroon's most important port city a healthy one for Europeans.[57]

German tropical doctors promoted their segregation plans by combining medical, economic and cultural arguments. Hans Ziemann specified in 1910 that the new "Negro town" was to be transformed into "an exemplary major port as a flagship of German colonial efforts," following the examples of other West African port cities such as

[55] Ludwig Külz, Guinée française und Kamerun, in: Amtsblatt für das Schutzgebiet Kamerun 13–16 (1909), p. 115–118, 133–144, 144–148, 163–168, here p. 133.

[56] Hans Ziemann, Zweiter Bericht über Malaria und Moskitos an der afrikanischen Westküste, in: Deutsche Medizinische Wochenzeitschrift 26 (1900), p. 753–756, 769–772, here p. 771.

[57] Andreas Eckert, Die Duala und die Kolonialmächte: Eine Untersuchung zu Widerstand, Protest und Protonationalismus in Kamerun vor dem Zweiten Weltkrieg, Münster 1991; Eckart, Medizin und Kolonialimperialismus, p. 217–231; Bauche, Medizin und Herrschaft, p. 274–310; Ulrike Hamann, Prekäre koloniale Ordnung: Rassistische Konjunkturen im Wiederspruch. Deutsches Kolonialregime 1884–1914, Bielefeld 2015, p. 219–274.

Conakry, Accra, Lagos and Freetown.[58] The hygienist Philalethes Kuhn, Cameroon's most prominent proponent of racial segregation, emphasised that it was for the Africans' own good, since contact with European culture had distorted their true nature.[59]

The colonial administration referred to these experts to justify their segregations policies.[60] The Duala received limited compensation for their land on the river bank and were forced to sell their property below value. The Basel Mission Committee assessed the situation in Douala in 1914, observing that the city was "probably the most advantageous harbour on the whole west coast of Africa" and that "the government therefore wants to expand the harbour and make the city the trading centre for the colony and the most important foothold of its rule on the West African Coast."[61] While colonial authorities relied on hygienic arguments to substantiate their segregation plans, their actions were fundamentally driven by economic and political motives, as contemporaries noted.[62]

The fact that hygienic rationales for racial segregation dovetailed with other European imperial goals made such measures all the more appealing. The expropriation and forced resettlement of the Duala opened up new building land on the shores of the Cameroon river, the capital's main trading and transport area, for administrative buildings and emergent colonial industries. Additionally, it undermined the Duala's role as key economic and political intermediaries.[63] Both the far-reaching implications of the segregation plan and the chronology of its ruthless

[58] Hans Ziemann, Gutachten über die Notwendigkeit der Entfernung der Eingeborenen aus der Nähe der Europäer in Duala, Duala, 28.05.1910, in: Denkschrift Enteignung, p. 3306–3307, BArch R 1001/4427.

[59] Philalethes Kuhn, Die Sanierung der Duala, April 1914, in: Denkschrift Enteignung, p. 3364–3366, BArch R 1001/5764.

[60] Kuhn was a co-founder and member of the *Deutsche Gesellschaft für Rassenhygiene*— German Society for Racial Hygiene—from 1905. He became one of the most eminent racial hygienist in Germany after WWI. See Eckart, Medizin und Kolonialimperialismus, p. 220–230.

[61] Evangelische Missionsgesellschaft zu Basel (ed.), Neunundneunzigster Jahresbericht, Basel 1914, p. 131.

[62] Wolfgang U. Eckart, Malariaprävention und Rassentrennung. Die ärztliche Vorbereitung und Rechtfertigung der Duala-Enteignung 1912–1914 in: History and Philosophy of the Life Sciences 10 (1988) 2, p. 363–378.

[63] Austen/Derrick, Middlemen of the Cameroons Rivers, p. 93–137; Eckert, Grundbesitz, Landkonflikte und kolonialer Wandel.

implementation led to the formation of a resistance movement among the African population in Douala. The Committee observed that it had "unleashed a storm of indignation among the Duala," who invoked that they had been assured in a contract with the colonial government in 1885 that they would never be displaced from their homes.[64]

The Basel Mission's annual report for 1914 illustrates that the mission society faced an ongoing dilemma in Cameroon, trapped between advocating for the rights of the Duala, who had been forcibly removed from their homeland, and the desire to improve hygienic conditions for their European staff in the colony:

> Our position has not been easy. On the one hand, we thought that a partial expropriation lies in the equal hygienic interest of blacks and whites; even perceptive Duala share this view. On the other hand, we think that an expansion of the dispossession of the whole tribe is unnecessary; the question of whether this is compatible with the pledges in the 1885 contract has been bothering us.[65]

The Duala, whose attitude had by no means been anti-German thus far, defended themselves by submitting numerous petitions to the colonial government and the Reichstag. They contacted German opposition leaders and solicited legal support in Germany.[66] They also "placed high hopes on the intervention of the mission," as the Committee admitted, but were bitterly disappointed by the mission's lack of assertiveness.[67] The Basel missionaries tried to appease the Duala by asking them to be forgiving and obedient towards the German rulers. When Rudolf Duala Manga Bell, a Basel Mission parishioner and church elder, applied to the mission leaders for support, they advised him to come to terms with the new reality.[68]

---

[64] Evangelische Missionsgesellschaft zu Basel (ed.), Neunundneunzigster Jahresbericht, Basel 1914, p. 131.

[65] Ibid., p. 131–132.

[66] Adolf Rüger, Die Widerstandsbewegung des Rudolf Manga Bell in Kamerun, in: Walter Markow (ed.), Études Africaines/African Studies/Afrika-Studien. Dem II. Internationalen Afrikanistenkongress in Dakar gewidmet, Leipzig 1967, p. 107–128.

[67] Evangelische Missionsgesellschaft zu Basel (ed.), Neunundneunzigster Jahresbericht, Basel 1914, p. 131.

[68] Gründer, Christliche Mission, p. 164.

The Duala's resistance eventually led to the condemnation and execution of the movement's alleged ringleaders, Rudolf Duala Manga Bell and his cousin Adolf Ngoso Din, who had been charged with high treason.[69] The Basel Mission, as well as other mission societies operating in Cameroon, had condemned the charges of high treason as unsubstantiated and repeatedly intervened on their behalf in Berlin and Douala. The Committee deplored that "the fall of the chief Manga Duala, who is accused of urging the King of Bamum to reject German rule, has led to a disastrous aggravation of the conflict" since "the Reichstag has taken this as a reason to endorse the full implementation of the expropriation, which had been temporarily suspended."[70]

The Basel Mission was directly affected by the dispossessions in Douala, losing some of their land at the river bank. Their protest, however, mainly arose from the fact that the relocation of the Duala meant that they had to follow them and establish new missionary facilities on the outskirts of the city.[71] Reflecting on the challenges caused by the spatial separation between their missionaries and the Duala, the Committee members openly expressed their worries:

> One thing is sadly certain: our work will be sensitively damaged by the expropriation. If the indigenous are truly moving into the resettlements, we will have to build one or two new stations there. [...] However, it looks like the people don't want to settle on the plots allocated to them by the government but prefer to move into the bush. Therefore, there is a serious risk that our communities, which have been laboriously gathered for decades, will be dispersed.[72]

The Basel Mission's hesitant and inconsistent position on the expropriation of the Duala left a bitter aftertaste.[73] The Committee members reported that a parishioner had proposed that "when the European uses

---

[69] Rüger, Die Widerstandsbewegung des Rudolf Manga Bell in Kamerun.

[70] Evangelische Missionsgesellschaft zu Basel (ed.), Neunundneunzigster Jahresbericht, Basel 1914, p. 132.

[71] Gründer, Christliche Mission, p. 162–163.

[72] Evangelische Missionsgesellschaft zu Basel (ed.), Neunundneunzigster Jahresbericht, Basel 1914, p. 132.

[73] Schlatter, Geschichte der Basler Mission, vol. 3, p. 309–310; Gründer, Christliche Mission, p. 159–169.

the word *bonate*—brothers—to address the Duala in his sermon, he should leave the service, since he is not serious about it," cautioning that "this proposal was very well received, and pastor Modi had trouble enough preventing it from becoming a resolution."[74] They also deplored that there had been "unpleasant disruptions during the Christmas celebration in Bonaduma" during which "the boys said, the Europeans come and proclaim 'Peace on Earth' and at the same time take away our property."[75] The Duala's fierce resistance against the German segregation policy and the outbreak of the First World War prevented more extensive expropriations.[76]

The relocation of schools, or even entire mission stations, for hygienic purposes remained highly controversial within the Basel Mission. The Committee asked the missionaries in West Africa in 1914: "Is it even possible to pursue missionary work in Africa if one keeps away from the indigenous?"[77] In their statement, the missionaries explained: "Despite all precaution towards the danger of malarial fevers, the missionary should not move away from the African community!"[78] The Committee members decided to separate the teachers' quarters from the schools and pupils' dorms, as Rudolf Fisch, Arthur Häberlin and Theodor Müller had required, yet left them on the same compound. They also refused the mission doctors' recommendation to segregate mission stations from adjacent villages, arguing that the missionary belonged in close proximity to the population.[79]

The conflicting views of the Basel Mission doctors and their non-medical colleagues on whether preventative measures to protect European lives should take precedence over the proclamation of the gospel in physical proximity to Africans indicate that scientific concepts of hygiene, colonial notions of cleanliness and religious ideas of purity presented fundamental tensions that proved difficult to reconcile. The missiologist

---

[74] Evangelische Missionsgesellschaft zu Basel (ed.), Neunundneunzigster Jahresbericht, Basel 1914, p. 132.

[75] Ibid.

[76] Eckert, Die Duala und die Kolonialmächte, p. 124.

[77] Committee report, 11.02.1914, BMA, Komitee-Protokoll 1914, §215.

[78] Committee report, 08.07.1914, BMA, Komitee-Protokoll 1914, §1082.

[79] Committee report, 06.04.1914, BMA, Komitee-Protokoll 1914, §479; Committee report, 08.07.1914, BMA, Komitee-Protokoll 1914, §1082.

Gustav Warneck stated in his reference work that "from a purely hygienic point of view, the avoidance of fever areas might be recommended" but that it "can never be the standpoint of the mission, which ought to walk in the footsteps of the man who gave his life as ransom."[80] The Basel Mission's evangelising agenda simply made it impossible to implement the isolation of European missionaries from their African clientele.

8.3   THE LOCALITY OF SCIENCE

The contributions of the Basel Mission doctors to the rise and consolidation of tropical medicine and hygiene were intimately tied to their long-term medical praxis in West Africa. The German Colonial Society conducted a survey on the climatology of the tropics by sending out a questionnaire to colonial officers, scientists and missionaries, the results of which were published in 1891. The sections on West Africa and Congo included Rudolf Fisch's research on the most prevalent diseases in the region.[81] Interestingly, the official report referred to him as a physician based in Aburi on the Gold Coast, completely omitting his role as a mission doctor. This detail highlights that the Basel medical missionaries earned scientific credibility through their occupation of specific locations abroad.[82]

The formation of tropical medicine and the growing body of knowledge about tropical hygiene fundamentally depended on experiences in specific geographical locations, often occupied by missionaries. Whether developing expertise on local pathologies, engaging in confrontations with African healers, adapting to regional ideas and practices of medicine or establishing systems of public health provision, the physical and cognitive spaces that the Basel Mission doctors inhabited shaped their contributions to medical knowledge. Their scientific studies and medical activities were quintessentially what David N. Livingstone has called a "spatial practice."[83]

---

[80] Warneck, Evangelische Missionslehre, p. 469–470.

[81] Otto Schellong, Die Klimatologie der Tropen (erster Bericht) nach den Ergebnissen des Fragebogenmaterials im Auftrage der Deutschen Kolonialgesellschaft, Berlin 1891, p. 17–23, BArch R 8023/1005.

[82] Chambers/Gillespie, Locality in the History of Science.

[83] By combining a knowledge-based approach with a space-based approach Livingstone has proposed an innovative concept for the history of science. Livingstone, Putting

Naturally, the Basel Mission doctors were not the only medical missionaries to establish themselves as experts in the field of tropical medicine and hygiene. Andrew Davidson, who took up a lectureship in oriental diseases at Edinburgh University after a stint as a London Mission Society medical missionary in Madagascar, was the author of the 1892 *Geographical Pathology* and the editor of *Hygiene and Diseases of Warm Climates* appearing in 1893. Others used their linguistic skills to work between their own and their hosts' medical traditions by translating European medical knowledge into Asian or African languages and vice-versa. Still others became experts in the treatment of conditions like leprosy and the therapies they advanced were intermingled with colonial development policies.[84]

Knowledge of tropical diseases and hygiene was negotiated across professional, linguistic and spatial borders to form what became an independent medical discipline at the turn of the twentieth century. Concurrently, it is difficult to conceptualise tropical medicine as a distinct scientific speciality in the sense that it did not have a well-defined research methodology of its own. Ronald Ross wrote in 1905 that "the term tropical medicine does not imply merely the treatment of tropical diseases" but a "science of medicine" and, more importantly, "a medicine for the Empire," where diseases were the "great enemies of civilisation."[85] Rather than producing a consistent and clearly circumscribed scientific methodology, tropical medicine served as a justification of colonialism and became part and parcel of the civilising mission.[86]

Tropical medicine and mission medicine were both conceived as a means of extending European influence in Africa but the religious agenda of the medical missionaries distinguished them from other actors in the colonial space. The first edition of the Basel Mission's medical journal

Science in Its Place; Ibid., Landscapes of Knowledge, in: Peter Meusburger/David N. Livingstone/Heike Jöns (eds.), Geographies of Science, London 2010, p. 3–22.

[84] Michael Worboys, The Colonial World as Mission and Mandate: Leprosy and Empire, 1900–1940, in: Osiris 15 (2000), p. 207–218; Richard Hölzl, Lepra als *entangled disease*. Leidende afrikanische Körper in Medien und Praxis der katholischen Mission in Ostafrika 1911–1945, in: Linda Ratschiller/Siegfried Weichlein (eds.), Der schwarze Körper als Missionsgebiet. Medizin, Ethnologie, Theologie in Afrika und Europa 1880–1960, Köln/Weimar/Wien 2016, p. 95–121.

[85] Ronald Ross, The Progress of Tropical Medicine, in: Journal of the Royal African Society 4 (1905) 15, p. 271–289, here p. 271–272.

[86] Neill, Science and Civilizing Missions.

clearly distanced the medical mission from worldly medical endeavours: "We believe that the medical mission is not humanitarian work but missionary work, whose ultimate objective it is to lead the heathens to the faith of Jesus Christ."[87] By 1900, Protestant medical missions had developed their own theology, which portrayed the alleviation of human suffering as a Christian duty that reflected the compassion that Christ had demonstrated by healing the sick.[88]

From the turn of the twentieth century, networks in tropical medicine became more impermeable with the foundation of laboratories, journals, public and private funding agencies and educational institutions. The Basel Mission doctors challenged the metropolitan developments in tropical medicine by pointing to their shortcomings, including a lack of in-the-field observation, indifference to cultural expertise and ignorance of social conditions. The scarcity of sources on African medicine before 1895 is indicative of a lack of intellectual interest and material incentives for systematic research into diseases affecting the population in Africa on the part of governments, doctors and colonial authorities.[89] Fisch's *Tropische Krankheiten*, first appearing in 1891, was one of the first medical handbooks that dealt with diseases mainly affecting the African population on the west coast of Africa.[90]

In contrast to colonial physicians, medical missionaries had very limited coercive powers and relied on gaining the approval of African societies. To a great extent, therefore, the medical practice of missionaries complied with the demands of the people they wished to convert. Michael Worboys has argued that "in certain ways, missionary medicine was the opposite of tropical medicine: clinical rather than laboratory-based, patient-centred rather than disease-centred and local rather than imperial."[91] In the foreword to the fourth edition of *Tropische Krankheiten* in 1912, Fisch explained:

---

[87] Basler Missionskomitee (ed.), An die Freunde des Ärztlichen Zweiges der Basler Mission, Basel 1891, p. 1.

[88] Ferngren, Medicine and Religion, p. 170.

[89] Bruchhausen/Roelcke, Categorising 'African Medicine', p. 78.

[90] Fisch, Tropische Krankheiten, 1st ed.

[91] Worboys, Colonial and Imperial Medicine, p. 232–233.

In the new edition of this book, which only pursues practical goals, namely to give guidance to missionaries, traders, planters and officials on how to recognise, prevent and treat tropical diseases, I have tried to put the main emphasis on their prevention, both in the introduction and also by describing the aetiologies of these diseases.[92]

By emphasising the purely practical aim of his handbook, Fisch distanced himself from metropolitan developments in tropical medicine. The Basel Mission doctors mostly operated in remote areas in West Africa with poor laboratory conditions. Their primary focus lay on practice-oriented solutions for concrete problems on the spot, as Fisch's statement clarifies: "I look on the results of my studies with satisfaction, and I am pleased that other doctors who work on the west coast acknowledge my results and my way of treatment as correct and apply them with satisfactory success."[93] In various ways, medical missionaries helped to define medical practice in tropical colonies in contradistinction to the discipline of tropical medicine developing in European metropolises with its shortage of prolonged practical experience.[94]

The institutionalisation of tropical medicine around 1900 took place in London, Liverpool, Hamburg, Paris, Antwerp, Brussels, Lisbon and Amsterdam. This disciplinary consolidation and professionalisation correlated with a change of scenery from the field in the tropics to the laboratory in European cities and a shift in scientific practice from practical experimentation to microscopic examinations. There was no similar institutional and cognitive development in tropical colonies at that time. Therefore, medical research in the colonies did not follow the strict paths of tropical medicine as institutionalised in early twentieth-century Europe, nor was it a simple derivative of the research agenda of any particular scientific school or tradition. Tropical medicine practised abroad remained an amalgam combining germ theory with environmental disease theories and laboratory medicine with field surveys.[95]

Ryan Johnson has argued for the British context that "the production of knowledge about tropical diseases might have taken place in medical schools in London and Liverpool, but the theatre for tropical

---

[92] Fisch, Tropische Krankheiten, 4th ed., p. 4.

[93] Fisch, Jahresbericht für 1893, p. 11.

[94] Livingstone, Scientific Inquiry and the Missionary Enterprise, p. 51.

[95] Chakrabarti, Medicine and Empire, p. 144–147.

medicine and hygiene was still the tropics."[96] The rise and increasing supremacy of laboratories for chemical, pharmaceutical, diagnostic and experimental purposes developed in tandem with the ascendancy of field sciences whose domain of expertise was often colonial terrain. Field scientists recognised that some kinds of phenomena could not be investigated or controlled in a confined space. While they evoked the authority of laboratory knowledge, they simultaneously challenged the physical boundaries and natural validity on which that authority was based, as Helen Tilley has demonstrated.[97]

Through serial medical examinations, lengthy observation processes, field collecting, cooperation with African knowledge brokers, statistical compilations, hands-on experience, linguistic expertise and global networking, the Basel Mission doctors greatly contributed to growing the body of knowledge about tropical diseases. Studies in the field highlighted interrelations, interdependence and a "bird's-eye-view," in contrast to laboratory study. Field sciences complied with the missionary agenda in the sense that they emphasised practical experimentation over laboratory testing and aspired to contribute to a larger cause by putting knowledge into practice.

The Basel Mission leaders encouraged their missionaries to produce topographical, geographical, botanical, medical and ethnological findings, since science was believed to improve missionary praxis. The importance attributed to ordered knowledge led to the compilation of detailed statistics published in the Basel Mission's annual reports. The Committee also promoted the exchange of scientific ideas by publishing the quarterly journal *Evangelisches Missionsmagazin,* which was aimed at experts in the missionary field to perfect evangelising approaches. Most articles dealt with research expeditions and exploration trips, discussing the establishment of potential new mission stations.[98] The *Missionsmagazin* was a precursor to the development of evangelical missiology in the 1870s.

Gustav Warneck held that missionaries were "born scientific pioneers" just as they were "cultural pioneers," encouraging them to pursue "a scientific occupation" since "their extended stay in foreign countries"

---

[96] Ryan Johnson, Commodity Culture. Tropical Health and Hygiene in the British Empire, in: Endeavour 32 (2008) 2, p. 70–74, here 71.

[97] Tilley, Africa as a Living Laboratory, p. 12.

[98] The *Missionsmagazin* was the Basel Mission's oldest journal going back to 1816. See Mack, Publikationen und Unterrichtsmaterialien, p. 119; Ibid., Menschenbiler, p. 75–82.

made them "the most natural consuls in the scientific realm."[99] Warneck played a seminal role in establishing evangelical missiology as a branch of theology in its own right, known as *Missionswissenschaft* in German-speaking Europe. The most important mouthpiece of the new discipline was the monthly journal *Allgemeine Missionszeitschrift*, which he founded with Theodor Christlieb in 1874. Warneck's three-volume *Evangelische Missionslehre*, appearing between 1892 and 1903 became the authoritative work on the science of missions. By 1910, sixteen professors were lecturing on Protestant missiology in twelve German universities.[100]

Johannes Fabian has argued that the supposedly scientific concept of method originated in religious praxis, stating that "much of the method in colonisation was the return of monastic rule by a detour."[101] He showed that colonial administrators in the Belgian Congo praised the missionaries' organisation and discipline and that method, therefore, was a "place of passage between religious and secular discourse."[102] This passage, however, was not one-way: when missions began to spread the gospel, they eagerly adopted military and bureaucratic models of organisation, they experimented with various funding strategies to assure their economic basis, they cultivated statistics in order to measure success and they employed scientific methods when it came to improving their medical practice.[103]

The Basel Mission doctors' scientific authority vitally depended on their location as long-term residents of the tropics. Many articles in the *Archiv für Schiffs- und Tropenhygiene* referred to their field studies, which highlights that scientists in Europe undoubtedly valued them as reliable informants.[104] They were equally esteemed as practical helpers in colonial

---

[99] Warneck, Evangelische Missionslehre, p. 604.

[100] Gladwin, Mission and Colonialism, p. 296.

[101] Fabian, Time and the Work of Anthropology, p. 166.

[102] Ibid.

[103] Ibid., p. 163–166.

[104] Hermann Vortisch's research was discussed in R. Bassenge, Besprechung von Vortisch Hermann, Ärztliche Erfahrungen und Beobachtungen auf der Goldküste, in: Archiv für Schiffs- und Tropenhygiene 11 (1907), p. 659; Karl Justi, Zur Methodik der Chinindarreichung bei Malaria, in: Archiv für Schiffs- und Tropenhygiene 15 (1913), p. 505–522; Dr. Scherer, Weisse Besiedlung im Norden des deutsch-südwestafrikanischen Schutzgebiets, in: Archiv für Schiffs- und Tropenhygiene 18 (1914), p. 198–206. Friedrich Hey's field work was quoted in Carl Mense, Syphilis und venerische Krankheiten in

medical service. The British colonial government, for example, solicited Rudolf Fisch during the bubonic plague epidemic on the Gold Coast in 1908.[105] During his two months of service, Fisch was deployed in several capacities. Initially, he inspected and reported on the situation in Christiansborg, La, Teschi and other towns on the eastern coast. Later, he gave lectures about the epidemic and appropriate prevention strategies in the parishes around Christiansborg and Accra.[106]

The career of Rudolf Fisch, who was seen as an expert in the field of tropical medicine and hygiene by colonial authorities and scientists alike, illustrates how the validity and authority of missionary knowledge was bound to the space of the tropics. Upon his return to Europe after twenty-six-years of performing surgeries and experimenting with quinine prophylaxis on the Gold Coast, he was not allowed to practise as a physician back home because he had not completed his secondary school degree and therefore never taken his medical state exam.[107] Similarly, Friedrich Hey had graduated as a medical doctor in 1894 with the distinction *cum laude* after eleven semesters at the University of Basel yet he

den neu der Kultur erschlossenen Ländern besonders in Afrika, in: Archiv für Schiffs- und Tropenhygiene 4 (1900), p. 86–109; Heinrich Botho Scheube, Die venerischen Krankheiten in den warmen Ländern (Fortsetzung), in: Archiv für Schiffs- und Tropenhygiene 6 (1902), p. 187–207; Dr. Friedrichsen, Die doppelseitige Nasengeschwulst der Tropenländer, in: Archiv für Schiffs- und Tropenhygiene 7 (1903), p. 1–18; E. Rothschuh, Die Syphilis in Zentralamerika, in: Archiv für Schiffs- und Tropenhygiene 12 (1908), p. 109–133. Rudolf Fisch's studies were reviewed in Karl Däubler, Über die gegenwärtige Stellung der Tropenpathologie, in: Archiv für Schiffs- und Tropenhygiene 1 (1897), p. 295–309; Otto Dempwolff, Aerztliche Erfahrung in Neu-Guinea, in: Archiv für Schiffs- und Tropenhygiene 2 (1898), p. 134–166; Heinrich Botho Scheube, Die venerischen Krankheiten in den warmen Ländern (Fortsetzung), in: Archiv für Schiffs- und Tropenhygiene 6 (1902), p. 187–207; Dr. Friedrichsen, Die doppelseitige Nasengeschwulst der Tropenländer, in: Archiv für Schiffs- und Tropenhygiene 7 (1903), p. 1–18; Dr. Zupitza, Über mechanischen Malariaschutz in den Tropen, in: Archiv für Schiffs- und Tropenhygiene 11 (1907), p. 257–272; H. Seiffert, Ein Beitrag zur Kenntnis des Porocephalus moniliformis, in: Archiv für Schiffs- und Tropenhygiene 14 (1910), p. 101–110; Karl Justi, Zur Methodik der Chinindarreichung bei Malaria, in: Archiv für Schiffs- und Tropenhygiene 15 (1913), p. 505–522.

[105] Ryan Johnson, *Mantsemei*, Interpreters, and the Successful Eradication of Plague. The 1908 Plague Epidemic in Colonial Accra, in: Ryan Johnson/Amna Khalid (eds.), Public Health in the British Empire. Intermediaries, Subordinates and the Practice of Public Health, 1850–1960, London 2011, p. 135–153.

[106] Fischer, Der Missionsarzt Rudolf Fisch, p. 420–434.

[107] Fisch, Diary Entry, 10.10.1912, BMA, D-10.24; Fischer, Der Missionsarzt Rudolf Fisch, p. 456.

could not take the state examination because, like Fisch, he had not gained a secondary school degree. Fisch and Hey were allowed to carry their doctorate title but banned from operating as physicians or opening a medical practice in Europe.[108]

Different rules applied to the praxis of medicine in tropical colonies and the formation of the medical profession in Europe. Whereas successful tropical doctors relied on experience and training in the field, the reputation of European scientists and physicians had to be acquired through institutions and degrees. Practitioners who lacked recognised training or qualification were marginalised as purveyors of irregular or unorthodox medicine.[109] Fisch nevertheless pursued his scientific activities once he returned to Switzerland aged fifty-five. He reworked his entire manuscript for the fourth edition of *Tropische Krankheiten*, appearing in 1912. The Committee also commissioned him to compile a statistical synopsis on the health conditions of the Basel Mission employees in all mission areas. After consulting with the head of the statistical department in Basel, Fisch designed a questionnaire, of which 3000 copies were sent out to all mission employees in 1913.[110]

Friedrich Hey published a medical self-help guide entitled *Der Tropenarzt* in 1906. His aim was to offer "a brief but complete, hopefully popular" book, which did not "tire the reader with scientific treatises," as he expounded in the preface.[111] Addressing "plantation owners, trading firms, colonial authorities and mission managements," the handbook offered practical advice on necessary gear, interaction with the "indigenous" and the prevention and treatment of tropical diseases. When the manual was published, Hey worked as a government doctor for the

---

[108] Wolters, Dr. Friedrich Hey, p. 335.

[109] Deborah Brunton, Introduction, in: ibid. (ed.), Medicine Transformed. Health, Disease and Society in Europe, 1800–1930, Manchester/New York 2004, p. xi–xviii, here p. xii.

[110] The outbreak of the First World War prevented Fisch from publishing the entirety of his results in a book. Parts of the results, such as the ones concerning quinine prophylaxis in Cameroon, appeared in the *Archiv für Schiffs- und Tropenhygiene*. Rudolf Fisch, Die Wirkung der Malariaprophylaxe bei den Missionsangestellten in Kamerun, in: Beihefte zum Archiv für Schiffs- und Tropenhygiene 18 (1914), p. 117–156.

[111] Hey, Der Tropenarzt, 1st ed., p. 1.

British in Akuse on the Gold Coast since he had left the Basel Mission in Cameroon after getting into a row with his fellow missionaries.[112]

In contrast to Rudolf Fisch's *Tropische Krankheiten*, which in many ways followed conventional scientific standards at that time, *Der Tropenarzt* openly praised that it "differed from usual approaches by emphasising Christian-natural healing."[113] Hey combined allopathic, homeopathic and naturopathic methods, since he was convinced that a sick person could only recover if "the whole, i.e. body, mind and soul is being treated with natural remedies."[114] This emphasis on natural remedies contradicted what metropolitan tropical medicine stood for: the search for pathogens under the microscope, the identification of vectors and the development of vaccines. Revealingly, while Hey's compendium sold well, it received bad reviews in scientific journals such as the *Archiv für Schiffs- und Tropenhygiene*.[115]

The Basel Mission doctors had to play by the rules, meaning their approaches and arguments had to comply with a set of approved criteria if they were to uphold their scientific reputation and disseminate their findings in scientific journals. Centrality and peripherality in the production of scientific knowledge were not only a matter of geographical location but also the combined effect of social and scientific power relations. Scientific knowledge depended on a specific set of procedures, academic institutions, growing disciplinary specialisation and professionalisation, patrolled and defined by metropolitan scientists themselves. Methods and techniques of medical science gradually became codified around 1900, allowing for less and less experimentation with approaches deemed unscientific.

By advocating a holistic, naturopathic approach to healing, Hey's *Tropenarzt* did not conform with the increasingly narrow self-conception of the scientific community dealing with tropical medicine and hygiene. Scientists delineated the boundaries of their research field by excluding

---

[112] Horst Gründer, Geschichte der deutschen Kolonien, 7th ed., Paderborn 2018, p. 238.

[113] Hey, Der Tropenarzt, 1st ed., p. 1.

[114] Ibid., p. 1–2.

[115] Carl Mense, Besprechung von Hey Fr., Der Tropenarzt, Offenbach 1906, in: Archiv für Schiffs- und Tropenhygiene 12 (1908), p. 204; Reinhold Ruge, Besprechung von: Hey Fr., Der Tropenarzt, 2. Aufl., Wismar i. M. 1912, in: Archiv für Schiffs- und Tropenhygiene 16 (1912), p. 409.

actors and bodies of knowledge that they perceived as a danger to their efforts to professionalise, differentiate and secularise. Nonetheless, the commercial success of Hey's handbook, leading to a second edition in 1912, indicates that it addressed the needs of laypeople. The chapter on hygiene, which was more than one hundred pages long, covered topics such as housing, nutrition, clothing, work, rest, social life and children's diet and education with an explicit religious message. This extensive advice on tropical hygiene manifestly spoke to the anxieties of a wider colonial audience, who did not look for health prevention and physical healing alone but for Christian guidance and moral support.[116]

REFERENCES

Warwick Anderson, Where Every Prospect Pleases and Only Man is Vile. Laboratory Medicine as Colonial Discourse, in: Critical Inquiry 18 (1992) 3, p. 506–529.

David Armstrong, Public Health Spaces and the Fabrication of Identity, in: Sociology 27 (1993) 3, p. 393–410.

Ralph A. Austen/Jonathan Derrick, Middlemen of the Cameroons Rivers. The Duala and their Hinterland c. 1600–c. 1960, Cambridge 1999.

Basler Missionskomitee (ed.), An die Freunde des Ärztlichen Zweiges der Basler Mission, Basel 1891.

R. Bassenge, Besprechung von Vortisch Hermann, Ärztliche Erfahrungen und Beobachtungen auf der Goldküste, in: Archiv für Schiffs- und Tropenhygiene 11 (1907), p. 659.

Manuela Bauche, Medizin und Herrschaft. Malariabekämpfung in Kamerun, Ostafrika und Ostfriesland 1890–1919, Frankfurt a. M. 2017.

Stephan Besser, Tropische Infektionsphantasmen. Zur kulturellen Typologie der Malaria um die Jahrhundertwende, in: Alexander Honold/Klaus R. Scherpe (eds.), Das Fremde. Reiseerfahrung, Schreibformen und kulturelles Wissen, Bern et al. 1999, p. 175–195.

Stephan Besser, Die hygienische Eroberung Afrikas. 9. Juni 1898: Robert Koch hält seinen Vortrag Ärztliche Beobachtungen in den Tropen, in: Alexander Honold/Klaus R. Scherpe (eds.), Mit Deutschland um die Welt. Eine Kulturgeschichte des Fremden in der Kolonialzeit, Stuttgart/Weimar 2004, p. 217–225.

[116] Hey's *Tropenarzt* was praised in a review in the German journal for medical mission *Die ärztliche Mission*, which referred to him as English government physician. Dr. Jungklaus, Bücherbesprechung von Hey Dr., englischer Regierungsarzt in Akuse, Goldküste: Der Tropenarzt, Offenbach 1906, in: Die ärztliche Mission 3 (1908), p. 63–64.

Olaf Briese, Angst in den Zeiten der Cholera. Über kulturelle Ursprünge des Bakteriums, Berlin 2003.

Thomas D. Brock, Robert Koch. A Life in Medicine and Bacteriology, New York 1988.

Walter Bruchhausen, Sind die "Primitiven" gesünder? Völkerkundliche Perspektiven um 1900, in: Céline Kaiser/Marie-Luise Wünsche (eds.), Die "Nervosität der Juden" und andere Leiden an der Zivilisation. Konstruktionen des Kollektiven und Konzepte individueller Krankheit im psychiatrischen Diskurs um 1900, Paderborn et al. 2003, p. 41–56.

Walter Bruchhausen/Volker Roelcke, Categorising 'African Medicine': The German Discourse on East African Healing Practices, 1885–1918, in: Waltraud Ernst (ed.), Plural Medicine, Tradition and Modernity, 1800–2000, London/New York 2002, p. 76–94.

Deborah Brunton, Introduction, in: ibid. (ed.), Medicine Transformed. Health, Disease and Society in Europe, 1800–1930, Manchester/New York 2004, p. xi–xviii.

Alexander Butchart, The Anatomy of Power. European Constructions of the African Body, London/New York 1998.

John Cell, Anglo-Indian Medical Theory and the Origins of Segregation in West Africa, in: American Historical Review 91 (1989) 2, p. 307–335.

Pratik Chakrabarti, Medicine and Empire, 1600–1960, Basingstoke 2014.

David Wade Chambers/Richard Gillespie, Locality in the History of Science. Colonial Science, Technoscience, and Indigenous Knowledge, in: Osiris 15 (2000), p. 221–240.

Philip D. Curtin, The Image of Africa: British Ideas and Action, 1780–1850, vol. 1, London 1964.

Philip D. Curtin, Medical Knowledge and Urban Planning in Tropical Africa, in: American Historical Review 90 (1985) 3, p. 594–613.

Philip D. Curtin, Death by Migration. Europe's Encounter with the Tropical World in the Nineteenth Century, Cambridge 1989.

Karl Däubler, Über die gegenwärtige Stellung der Tropenpathologie, in: Archiv für Schiffs- und Tropenhygiene 1 (1897), p. 295–309.

Otto Dempwolff, Aerztliche Erfahrung in Neu-Guinea, in: Archiv für Schiffs- und Tropenhygiene 2 (1898), p. 134–166.

Wolfgang U. Eckart, Malariaprävention und Rassentrennung. Die ärztliche Vorbereitung und Rechtfertigung der Duala-Enteignung 1912–1914, in: History and Philosophy of the Life Sciences 10 (1988) 2, p. 363–378.

Wolfgang U. Eckart, Medizin und Kolonialimperialismus. Deutschland 1884–1945, Paderborn 1997.

Wolfgang U. Eckart, Robert Koch. Ein Bakteriologe für die Kolonien, in: Ulrich van der Heyden/Joachim Zeller (eds.) Kolonialmetropole Berlin. Eine Spurensuche, Berlin 2002, p. 102–106.

Andreas Eckert, Die Duala und die Kolonialmächte: Eine Untersuchung zu Widerstand, Protest und Protonationalismus in Kamerun vor dem Zweiten Weltkrieg, Münster 1991.

Andreas Eckert, Grundbesitz, Landkonflikte und kolonialer Wandel. Douala 1880 bis 1960, Stuttgart 1999.

Alfred Eckhardt, Ärztliche Missionsarbeit in Christiansborg, in: An die Freunde des Ärztlichen Zweiges der Basler Mission, Basel 1891, p. 8–19.

Rod Edmond, Returning Fears: Tropical Disease and the Metropolis, in: Felix Driver/Luciana Martins (eds.), Tropical Visions in the Age of Empire, Chicago 2005, p. 175–194.

Evangelische Missionsgesellschaft zu Basel (ed.), Neunundneunzigster Jahresbericht, Basel 1914.

Johannes Fabian, Time and the Work of Anthropology. Critical Essays 1971–1991, Chur et al. 1991.

Gary B. Ferngren, Medicine and Religion. A Historical Introduction, Baltimore 2014.

Rudolf Fisch, Jahresbericht für 1893, in: An die Freunde des Ärztlichen Zweiges der Basler Mission, Basel 1894, p. 10–13.

Rudolf Fisch, Das Schwarzwasserfieber, in: Deutsche Kolonialzeitung 9 (1896), p. 139–141.

Rudolf Fisch, Das Schwarzwasserfieber nach den Beobachtungen und Erfahrungen auf der Goldküste Westafrikas, in: Deutsche Medizinal-Zeitung 17 (1896), p. 223–225, 235–236, 247–249.

Rudolf Fisch, Über Schwarzwasserfieber, in: Correspondenz-Blatt für Schweizer Ärzte 26 (1896), p. 271–276.

Rudolf Fisch, Ist Schwarzwasserfieber Chininvergiftung? in: Afrika-Post 2 (1899), p. 277–278.

Rudolf Fisch, Tropische Krankheiten. Anleitung zu ihrer Verhütung und Behandlung speziell für die Westküste von Afrika, für Missionare, Kaufleute, Pflanzer und Beamte, 1st ed., Basel 1891; 2nd ed., Basel 1894; 3rd ed., Basel 1903; 4th ed., Basel 1912.

Rudolf Fisch, Die Wirkung der Malariaprophylaxe bei den Missionsangestellten in Kamerun, in: Beihefte zum Archiv für Schiffs- und Tropenhygiene 18 (1914), p. 117–156.

Friedrich Hermann Fischer, Der Missionsarzt Rudolf Fisch und die Anfänge medizinischer Arbeit der Basler Mission an der Goldküste (Ghana), Herzogenrath 1991.

Dr. Friedrichsen, Die doppelseitige Nasengeschwulst der Tropenländer, in: Archiv für Schiffs- und Tropenhygiene 7 (1903), p. 1–18.

Thomas S. Gale, Segregation in British West Africa, in: Cahiers d'Études Africaines 20 (1980) 80, p. 495–507.

Michael Gladwin, Mission and Colonialism, in: Joel D. S. Rasmussen/Judith Wolfe/Johannes Zachhuber (eds.), The Oxford Handbook of Nineteenth-Century Christian Thought, Oxford 2017, p. 282–304.

Christoph Gradmann, Laboratory Disease. Robert Koch's Medical Bacteriology, Baltimore 2009.

Christoph Gradmann, Robert Koch and the Invention of the Carrier State: Tropical Medicine, Veterinary Infections and Epidemiology around 1900, in: Studies in History and Philosophy of Biological and Biomedical Sciences 41 (2010) 3, p. 232–240.

Charles Scovell Grant, West African Hygiene. Or, Hints on the Preservation of Health, and the Treatment of Disease on the West Coast of Africa, London 1882, 1884, 1887.

Horst Gründer, Christliche Mission und deutscher Imperialismus. Eine politische Geschichte ihrer Beziehung während der deutschen Kolonialzeit (1884–1914) unter besonderer Berücksichtigung Afrikas und Chinas, Paderborn 1982.

Horst Gründer, Geschichte der deutschen Kolonien, 7th ed., Paderborn 2018.

Ulrike Hamann, Prekäre koloniale Ordnung: Rassistische Konjunkturen im Wiederspruch. Deutsches Kolonialregime 1884–1914, Bielefeld 2015.

Mark Harrison, Tropical Medicine in Nineteenth-Century India, in: The British Journal for the History of Science 25 (1992) 3, p. 299–318.

Douglas Melvin Haynes, Imperial Medicine. Patrick Manson and the Conquest of Tropical Disease, Philadelphia 2001.

Daniel R. Headrick, The Tools of Empire. Technology and European Imperialism in the Nineteenth Century, Oxford 1981.

Friedrich Hey, Der Tropenarzt. Ausführlicher Ratgeber für Europäer in den Tropen, sowie für Besitzer von Plantagen und Handelshäusern, Kolonialbehörden und Missionsverwaltungen, 1st ed., Offenbach 1906.

Richard Hölzl, Lepra als *entangled disease*. Leidende afrikanische Körper in Medien und Praxis der katholischen Mission in Ostafrika 1911–1945, in: Linda Ratschiller/Siegfried Weichlein (eds.), Der schwarze Körper als Missionsgebiet. Medizin, Ethnologie, Theologie in Afrika und Europa 1880–1960, Köln/Weimar/Wien 2016, p. 95–121.

Valesca Huber, The Unification of the Globe by Disease? The International Sanitary Conferences on Cholera, 1851–1894, in: The Historical Journal 49 (2006) 2, p. 453–476.

Ryan Johnson, Commodity Culture. Tropical Health and Hygiene in the British Empire, in: Endeavour 32 (2008) 2, p. 70–74.

Ryan Johnson, *Mantsemei*, Interpreters, and the Successful Eradication of Plague. The 1908 Plague Epidemic in Colonial Accra, in: Ryan Johnson/Amna Khalid (eds.), Public Health in the British Empire. Intermediaries, Subordinates and the Practice of Public Health, 1850–1960, London 2011, p. 135–153.

Anna Johnston, Missionary Writing and Empire, 1800–1860, Cambridge 2003.

Dr. Jungklaus, Bücherbesprechung von Hey Dr., englischer Regierungsarzt in Akuse, Goldküste: Der Tropenarzt, Offenbach 1906, in: Die ärztliche Mission 3 (1908), p. 63–64.

Karl Justi, Zur Methodik der Chinindarreichung bei Malaria, in: Archiv für Schiffs- und Tropenhygiene 15 (1913), p. 505–522.

Robert Koch, Ergebnisse der vom Deutschen Reich ausgesandten Malariaexpeditionen. Vortrag vom 05.11.1900, in: Julius Schwalbe (ed.), Gesammelte Werke von Robert Koch, Leipzig 1912, vol. 2, p. 435–447.

Robert Koch, Über Schwarzwasserfieber (Hämoglobinurie), in: Julius Schwalbe (ed.), Gesammelte Werke von Robert Koch, Leipzig 1912, vol. 2, p. 348–370.

Ludwig Külz, Guinée française und Kamerun, in: Amtsblatt für das Schutzgebiet Kamerun 13–16 (1909), p. 115–118, 133–144, 144–148, 163–168.

Birthe Kundrus, Moderne Imperialisten. Das Kaiserreich im Spiegel seiner Kolonien, Köln et al. 2003.

David N. Livingstone, Putting Science in Its Place: Geographies of Scientific Knowledge, Chicago/London 2003.

David N. Livingstone, Scientific Inquiry and the Missionary Enterprise, in: Ruth Finnegan (ed.), Participating in the Knowledge Society. Researchers Beyond the University Walls, Basingstoke 2005, p. 50–64.

David N. Livingstone, Landscapes of Knowledge, in: Peter Meusburger/David N. Livingstone/Heike Jöns (eds.), Geographies of Science, London 2010, p. 3–22.

Maryinez Lyons, The Colonial Disease. A Social History of Sleeping Sickness in Northern Zaire, 1900–1940, Cambridge/New York 1992.

Julia Mack, Publikationen und Unterrichtsmaterialien, in: Christine Christ-von Wedel/Thomas K. Kuhn (ed.), Basler Mission. Menschen, Geschichte, Perspektiven 1815–2015, Basel 2015, p. 119–124.

Julia Ulrike Mack, Menschenbilder. Anthropologische Konzepte und stereotype Vorstellungen vom Menschen in der Publizistik der Basler Mission 1816–1914, Zürich 2013.

Ernst Mähly, Über das sogenannte "Gallenfieber" an der Goldküste, in: Correspondenz-Blatt für Schweizer Ärzte 15 (1885), p. 73–79, 108–116.

Ernst Mähly, Akklimatisation und Klimafieber, in: Deutsche Kolonialzeitung 3 (1886), p. 72–83.

Carl Mense, Syphilis und venerische Krankheiten in den neu der Kultur erschlossenen Ländern besonders in Afrika, in: Archiv für Schiffs- und Tropenhygiene 4 (1900), p. 86–109.

Carl Mense, Besprechung von Hey Fr., Der Tropenarzt, Offenbach 1906, in: Archiv für Schiffs- und Tropenhygiene 12 (1908), p. 204.

Walter Myers, Seventy Second Annual Meeting of the British Medical Association, in: British Medical Journal, 1904, p. 631.

Deborah J. Neill, Science and Civilizing Missions. Germans and the Transnational Community of Tropical Medicine, in: Bradley Naranch/Geoff Eley (eds.), German Colonialism in a Global Age, Durham/London 2014, p. 74–92.

Carl Nightingale, Segregation: A Global History of Divided Cities, Chicago 2012.

Karl David Patterson, Health in Colonial Ghana. Disease, Medicine, and Socio-Economic Change, 1900–1955, Waltham 1981.

Albert Plehn, Beitrag zur Kenntnis von Verlauf und Behandlung der tropischen Malaria in Kamerun, Berlin 1896.

Albert Plehn, Besprechung des Artikels von R. Fisch: Ist Schwarzwasserfieber Chininvergiftung? in: Archiv für Schiffs- und Tropenhygiene 4 (1900), p. 63–65.

Albert Plehn, Zur Chininprophylaxe der Malaria nebst Bemerkungen zur Schwarzwasserfieberfrage, in: Archiv für Schiffs- und Tropenhygiene 5 (1901), p. 380–393.

Friedrich Plehn, Über das Schwarzwasserfieber an der afrikanischen Westküste, in: Deutsche medizinische Wochenschrift 21 (1895), p. 397–400, 416–418, 434–437.

Friedrich Plehn, Bericht über eine Informationsreise nach Ceylon und Indien, in: Archiv für Schiffs- und Tropenhygiene 3 (1899), p. 273–311.

Ronald Ross, The Progress of Tropical Medicine, in: Journal of the Royal African Society 4 (1905) 15, p. 271–289.

E. Rothschuh, Die Syphilis in Zentralamerika, in: Archiv für Schiffs- und Tropenhygiene 12 (1908), p. 109–133.

Reinhold Ruge, Besprechung von: Hey Fr., Der Tropenarzt, 2. Aufl., Wismar i. M. 1912, in: Archiv für Schiffs- und Tropenhygiene 16 (1912), p. 409.

Adolf Rüger, Die Widerstandsbewegung des Rudolf Manga Bell in Kamerun, in: Walter Markow (ed.), Études Africaines/African Studies/Afrika-Studien. Dem II. Internationalen Afrikanistenkongress in Dakar gewidmet, Leipzig 1967, p. 107–128.

Thomas Rütten/Martina King (eds.), Contagionism and Contagious Diseases. Medicine and Literature 1880–1933, Berlin/Boston 2013.

Philipp Sarasin/Silvia Berger/Marianne Hänseler/Myriam Spörri (eds.), Bakteriologie und Moderne. Studien zur Biopolitik des Unsichtbaren 1870–1920, Frankfurt a. M. 2007.

Dr. Scherer, Weisse Besiedlung im Norden des deutsch-südwestafrikanischen Schutzgebiets, in: Archiv für Schiffs- und Tropenhygiene 18 (1914), p. 198–206.

Heinrich Botho Scheube, Die venerischen Krankheiten in den warmen Ländern (Fortsetzung), in: Archiv für Schiffs- und Tropenhygiene 6 (1902), p. 187–207.

Wilhelm Schlatter, Geschichte der Basler Mission 1815–1915, 3 vol., Basel 1916.

H. Seiffert, Ein Beitrag zur Kenntnis des Porocephalus moniliformis, in: Archiv für Schiffs- und Tropenhygiene 14 (1910), p. 101–110.

Maynard Swanson, The Sanitation Syndrome: Bubonic Plague and Urban Native Policy in the Cape Colony, 1900–1909, in: The Journal of African History 18 (1977) 3, p. 387–410.

Helen Tilley, Africa as a Living Laboratory. Empire, Development, and the Problem of Scientific Knowledge, 1870–1950, Chicago 2011.

Helen Tilley, Medicine, Empires, and Ethics in Colonial Africa, in: AMA Journal of Ethics 18 (2016) 7, p. 743–753.

Gustav Warneck, Evangelische Missionslehre. Ein missionstheoretischer Versuch, ed. by Friedemann Knödler, Bonn 2015.

Paul Weindling, Epidemics and Genocide in Eastern Europe, 1890–1945, Oxford 2000.

Christine Wolters, Dr. Friedrich Hey (1864–1960), Missionsarzt und Bückeburger Unternehmer, in: Hubert Höing (ed.), Strukturen und Konjunkturen. Faktoren in der schaumburgischen Wirtschaftsgeschichte, Bielefeld 2004, p. 328–366.

Michael Worboys, Germs, Malaria and the Invention of Mansonian Tropical Medicine. From "Diseases in the Tropics" to "Tropical Diseases", in: David Arnold, (ed.) Warm Climates and Western Medicine. The Emergence of Tropical Medicine 1500–1900, Amsterdam/Atlanta 1996, p. 181–207.

Michael Worboys, The Colonial World as Mission and Mandate: Leprosy and Empire, 1900–1940, in: Osiris 15 (2000), p. 207–218.

Michael Worboys, Colonial and Imperial Medicine, in: Deborah Brunton (ed.), Medicine Transformed. Health, Disease and Society in Europe 1880–1930, Manchester/New York 2004, p. 211–238.

Hans Ziemann, Zweiter Bericht über Malaria und Moskitos an der afrikanischen Westküste, in: Deutsche Medizinische Wochenzeitschrift 26 (1900), p. 753–756, 769–772.

Dr. Zupitza, Über mechanischen Malariaschutz in den Tropen, in: Archiv für Schiffs- und Tropenhygiene 11 (1907), p. 257–272.

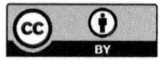

CHAPTER 9

Soothing Weak Nerves: Tropical Anxieties, Missionary Guidance and Moral Hygiene

Tropical hygiene was a concept with deeper and wider meaning than later usage of the word "hygiene" would suggest. It evoked a spiritual, ascetic ideal of purity and self-control, a quality that conquered the dangers of a hostile physical and social environment through the mastery of mind over body. This puritan dimension of tropical hygiene allowed the Basel medical missionaries to position themselves as experts on the matter and mould scientific and colonial debates with their religious logic. They enjoyed extensive moral authority among the colonial public, not only advising how the sick should be treated but also prescribing healthy diets, behaviours and lifestyles. Although many of the debates surrounding tropical hygiene were carried out in medical journals and other specialised publications, their influence ranged far beyond the disciplinary boundaries of tropical medicine, gaining currency in wider social and political contexts.

© The Author(s) 2023   347
L. M. Ratschiller Nasim, *Medical Missionaries and Colonial Knowledge in West Africa and Europe, 1885–1914*,
Cambridge Imperial and Post-Colonial Studies,
https://doi.org/10.1007/978-3-031-27128-1_9

9.1   Resurging Climatic Fears

Advice on tropical hygiene and the treatment of tropical diseases had only played a minor role in travel guidebooks in the first half of the nineteenth century.[1] One of the first handbooks dealing with such questions explicitly with regard to Africa was authored by James Africanus Beale Horton.[2] Born as a son of a former slave in Sierra Leone in 1835, he was one of the first Africans to train as a physician at a British university in the nineteenth century. He served as a doctor in the West India Regiment on the Gold Coast in 1860 and published his medical compendium advising Europeans on how to stay in good health in the tropics in 1867.[3] Horton asserted that the tropical climate and the unfamiliar environment posed a great threat to the physical and mental health of Europeans. "Maladies peculiar to tropical climates," he argued, "have the most mischievous effect in checking the progress of true civilisation."[4]

Despite a considerable decline in death rates among Europeans in West Africa from 1875, optimism regarding the adaptability of Europeans to the tropics gradually vanished.[5] The late nineteenth century saw a resurgence of climatic fears as theories became charged with new and sophisticated explanatory models. The notion that climate and physiology affected one's resistance to illness was in many ways inconsistent with the teachings of germ theory and the new understanding of parasitology. Experts in the field of tropical medicine now argued, however, that even if the tropical climate did not actually cause disease, it had grievous effects

---

[1] Michael Pesek, Vom richtigen Reisen und Beobachten: Ratgeberliteratur für Forschungsreisende nach Übersee im 19. Jahrhundert, in: Berichte zur Wissenschaftsgeschichte 40 (2017) 1, p. 17–38.

[2] For a biography of James Africanus Beale Horton, see Andrea Graf, James Africanus Beale Horton, Medizinaltopographien und wissenschaftliche Selbstlegitimierung vor der mikrobiologischen Revolution (ca. 1835–1885), Master Thesis, University of Basel, 2019.

[3] James Africanus Beale Horton, Physical and Medical Climate and Meteorology of the West Coast of Africa with Valuable Hints to Europeans for the Preservation of Health in the Tropics, London 1867.

[4] Ibid., p. v.

[5] Philip D. Curtin, The End of the "White Man's Grave"? Nineteenth-Century Mortality in West Africa, in: Journal of Interdisciplinary History 21 (1990), p. 63–88; Ibid., Disease and Empire: The Health of European Troops in the Conquest of Africa, Cambridge 1998.

on the constitution of Europeans and predisposed them to contagion.[6] Individual hygiene and the internalisation of a catalogue of appropriate measures were thus regarded as essential for survival, and discipline took on an important role in the understanding of suitability for the tropics.

Patrick Manson delivered an address on *Tropical Research in its Relation to the Missionary Enterprise* at Livingstone College in 1908, which the Society for Medical Mission in Stuttgart translated and published in German in 1909. He opened his lecture by recalling that "thirty years ago no man knew what Malaria was; no man had the slightest conception of how it was caused, how it was transmitted, nor what was the nature of the germ."[7] He proceeded by enumerating a number of disease pathogens that had been identified and could now be curbed by medical science. "One important deduction from this modern knowledge", he concluded was "that Tropical diseases are not produced, as formerly supposed, by climate." Instead, disease depended "upon the intermediaries through which the germ cause of the disease is transmitted and these intermediaries are prevalent in the Tropics."[8]

Manson's statement illustrates that while the discovery of the pathogens involved in diseases such as malaria, cholera, plague or typhoid and the gradual development of vaccines brought new hope to medical research in tropical colonies, it also complicated the understanding of diseases there. The tropical environment, which for much of the nineteenth century appeared to Europeans to be full of noxious, foul air, henceforth seemed to be infested with invisible germs.[9] By 1900, the tropics and tropical bodies were seen as the natural home of deadly

---

[6] Worboys, Germs, Malaria and the Invention of Mansonian Tropical Medicine; Gregory H. Maddox, Disease and Environment in Africa. Imputed Dynamics and Unresolved Issues, in: Karl Ittman/Dennis D. Cordell/Gregory H. Maddox (eds.), The Demographics of Empire. The Colonial Order and the Creation of Knowledge, Athens 2010, p. 198–216.

[7] Manson, Tropical Research in its Relation to the Missionary Enterprise, p. 3–4.

[8] Ibid., p. 10.

[9] Dane Kennedy, The Perils of the Midday Sun: Climatic Anxieties in the Colonial Tropics, in: John M. MacKenzie (ed.), Imperialism and the Natural World, Manchester/New York 1990, p. 118–140.

pathogens, which scientists thought to combat with the help of germ theory and laboratory medicine.[10]

Medical and travel guides for tropical territories around 1900 were replete with warnings about the climate and advice on preventive measures, collectively referred to as tropical hygiene.[11] Michael Pesek has characterised these publications as "mobile education institutions" that tried to transfer the ideal of the laboratory onto the field.[12] As knowledge on tropical diseases grew, medical scientists formulated ever more detailed guidelines of behaviour, lifestyle and equipment. The discovery of the transmission paths of malaria, for instance, led to new recommendations on protective clothing and nets, means of transport and construction away from mosquito breeding sites. The Basel Mission doctors' advice on house building in West Africa according to the newest hygiene standards aroused considerable interest in the contemporary colonial press.[13]

The physician Alexander Lion, who served as medical officer in German South-West Africa between 1904 and 1906, published a book with advice on tropical hygiene in 1907 that found wide recognition and was also part of the Basel Mission library. He stated that a "reasonable lifestyle protects against tropical diseases or reduces their danger." Therefore, he instructed: "Do not drink too much, never get drunk, ideally practise sexual abstinence, take daily baths and do not get angry."[14] The personal regimen recommended in the medical literature

---

[10] Stepan, Picturing Tropical Nature, p. 149–179; Warwick Anderson, Immunities of Empire: Race, Disease and the New Tropical Medicine, 1900–1920, in: Bulletin of the History of Medicine 70 (1996) 1, p. 94–118.

[11] See selectively Carl Mense, Tropische Gesundheitslehre und Heilkunde, Berlin 1902; William John Simpson, The Maintenance of Health in the Tropics, London 1905; Friedrich Plehn, Tropenhygiene. Mit spezieller Berücksichtigung der deutschen Kolonien. Ärztliche Ratschläge für Kolonialbeamte, Offiziere, Missionare, Expeditionsführer, Pflanzer und Faktoristen, Jena 1906; Alexander Lion, Tropenhygienische Ratschläge, München 1907; Hans Ziemann, Hints to Europeans in Tropical Stations, London 1910.

[12] Pesek, Vom richtigen Reisen und Beobachten, p. 33.

[13] Eckhardt, Häuserbau in Westafrika und die Station Ho; Ibid., Land, Leute und ärztliche Mission auf der Goldküste, p. 15–18; Hey, Der Tropenarzt, 1st ed., p. 91–104; Fisch, Tropische Krankheiten, 1st ed., p. 10–13; Ibid., Tropische Krankheiten, 4th ed., p. 29–44.

[14] Lion, Tropenhygienische Ratschläge, p. 17. Lion met Maximilian Bayer during his time in South-West Africa with whom he would later go on to found the *Pfadpfinder* —the German branch of the Scout Movement. See Hartmut Bartmuss, Alexander Lion. Arzt, Sanitätsoffizier, Pfadfinder, Berlin 2017.

focussed on asceticism, self-discipline and temperance. These measures were congruent with the proscriptions of Pietist purity, underlining the continued belief in a connection between morality and disease.[15]

The question of whether Europeans could cope with the health and moral challenges posed by the tropical climate was a key aspect of virtually every debate about the viability of the colonial project between 1885 and 1914. It had this larger resonance because, on the one hand, it spoke to the deep-felt anxieties of Europeans residing in tropical colonies. For them, advice on tropical hygiene possessed an immediacy that derived from personal worries about maintaining health and sanity in an alien climate. It gave scientifically legitimised meaning to their experience and prescribed a specific code of conduct, allowing them to define and assert their cultural and racial identities in contrast to the people native to the colonies. What tropical hygiene offered was an "oddly satisfying diagnosis of these concerns, at once prescriptive and proscriptive in its recommendations," as Dane Kennedy argued.[16]

On the other hand, tropical hygiene addressed broader concerns of imperial policy-makers about the very shape and future of European colonialism. Metropolitan authorities looked at tropical colonies as potential homelands in reaction to fears of overpopulation in Europe. However, at the same time, the future of these recently acquired possessions in Africa and elsewhere raised crucial issues about the role and position of white men and women in that future, revealing fundamental political uncertainties.[17] They implemented a rigorous and highly restrictive selection process to ensure that only able-bodied and mentally stable Europeans relocated to the colonies. Potential emigrants, military recruits and administrative personnel had to undergo regular medical check-ups and preparatory measures to assess whether they were suited for life in a tropical colony or not.[18]

---

[15] Curtin, The Image of Africa, p. 177–197; Fabian, Time and the Work of Anthropology, p. 158–163; David. N. Livingstone, Tropical Climate and Moral Hygiene: The Anatomy of a Victorian Debate, in: The British Journal for the History of Science 32 (1999) 1, p. 93–110; Endfield/Nash, Missionaries and Morals.

[16] Kennedy, The Perils of the Midday Sun, p. 136.

[17] Edmond, Returning Fears.

[18] This assessment was known as *Tropentauglichkeit* in the German context. See Pascal Grosse, Kolonialismus, Eugenik und bürgerliche Gesellschaft in Deutschland 1850–1918, Frankfurt a. M. 2000, p. 53–95; Hartmann, Tropical Soldiers?

Europeans' colonial experience was substantially shaped by negative emotions such as anxiety, insecurity and fear, as recent studies have emphasised.[19] The debate on the difficulty for Europeans to acclimatise in tropical colonies subtly called into question European supremacy, exposing the colonial situation as an experience of permanent scientific and political crisis as well as imperial helplessness. New theories of race emerging in the late nineteenth century increasingly drew upon evolutionary arguments and implied that European bodies were unfit for African conditions.[20] Tropical hygiene consequently was an enduring concern of colonial rule and an essential aspect of imperial expansion. Instead of reducing climatic fears, most scientific discoveries in the late nineteenth and early twentieth centuries triggered the development of deeper tropical anxieties, with a new vocabulary through which they could be expressed.

9.2   Missionary Advice on Moral Hygiene

The contemporary image of the tropics as a site of jeopardy and trial offered an effective framework to preach the Basel Mission's Pietist code of conduct to a broader audience. The evangelical struggle against filth, alcoholism and sexual immorality at home gained significance abroad due to the tropical setting, which was commonly conceived of as a perilous place for Europeans. Tropical colonies exerted moral pressure on potential immigrants by magnifying the serious repercussions of ignoring hygiene guidelines. They demanded a regime of moral hygiene every bit as rigorous as physical hygiene measures. All guidebooks on tropical hygiene appearing after 1900 saw mental strength and emotional resilience as an imperative prerequisite for Europeans who planned on

---

[19] Ulrike Lindner et al. (eds.), Hybrid Cultures—Nervous States. Britain and Germany in a Post(Colonial) World, Amsterdam/New York 2010; Maurus Reinkowski/Gregor Thum (eds.), Helpless Imperialists: Imperial Failure, Fear and Radicalization, Göttingen 2013; Robert Peckham (ed.), Empires of Panic: Epidemics and Colonial Anxieties, Hong Kong 2015; Harald Fischer-Tiné (ed.), Anxieties, Fear and Panic in Colonial Settings. Empires on the Verge of a Nervous Breakdown, Basingstoke 2016; Hunt, A Nervous State.

[20] Grosse, Kolonialismus, Eugenik und bürgerliche Gesellschaft in Deutschland, p. 53–95; Kundrus, Moderne Imperialisten, p. 162–173; Eckart, Medizin und Kolonialimperialismus, p. 73–85.

staying in the tropics. Already in 1891, Fisch had made clear in the foreword of *Tropische Krankheiten* that the tropics were only feasible for the scientifically enlightened and morally disciplined:

> The main purpose of the manual is to initiate a rational treatment of malaria and, besides the various advice on the prevention and treatment of diseases, to demonstrate that the surrender of many Europeans to debauchery poses a grave danger to their lives. [...] May the booklet fulfil its purpose and thus encourage the true civilisation, i.e. Christianisation of the Dark Continent.[21]

Fisch intertwined scientific and sermonic modes of speech to warn his readers of the serious consequences of moral misconduct. He cautioned how much a lack of self-discipline was a risk to the civilising project in Africa and left no doubt that progress could only be achieved by the spread of Christian values and behaviour. By combining moral purity with physical discipline, his book not only offered practical advice for survival in the tropics but also depicted the individual European as an agent of imperial, rational and, above all, Christian Europe. Fisch turned the medical and colonial discourse on tropical hygiene into a religious responsibility by emphasising that "true civilisation" meant Christian civilisation. In order to advance this civilising mission, Europeans had to comply with detailed rules of personal hygiene, not only to preserve their own health but also to uplift the population in the colonies.

The medical discourse on Africa shows that environmental, social and cultural lines of explanation continued to dominate scientific knowledge.[22] From 1913, the influential magazine *Koloniale Rundschau*, published by the German Colonial Society, included a specialised quarterly dedicated to tropical hygiene, the *Tropenhygienische Rundschau*, edited by Gottlieb Olpp, the director of the Institute for Medical Mission in Tubingen. Reports published in the *Tropenhygienische Rundschau* compared figures released by state institutions, such as the medical services, with statistics issued by mission societies. They frequently underscored the point that the latter promised a lower infant mortality rate, a higher life expectancy for Africans and Europeans, and overall improved

---

[21] Fisch, Tropische Krankheiten, 1st ed., p. viii.
[22] Vaughan, Curing Their Ills, p. 6.

the practice of hygiene.[23] Mission medicine, which was aimed at treating body, mind and soul, offered a holistic approach in dealing with the health and moral challenges posed by life in tropical colonies.

The familiarity of the Basel medical missionaries with tropical climates ensured that their wide-ranging studies on tropical hygiene captured the attention of a general public concerned with the colonial question. They offered extensive advice on anatomy and physiology, air and ventilation, water and sanitation, house and school building, drainage and plumbing, gear and means of transport, diet and cooking, washing and personal cleanliness, maternal and child health, social and work life, sleep patterns and physical activity, and diseases and their prevention. Such a list indicates the degree to which hygiene was thought to have a potentially revolutionary impact on all aspects of personal and public life. Their articles appeared in the *Deutsche Kolonialzeitung*, in a range of missionary magazines, in the *Archiv- für Schiffs- und Tropenhygiene* and in other medical publications.[24]

---

[23] Gottlieb Olpp (ed.), Tropenhygienische Rundschau, in: Sonderbadruck aus der "Kolonialen Rundschau" (1913) 3, p. 178–184; Ibid. (ed.), Tropenhygienische Rundschau, in: Sonderbadruck aus der "Kolonialen Rundschau" (1913) 6, p. 374–380; Ibid. (ed.), Tropenhygienische Rundschau, in: Sonderbadruck aus der "Kolonialen Rundschau" (1913) 9, p. 551–559; Ibid. (ed.), Tropenhygienische Rundschau, in: Sonderbadruck aus der "Kolonialen Rundschau" (1913) 12, p. 745–753; Ibid. (ed.), Tropenhygienische Rundschau, in: Sonderbadruck aus der "Kolonialen Rundschau" (1914) 3, p. 171–181; Ibid. (ed.), Tropenhygienische Rundschau, in: Sonderbadruck aus der "Kolonialen Rundschau" (1914) 6, p. 359–368.

[24] See selectively Eckhardt, Häuserbau in Westafrika und die Station Ho, in: Deutsche Kolonialzeitung 4 (1891), p. 43–46; Rudolf Fisch, Die Malaria und ihre Behandlung auf der Goldküste, in: Allgemeine Missionszeitschrift 16 (1889), p. 553–569; Ibid., Zur Prophylaxe des Schwarzwasserfiebers, in: Archiv für Schiffs- und Tropenhygiene 6 (1902), p. 10–14; Ibid., Über die Ätiologie der Tuberkulose auf der Goldküste, in: Correspondenz-Blatt für Schweizer Ärzte 34 (1904), p. 761–763; Ibid., Über die Behandlung der Amöbendysentrie und einige andere tropenmedizinische Fragen, in: Archiv für Schiffs- und Tropenhygiene 8 (1904), p. 207–212; Ibid., Über Stoffe zur Moskitosicherung, in: Archiv für Schiffs- und Tropenhygiene 10 (1906), p. 172–175; Ibid., Die Wurmkrankheit auf der Goldküste, in: Die ärztliche Mission 3 (1908), p. 89–90; Ibid., Behandlung der Malaria mit fraktionierten Chinindosen, in: Archiv für Schiffs- und Tropenhygiene 13 (1909), p. 309–312; Ibid., Über Nachteile in der Säuglingsernährung in den Tropen durch homogenisierte Milch und deren Vermeidung, in: Archiv für Schiffs- und Tropenhygiene 16 (1912), p. 220–222; Theodor Müller, Krankheitsbilder von der Goldküste, in: Die ärztliche Mission 7 (1912), p. 131–136; Ibid., Westafrikanische Krankheiten, in: Die ärztliche Mission 8 (1913), p. 85–89; Ibid., Über Gelbfieber in Westafrika, in: Die ärztliche Mission 9 (1914), p. 15–22, 40–41; Hermann Vortisch,

Tropical hygiene enjoyed considerable influence among Europeans in the colonies and metropolitan interest groups because it spoke the language of medical science and carried the authority of doctors' expertise. At the same time, the tropics constituted a moral arena, a risky space in which circumspection and self-control were as essential to survival as physical vigour and medication.[25] The Basel Mission doctors used their credibility in the field of tropical hygiene to promote their Pietist beliefs beyond evangelical circles. Their hygiene guidelines did not simply comprise measures to maintain health but actively sought to establish new behavioural norms in line with their purity ideals. In this sense, hygiene was not merely the absence of illness but a positive power to control oneself and one's environment. The popularity of their articles and handbooks on tropical hygiene indicates that hygienic knowledge around 1900 was infused with pious notions of purity.[26]

Most scientists, missionaries and colonialists agreed that hygiene in Africa was first and foremost a question of upholding discipline in the absence of the habitual societal pressures and amenities of civilisation. Such discipline was all the more important because self-control was generally believed to be a precondition for the control of others.[27] Hey clearly stated that "the biggest difficulty in the education of subordinates" lay in "the ill-breeding of the Europeans themselves," since people who were not "properly educated themselves" could "obviously not educate others." He emphasised that "the correct influence of Europeans and particularly of every individual must help to lay the foundation on which a fruitful colonial policy can be built."[28] From this point of view, the

Erfahrungen über einige spezifische Krankheiten an der Goldküste, in: Archiv für Schiffs- und Tropenhygiene 10 (1906), p. 537–539; Ärztliche Beobachtungen und Erfahrungen auf der Goldküste, in: Deutsche Medizinische Wochenschrift 33 (1907), p. 110–111; Ibid., Über Säuglingsernährung in den Tropen, in: Archiv für Schiffs- und Tropenhygiene 16 (1912), p. 69–77.

[25] David N. Livingstone, Race, Space and Moral Climatology: Notes Toward a Genealogy, in: Journal of Historical Geography 28 (2002) 2, p. 159–180.

[26] Fisch's *Tropische Krankheiten* consistently received good reviews in the *Archiv für Schiffs- und Tropenhygiene*. See Carl Mense, Besprechung von Tropische Krankheiten, in: Archiv für Schiffs- und Tropenhygiene 7 (1903), p. 525–526; Ibid., Besprechung von Tropische Krankheiten, in: Archiv für Schiffs- und Tropenhygiene 16 (1913), p. 569.

[27] Fabian, Out of Our Minds, p. 59.

[28] Hey, 1st ed., p. 392.

greatest threat to the success of the colonial project lay in the moral integrity of the people assigned to carry out colonial rule.

Two topics in particular highlight that tropical hygiene played into the Basel Mission doctors' hands: alcohol consumption and sexual transgression. As early as 1894, at the International Congress for Hygiene and Demography in Budapest, British surgeon general Charles Richard Francis warned Europeans against the intake of alcohol in tropical countries.[29] In the following years, many German experts in tropical medicine concurred with this advice.[30] Drinking habits were seen as a major impediment to the colonial project in West Africa, not only damaging the health of Europeans but also "the reputation of the white race."[31] It was believed that the misuse of alcohol provoked moral transgressions, thereby undermining the civilising mission amongst the African population. The Basel missionaries, and alcohol abstainers more generally, appreciated this line of argument because it supported their agenda.[32]

Rudolf Fisch addressed the "moral behaviour of Europeans in the tropics" explicitly in a chapter of *Tropische Krankheiten*, describing it as "a blot that clings to the Christian name and impedes the true civilisation of the Black Continent."[33] His main concern was the promiscuity of white men in West Africa, which in his view inevitably led to death or a forced journey home. Once home, Fisch warned, these "corrupt people without true honour" would have to deal with "the stigma on their conscience" and a "shattered body as the punishment of disdainful pleasure, which the righteous God allots to them."[34] Along with scientific arguments and carefully reviewed medical findings, Fisch's *Tropische Krankheiten* conveyed the idea that "fornication" posed as much of a

---

[29] Charles Richard Francis, On Opium, Narcotics and Alcohol in the Tropics, in: VIIIème Congrès International d'Hygiène et de démographie, tenu à Budapest du 1er au 9 septembre 1894. Comptes-rendus et mémoires, Budapest 1896, p. 722–729.

[30] See for instance, Ludwig Külz, Zur Hygiene des Trinkens in den Tropen, Flensburg 1904; Max Fiebig, Die Bedeutung der Alkoholfrage für unsere Kolonien, Berlin 1908; Ibid., Über den Einfluss des Alkohols auf den Europäer in den Tropen, in: Archiv für Schiffs- und Tropenhygiene 5 (1901), p. 14–26, 59–66, 92–106.

[31] Fiebig, Die Bedeutung der Alkoholfrage, p. 14; Hans Paasche, Was ich als Abstinent in den afrikanischen Kolonien erlebte, Reutlingen 1911, p. 12.

[32] Spöring, Mission und Sozialhygiene.

[33] Fisch, Tropische Krankheiten, 1st ed., p. 33.

[34] Ibid., p. 34.

risk to the health of Europeans as malaria or black water fever. From his perspective, diseases caused by alcohol indulgence and sexual promiscuity were the visible manifestations of both religious sin and social deviance.

9.3 WEAK NERVES AND MISSIONARY RESILIENCE

Rudolf Fisch drafted a manuscript entitled "How do I make myself suitable for service in the tropics?" for the students at the Basel Mission seminary. He reminded them that "the missionary profession" posed "manifold challenges to body and soul," unmatched by any other profession.[35] The tropical climate demanded a "considerable measure of energy," which Fisch defined as a "capacity of the soul." He concluded: "Anyone who wants to prepare for service in the tropics with prospects of success must be free from any physical ailments and especially free from pathological mental dispossessions."[36] The latter included what Fisch called "hysteria" and "neurasthenia," a term coined by the American neurologist George M. Beard in the 1870s. Neurasthenia was described as a form of nervous exhaustion induced by the pressures of modern civilisation and developed into a widespread diagnosis in Europe and America.[37]

The late nineteenth century saw the identification of tropical neurasthenia, which according to some sources existed in near epidemic proportions among Europeans abroad. On the Gold Coast, the number of colonial officials sent home as medical invalids based on the diagnosis of tropical neurasthenia was nearly on a par with malaria.[38] Like its metropolitan namesake, tropical neurasthenia was viewed to be a form of

---

[35] Rudolf Fisch, Wie mache ich mich tauglich für den Tropendienst, p. 3, BMA, G.II.22.

[36] Ibid., p. 4.

[37] Joachim Radkau, Das Zeitalter der Nervosität. Deutschland zwischen Bismarck und Hitler, München 1998; Marijke Gijswijt-Hofstra/Roy Porter (eds.), Cultures of Neurasthenia from George Beard to the First World War, Amsterdam/New York 2001; Wolfgang U. Eckart, Nervös in den Untergang. Zu einem medizinisch-kulturellen Diskurs um 1900, in: Zeitschrift für Ideengeschichte 3 (2009) 1, p. 64–79; Patrick Kury, Der überforderte Mensch. Eine Wissensgeschichte vom Stress zum Burnout, Frankfurt a. M./New York 2012, p. 37–54.

[38] Barbara Busch, Imperialism, Race and Resistance: Africa and Britain 1919–1945, London/New York 1999, p. 61.

nerve damage or exhaustion, presenting many similar symptoms.[39] Unlike neurasthenia at home, however, it was not considered to be caused by the burdens of modern civilisation.[40] Au contraire, the root of tropical neurasthenia was seen to lie in the combined effect of the tropical climate, physical exertion and mental strain in the face of seclusion from modern society, which corrupted the nervous system of the white male body.[41]

By relocating the diagnosis of neurasthenia to colonial contexts, physicians applied the authority of medical knowledge to a disorder that had been described by Europeans in the tropics for decades as "tropical inertia," "tropical amnesia," "Punjab head," "Burmah head" or "*Tropenkoller*" in German-speaking circles.[42] In his 1906 publication, the colonial doctor Ludwig Külz recalled a feverish episode in northern Togo, where he almost shot his African companions suspecting them of projecting arrows at him after hearing a number of noises. In retrospect, he considered his irrational behaviour a typical example of the neurological condition many white men developed in the tropics, *Tropenkoller*.[43]

Both adversaries and advocates of colonialism used the condition to describe a dramatic loss of self-control, suffered by white men in the tropics, causing them to transgress sexual boundaries and exert excessive

---

[39] They included irritability, insomnia, lack of appetite, loss of memory, headaches, heart palpitations, phobias, sexual disorders, alcoholism, depression and, in severe cases, insanity and suicide. See Dane Kennedy, Minds in Crisis: Medico-moral Theories of Disorder in the Late Colonial World, in: Harald Fischer-Tiné (ed.), Anxieties, Fear and Panic in Colonial Settings. Empires on the Verge of a Nervous Breakdown, Basingstoke 2016, p. 27–47, here p. 32.

[40] Radkau, Das Zeitalter der Nervosität, p. 296–318, 407–421; Sarasin, Reizbare Maschinen, p. 197–207.

[41] Albert Plehn, Über Hirnstörungen in den heissen Ländern und ihre Beurteilung, in: Archiv für Schiffs- und Tropenhygiene 10 (1906), p. 220–230.

[42] Stephan Besser, Tropenkoller: The Interdiscursive Career of a German Colonial Syndrome, in: George S. Rousseau (ed.), Framing and Imagining Disease in Cultural History, Basingstoke 2003, p. 303–320; Eva Bischoff, Tropenkoller: Male Self-Control and the Loss of Colonial Rule, in: Maurus Reinkowski/Gregor Thum (eds.), Helpless Imperialists: Imperial Failure, Fear and Radicalization, Göttingen 2013, p. 117–136; Stephan Besser, Pathographie der Tropen. Literatur, Medizin und Kolonialismus um 1900, Würzburg 2013; Ulrike Schaper, Tropenkoller. States of Agitation and Mood Swings in Colonial Jurisdiction in the German Colonies, in: InterDisciplines 6 (2015) 2, p. 75–100.

[43] Ludwig Külz, Blätter und Briefe eines Arztes aus dem tropischen Deutschafrika, Berlin 1906, p. 158.

violence.[44] Early warning signs included indolence, lack of initiative, a drift into alcoholism and a disregard for the rules of personal hygiene and moral conduct. Most medical and psychiatric experts agreed that tropical neurasthenia occurred most often where the "cultural straitjacket" was loosened and, in contrast to the situation in the motherland, neither the "watchful eye of the law and the general public" nor the customs and conventions of civilisation restricted the individual's conduct.[45] Thus an explosive combination of lack of restraint and an inclination to violence materialised, which erupted in inconsiderate and cruel behaviour that contradicted "common moral and juridical opinion."[46]

Fisch elaborated on neurasthenia in his manuscript on suitability for service in the tropics, arguing that tropical neurasthenia was not a distinct condition to the one found in Europe. While he admitted that the tropical world certainly posed greater challenges to Europeans in both physical and moral terms than more temperate regions, neurasthenia was ultimately a mental condition originating from a lack of modesty and a failure of mastery of mind over body. According to him, the condition known as *Nervenschwäche*—weakness of the nerves—in German medical literature bore the wrong name, since "it is not the nerves but the part of consciousness that we call the soul which is altered by the disease."[47]

Fisch characterised neurasthenia as a form of egocentrism or narcissism that resulted from a lack of Christian asceticism, devotion and sacrifice. He believed that "almost all of us suffer from this condition" in which "the I has taken centre stage of thinking, wanting and feeling."[48] Therefore, if prospective missionaries wished to serve in the tropics, they had "to recognise their enemy" and resolutely oppose it from the beginning.[49] The only way to avoid neurasthenia in Fisch's view was "to practise selfless love," "to devotedly live for others and serve them."[50] He

[44] On colonial critique in the German context, see Benedict Stuchtey, Die europäische Expansion und ihre Feinde. Kolonialismuskritik vom 18. bis in das 20. Jahrhundert, München 2010, p. 232–287.

[45] Mense, Tropische Gesundheitslehre, p. 23.

[46] Plehn, Tropenhygiene, p. 37.

[47] Rudolf Fisch, Wie mache ich mich tauglich für den Tropendienst, p. 4, BMA, G.II.22.

[48] Ibid., p. 4.

[49] Ibid., p. 5.

[50] Ibid., p. 4.

concluded that no disease was "as incompatible with powerful, pneumatic Christianity as neurasthenia."[51]

Like Fisch, a number of tropical doctors refused to accept *Tropenkoller* as a medical diagnosis, arguing that while moving from a temperate into a tropical climate certainly contributed to nervous irritability, people with weak nerves tended to behave impulsively in all climatic zones. Heinrich Botho Scheube, the author of a medical textbook on "diseases in warm countries," firmly rejected tropical frenzy, calling it a "political disease."[52] The tropical physician Carl Mense held that the tropical climate, boredom, loneliness and disappointment of not finding "oriental opulence and paradisiacal freedom" could indeed cause neurasthenia. Nonetheless, he refused to accept that nervous disturbance was an inevitable side effect of colonial service because some men "learned to love tropical nature" and enjoyed the recreation of nature study and collecting while others even found the privations of colonial life conducive to mental health.[53]

Friedrich Hey's *Tropenarzt* included a chapter on "*Tropenkoller und Geisteskrankheiten*"—tropical frenzy and mental illnesses.[54] He explained that the title merely reflected an established expression and not his view, clarifying that "there are no mental diseases." He elaborated on his statement by arguing that "the mind can never fall ill but it can certainly be clouded and hindered in its actions when a person has weak nerves or a weak brain."[55] According to Hey, tropical influences were not the actual root cause of the widespread diagnosis of *Tropenkoller*: "It is mostly, or we may safely say always, people who already at home get irritated easily and suffer from neurasthenia."[56] Once in the tropics, however, the condition was exacerbated due to the "harmful influence of the tropical climate on the central nervous system," malaria infections, alcohol abuse and

---

[51] Ibid., p. 8.

[52] Heinrich Botho Scheube, Krankheiten der warmen Länder, 1st ed., Jena 1896; 2nd ed., Jena 1900; 3rd ed., Jena 1903; 4th ed., Jena 1910.

[53] Mense, Tropische Gesundheitslehre, p. 21–23.

[54] Hey, Der Tropenarzt, 1st ed. p. 346–355.

[55] Ibid., p. 346.

[56] Ibid., p. 348.

"unedifying cases of mental depressions" caused by "detrimental social interactions."[57]

The German pastor Philipp Horbach picked up on the controversy surrounding tropical neurasthenia in 1904 by asking: "If the climate has an influence on such excesses, why do they not occur among missionaries who live in the same climate as their fellow European countrymen?"[58] Horbach's rhetorical question highlights that missionaries were commonly regarded as less susceptible to tropical neurasthenia than other Europeans, although a pre-First World War study of 1479 stricken British missionaries found that "nervous conditions of a neurasthenic type" were the largest single cause of medical repatriation, accounting for 20.8 per cent from Africa.[59] Nonetheless, missionaries appeared to be better prepared for the physical and mental challenges that awaited them abroad than most military and colonial personnel.

A look at the external influences that were considered to cause or aggravate nervous conditions explains why the Basel missionaries might have been less likely to be diagnosed with tropical neurasthenia than other groups of Europeans: they included alcohol indulgence, overemphasis of material goods, deprivation of familiar conviviality and comfortable consumer goods, physical and mental adjustment problems, morphine abuse and sexual excesses.[60] The Basel Mission's behavioural norms represented the polar opposite of these trigger factors by emphasising the importance of temperance, spirituality, a strong community bond, asceticism, intensive preparation, sobriety and Christian marriage. "Missionary service" was a "school of self-renunciation" as Fisch put it.[61]

The Basel Mission did everything in their power to prevent being associated with cases of tropical neurasthenia. By the time the Basel missionaries arrived in the tropics, they had acquired a great deal of experience in discipline, asceticism and self-control under the supervision of

---

[57] Ibid.

[58] Philipp Horbach, Reichskanzler, Missionare und Herero-Aufstand, Bonn 1904, p. 23–24.

[59] George Basil Price, Discussion on The Causes of Invaliding from the Tropics, in: The British Medical Journal, 15.11.1913, p. 1290–1293.

[60] Fiebig, Die Bedeutung der Alkoholfrage für unsere Kolonien, p. 13; Mense, Tropische Gesundheitslehre, p. 22–23; Plehn, Tropenhygiene, p. 37.

[61] Rudolf Fisch, Wie mache ich mich tauglich für den Tropendienst, p. 21, BMA, G.II.22.

their instructors and fellow students in Basel. The Basel Mission's official regulations laid down that it was "a duty to God, who bestows life and health, to do what is necessary to maintain these gifts." The Committee expected every missionary to "conscientiously observe the rules for the protection and conservation of his health, gained from experience and science" as "proof of his diligence and faith to his calling." They cautioned that "the reckless and stubborn disregard of these rules" would be seen "as a sign of the lack of the right spirit of obedience and humility, of simplicity and sobriety, which accounts for an essential part of the suitability for missionary service."[62]

Eva Bischoff demonstrated that the diagnosis of *Tropenkoller*, which simultaneously gained currency in public debates, literary representations and judicial practice, "was successful not because it accurately described what had happened in the colonies, but because it enabled historical actors to further their scientific, political, and personal agendas."[63] Rudolf Fisch and Friedrich Hey denied that the tropical climate actually caused neurasthenia but nevertheless cautioned against moral recklessness if one was to avoid falling prey to tropical frenzy. They used the controversial issue to push a distinctly religious agenda in which moral purity and bodily chastity were inextricably linked. Their message gained the approval of colonial enthusiasts, who emphasised that the demographic weakness of European communities in tropical colonies required maintaining behavioural norms and patrolling cultural boundaries.

9.4   Boundaries of Colonial Rule

The Basel Mission doctors did not differentiate between neurasthenia at home and abroad because, according to them, the condition reflected an individual's mental disposition and spiritual health, regardless of climatic and environmental factors. They were, nevertheless, heavily engaged in debating neurasthenic cases occurring in the tropics, arguing that it was only through strict discipline of the individual that a complete moral collapse of colonial society could be avoided. They cautioned the colonial

---

[62] Verordnungen über die persönliche Stellung der Missionare, Basel 1914, p. 28, BMA Q-09.26.

[63] Bischoff, Tropenkoller, p. 136.

public about the dangers of involving mentally unstable or neurasthenic people into the colonial enterprise, as Friedrich Hey's warning illustrates:

> Anyone who tends to have mental breakdowns at home, who is easily irritable or nervous, should not be allowed in the tropics and if it becomes apparent only when in the tropics, he has to be sent home immediately for his own and other people's sake. For the colonies, only the best is just about good enough. Colonial authorities, trading firms etc. should keep this in mind.[64]

By stressing the importance of self-control in upholding colonial rule, Hey argued that nervous conditions represented not only a lack of self-discipline but a risk to the body politic. Anne Crozier showed that neurasthenic diagnoses were used to confine and deport Europeans seen as weak and irrational for fear that their behaviour would tarnish the image of colonial officials and therefore undermine European claims of cultural and racial superiority.[65] The concern for the mental disposition of Europeans in the tropics not only preoccupied imperial stakeholders but became a key feature in the popular imagination of the colonial world, raising fundamental questions about the feasibility of the colonial project and the place of Europeans in the world.[66]

White men appeared to be at particular risk of nervous breakdowns because they spent more time on the colonial front lines, making them susceptible to alcoholism, sexual excesses and neurasthenic conditions.[67] The medical discourse on mental illnesses induced by life in the tropics excused the behaviour of white men in tropical colonies. It relieved them

[64] Hey, Der Tropenarzt, 1st ed., p. 354.

[65] Anna Crozier, What Was Tropical about Tropical Neurasthenia? The Utility of the Diagnosis in the Management of British East Africa, in: Journal of the History of Medicine and Allied Sciences 64 (2009) 4, p. 518–548.

[66] See, for instance, the popular colonial novel by Frieda von Bülow, Tropenkoller. Episode aus dem deutschen Kolonialleben, Berlin 1896.

[67] Warwick Anderson suggested that tropical frenzy served as a means to delineate the boundaries of colonial masculinity while Sandra Mass interpreted the diagnosis as an effort to characterise and reify European manliness against the figure of the helpless imperialist. See Warwick Anderson, The Trespass Speaks: White Masculinity and Colonial Breakdown, in: American Historical Review 102 (1997) 5, p. 1343–1370; Sandra Mass, Welcome to the Jungle: Imperial Men, "Inner Africa", and Mental Disorder in Colonial Discourse, in: Maurus Reinkowski/Gregor Thum (eds.), Helpless Imperialists: Imperial Failure, Fear and Radicalization, Göttingen 2013, p. 92–116, here p. 93.

of their accountability, for example in cases where criminals were sent back to the "moderate" European climate instead of being sent to prison. Supporters of colonialism employed the idea that mental disorders were responsible for colonial violence and sexual transgressions to disguise and trivialise the system's inherently violent nature.[68]

Moreover, the substantial research into mental disorders reassured Europeans in the tropics that their discomfort was taken seriously and therapies were being developed. The neurasthenic cases described in medical and travel guides around 1900 provided scientific explanations for a wide array of symptoms many white men experienced in tropical colonies. Handbooks on tropical hygiene offered them support for their nervous conditions while simultaneously demanding that they exhibit the moral discipline necessary to maintain the stability of the colonial order.[69]

The large number of single men in the colonies constituted an ongoing concern for colonial rule.[70] Medical and popular debates substantially revolved around sexual issues such as impotence, concupiscence and miscegenation. It was feared that white men would either turn to black women for sexual gratification, thereby fathering mixed-race progeny and eroding racial purity or cultural identity, or give up sex altogether, thereby generating various neuroses and undermining their masculine sense of self.[71] Marriage to European women clearly offered the most suitable solution to this problem but for the majority of white men in the tropics, this was not a viable option. In contrast to the Basel missionaries, their

---

[68] Steven Pierce/Anupama Rao (eds.), Discipline and the Other Body. Correction, Corporeality, Colonialism, Durham 2006; Thomas Schwarz, Kolonialer Ekel und die Kultur der Gewalt. Zur strategischen Allianz von Tropen- und Rassenhygiene mit der deutschen Kolonialliteratur, in: Sven Halse (ed.), Worte, Blicke, Träume. Beiträge zum deutschen Kolonialismus in Literatur, Fotografie und Ausbildung, Kopenhagen 2007, p. 23–50; Rebekka Habermas, Skandal in Togo. Ein Kapitel deutscher Kolonialherrschaft, Frankfurt a. M. 2016.

[69] Grosse, Kolonialismus, Eugenik und bürgerliche Gesellschaft in Deutschland, p. 88–89; Kennedy, Minds in Crisis, p. 34; Will Jackson, Madness and Marginality: The Lives of Kenya's White Insane, Manchester 2013.

[70] Ronald Hyam, Empire and Sexuality. The British Experience, Manchester 1991; Robert J. C Young, Colonial Desire: Hybridity in Theory, Culture and Race, London 1995; Sandra Mass, Weisse Helden, schwarze Krieger. Zur Geschichte kolonialer Männlichkeit in Deutschland, 1918–1964, Köln 2006.

[71] Daniel J. Walther, Creating Germans Abroad: Cultural Policies and National Identity in Namibia, Athens 2002, p. 41.

employers or incomes prevented them from bringing their wives to the colonies.[72]

Fisch called on politicians and directors to increase the wages of colonial administrators and traders so they could afford to bring their European wives to the tropics: "A lot would be gained because a noble woman is a more effective protection against the reckless life around her than anything else, except true fear of God and unfeigned piety."[73] However, for those white women who did take up residence in the tropics, as wives or in other capacities, such as deaconesses, teachers and nurses, the disease environment was thought to be no less threatening.[74] In addition to contracting the standard array of neurasthenic ills, these women were warned that they would likely suffer from irregular menstrual cycles and frequent miscarriages. Virchow went so far as to pin the future of European communities in the colonies on the health of the female body, formulating the bleak prospect that the tropics would make white women infertile.[75]

Anxieties over racial and gender boundaries were frequently sexualised, particularly on imperial frontiers.[76] The debates on the sexuality of white men in tropical colonies not only reflected worries for their physical well-being but centred on the importance of maintaining their racial and cultural integrity. The danger of too much acculturation was considered particularly acute if they shared their lives with a non-European concubine or wife, for this put them in peril of adopting an "indigenous" lifestyle; in short, of "going native" or "*verkaffern*" as it was coined in

[72] Luigi Westenra Sambon, Remarks on the Possibility of the Acclimatisation of Europeans in Tropical Regions, in: British Medical Journal 1 (1897), p. 61–66, here p. 66.

[73] Fisch, Tropische Krankheiten, 3rd ed., p. 176.

[74] Georgina H. Endfield/David J. Nash, "Happy Is The Bride the Rain Falls on": Climate, Health and "the Woman Question" in Nineteenth Century Missionary Documentation, in: Transactions of the Institute of British Geographers 30 (2005) 3, p. 368–386.

[75] Virchow, Über Acclimatisation, p. 542.

[76] McClintock, Imperial Leather; Stoler, Carnal Knowledge and Imperial Power; Bashford, Medicine, Gender and Empire; Anette Dietrich, Weisse Weiblichkeiten. Konstruktionen von "Rasse" und Geschlecht im deutschen Kolonialismus, Bielefeld 2007, p. 243–250; Oliver Philips, The "Perils" of Sex and the Panics of Race: The Dangers of Interracial Sex in Colonial Southern Rhodesia, in: Sylvia Tamale (ed.), African Sexualities. A Reader, Cape Town et al. 2011, p. 101–115.

Germany.[77] These apprehensions found their clearest expression in the rejection of marriages between colonisers and colonised.[78]

Although the Basel Mission principally opposed miscegenation and cohabitation, interracial marriages constituted a complex subject. The Committee feared that by declaring marriages to African women invalid and banning future marriages, white men would be encouraged to cohabit with black women, fathering their children, without having to take responsibility for their actions. In his 1891 edition of *Tropische Krankheiten*, Fisch wrote that instead of allowing men to lead a life of debauchery by outlawing interracial marriages, colonial administrations should hold such men accountable and not punish those who acted honourably and lived conjugally with African women.[79] In West Africa, extramarital relationships between European colonists and African women were part of everyday life while legally binding marriages remained the exception.[80]

Fisch stated that most white men in West Africa behaved "like animals," paid prostitutes, abandoned the children they fathered abroad and passed on syphilis to their children at home. Ultimately, he saw it as the government's responsibility to ensure that the children begotten by Europeans in West Africa received support from their fathers and a proper

[77] Pascal Grosse, Turning Native? Anthropology, German Colonialism and the Paradoxes of the "Acclimatization Question", 1885–1914, in: Matti Bunzl/Glenn Penny (eds.), Worldly Provincialism. German Anthropology in the Age of Empire, Ann Arbor 2003, 179–197; Bischoff, Tropenkoller, p. 123–124.

[78] Interracial marriages between white men and black women, so-called *Mischehen*, became illegal in some German colonies such as German South-West Africa in 1905 and German East Africa in 1906. See Lora Wildenthal, Race, Gender, and Citizenship in the German Colonial Empire, in: Frederick Cooper/Ann Laura Stoler (eds.), Tensions of Empire. Colonial Cultures in a Bourgeois World, Berkeley et al. 1997, p. 263–283; Ibid., German Women for Empire, Durham/London 2001, p. 79–130, 139–145; Kundrus, Moderne Imperialisten, p. 219–280; Ibid., Von Windhoek nach Nürnberg? Koloniale "Mischehenverbote" und die nationalsozialistische Rassengesetzgebung, in: ibid. (ed.), Phantasiereiche. Zur Kulturgeschichte des deutschen Kolonialismus, Frankfurt a. M. 2003, p. 110–131; Frank Becker (ed.), Rassenmischehen—Mischlinge—Rassentrennung. Zur Politik der Rasse im deutschen Kolonialreich, Stuttgart 2004; Lindner, Koloniale Begegnungen, p. 317–361.

[79] Fisch, Tropische Krankheiten, 1st ed., p. 34.

[80] Carina E. Ray, Crossing the Color Line. Race, Sex, and the Contested Politics of Colonialism in Ghana, Athens 2015.

school education.[81] To evangelicals, the promiscuity of large numbers of European men in the tropics was not simply sinful but also smeared the Christian reputation and undercut the progress of the civilising mission.[82] In 1912, Fisch painted a dark picture of the legacy that European men would leave in tropical colonies, if they did not control their sexual urges: "How horrible it will be, when heathen women will sue Christians one day because instead of bringing them the word of life, which made us civilised, they brought them moral ruin, venereal diseases and decay."[83]

Non-marital sexual interactions between a black woman and a white man did not question the existing racial and sexual balance of power, as Philippa Levine has argued.[84] While they certainly went against contemporary concerns expressed in the field of tropical medicine and hygiene, they actually reinforced the established power dynamics in the colonies: the rule of Europeans over Africans and their bodies.[85] Interracial marriages and particularly the offspring resulting from these unions, by contrast, posed a danger to the status quo in the colonies by undermining cultural and racial distinctions. A handful of Basel missionaries transgressed these boundaries by marrying African women, the most famous example being that of Johannes Zimmermann marrying Catherine Mulgrave, originally from the West Indies, in 1851. The Committee, however, denied such couples the right to move to Europe with their families.[86]

"Going native" was a highly charged issue since it diluted the idea of European cultural hegemony and racial superiority. Government physicians, colonial authorities and mission boards insisted that if Europeans hoped to retain their health, sanity and cultural identity, they had to restore themselves with occasional visits to cooler, more familiar

---

[81] Fisch, Tropische Krankheiten, 3rd ed., p. 175–177.

[82] Gottlob Haussleiter, Zur Eingeborenen-Frage in Deutsch-Südwest-Afrika. Erwägungen und Vorschläge, Berlin 1906, p. 36–37.

[83] Fisch, Tropische Krankheiten, 4th ed., p. 69.

[84] Philippa Levine, Sexuality, Gender, and Empire, in: ibid. (ed.), Gender and Empire, Oxford 2004, p. 134–155, here p. 140.

[85] Lora Wildenthal, German Women for Empire, p. 79–86; Stoler, Race and the Education of Desire, p. 95–136.

[86] Schlatter, Geschichte der Basel Mission, vol. 3, p. 51; Miller, Missionary Zeal and Institutional Control, p. 141–150.

surroundings.[87] Albert Plehn emphasised the importance of home leaves not only to retain health but aslo a "national sense of belonging," urging colonists "to stay acclimatised at home and repeatedly gather fresh powers from home for the victorious battle against the foreign climate abroad."[88] The Committee prescribed extended home leaves and regular visits to hill stations during hot and humid months. Hill stations were a central feature of European life in tropical colonies, forming spatial enclaves that symbolised European unity and demarcation from the climatically and culturally alien environment.[89]

On the Gold Coast, the Basel Mission's sanatorium, located on the hill station in Aburi, accommodated a range of Europeans from different backgrounds, including British administrators, German traders, French explorers and Catholic priests, offering them recreation from the exertions of life in the tropics and a place of exchange.[90] In Cameroon, the Basel Mission opened a health resort in 1903 at the hill station Buea at Mount Cameroon, where Europeans received medical assistance and were hosted with fresh vegetables, milk, butter and cheese.[91] David N. Livingstone has argued for hill stations in British colonies that "the carving out of such spaces can be seen as symptomatic of a more general Victorian preoccupation with a bi-polar classifying of places into the sickly and the salubrious."[92] At the same time, these European sanctuaries highlighted the limits of the European presence in tropical colonies.

The tropical world had its own moral economy, not only threatening Europeans' physical and mental health but also their cultural heritage. Handbooks on tropical hygiene recommended cultural commodities and spaces such as gramophones, pianos, reading rooms and skittle alleys, in

---

[87] Mense, Tropische Gesundheitslehre, p. 208.

[88] Albert Plehn, Die Akklimatisationsaussichten der Germanen im tropischen Afrika, in: Verhandlungen des Deutschen Kolonialkongresses 1910, Berlin 1910, p. 888–904, here p. 901.

[89] See Eric C. Jennings, Curing the Colonizers. Hydrotherapy, Climatology, and French Colonial Spas, London 2006.

[90] In 1893, Fisch reported that the sanatorium had seen a total of 40 patients obtaining 1184 days of treatment, including "a brother from Cameroon, one brother and three sisters from the Bremen Mission, two Englishmen from the Coast, one Catholic priests from Elmina and two traders." Fisch, Jahresbericht für 1893, p. 13.

[91] Eckart, Medizin und Kolonialimperialismus, p. 248.

[92] Livingstone, Tropical Climate and Moral Hygiene, p. 108.

short "a somewhat higher kind of conviviality," to distract white men from the dangers lurking in the tropics such as alcohol and women.[93] Self-control required the control of one's environment, which above all meant maintaining distance from the country to be ruled and its people. Therefore, experts in the field of tropical hygiene exhorted Europeans to set themselves apart from their environment in the colonies with the help of protective equipment and practices of withdrawal.[94]

Friedrich Plehn recommended a rigorous daily routine, particularly in "an uncivilised environment" where one needed disciplining signals such as the changing of clothes before meals to remind oneself where one came from.[95] Carl Mense argued that hobbies such as collecting, scientific observations and photography were indispensable to tackle monotony and solitude, and make life in the tropics bearable.[96] Scientists, administrators and missionaries made the chores of knowledge production, including taking regular observations and measurements, collecting zoological, botanical and geological specimens, acquiring ethnographic objects, drawing maps, gathering information, and keeping logs and diaries, a form of hygiene and often a question of preserving European cultural identity.[97]

The controversial debates about European acclimatisation and acculturation depicted the tropics as a site of a racial struggle for survival.[98] However, against a backdrop of what were at times catastrophic experiences of illness and mortality suffered by white settlers, missionaries and officers, the biological argument of racial superiority could hardly

---

[93] Fiebig, Bedeutung der Alkoholfrage, p. 12; Plehn, Tropenhygiene, p. 235; Hermann von Wissmann, Afrika. Schilderungen und Rathschläge zur Vorbereitung für den Aufenthalt und Dienst in den Deutschen Schutzgebieten, Berlin 1895, p. 3.

[94] Ryan Johnson, European Clothes and "Tropical" Skin: Clothing Material and British Ideas of Health and Hygiene in Tropical Climates, in: Bulletin of the History of Medicine 83 (2009), p. 530–560; Ibid., Commodity Culture.

[95] Plehn, Tropenhygiene, p. 234.

[96] Mense, Tropische Gesundheitslehre, p. 22.

[97] Fabian, Out of Our Minds, p. 60.

[98] Ernst Below, Impaludismus, Bakteriologie und Rassenresistenz, in: Archiv für Schiffs- und Tropenhygiene 1 (1897), p. 101–113; Hans Ziemann, Wie erobert man Afrika für die weisse und farbige Rasse? in: Beihefte zum Archiv für Schiffs- und Tropenhygiene 11 (1907), p. 235–259; Paul Schmidt, Über die Anpassungsfähigkeit der weissen Rasse an das Tropenklima, in: Archiv für Schiffs- und Tropenhygiene 14 (1910), p. 397–417.

be sustained.[99] A purely physical definition of tropical fitness, portraying colonial rule as a consequence of racial supremacy, did not prevail in colonial campaigns. In the end, arguments for the superiority of European civilisation had to take a circuitous route by appealing to cultural values and regulated patterns of behaviour.[100]

Handbooks on tropical hygiene prescribed a set of guidelines, which promised to uphold the moral and cultural integrity of Europeans in tropical colonies by combining physical fitness with mental and political self-possession. They were not reflections of commonly shared knowledge but creative sites of a new type of knowledge that tied personal conduct to the success of the colonial project. This was reinforced via the legitimising discourse of medical science. The very precise guidance and advice for tropical hygiene "seemed to have been a psychological necessity," as Philipp Curtin argued. According to him, "to think that life and death were pure chance beyond human knowledge would have been intolerable," especially in areas where Europeans suffered high mortality, like in West Africa: "It was much more satisfying to believe the dead had broken one or another of a numerous and complex system of taboos."[101]

The history of tropical hygiene shows that anxiety, fear and unease often lurked behind European colonial rule, or as Mark Harrison phrased it, "feelings of superiority and vulnerability were two sides of the same imperial coin."[102] The Basel Mission doctors argued that the exercise of effective self-control, as a basis for realising the civilising mission, called for religious virtues such as self-examination and asceticism. The self-techniques and renunciation practices engrained in Pietist purity rituals fell onto fertile soil in tropical colonies because these places were construed as a world in extremis, where a high price would be paid for indulgence, carelessness and misconduct. The Basel Mission doctors' publications on tropical hygiene formed a trusted source of information through which Europeans interpreted their experience in

---

[99] Anderson, Immunities of Empire.

[100] Tilley, Africa as a Living Laboratory, p. 223–224; Hartmann, Tropical Soldiers? p. 130–131.

[101] Curtin, The Image of Africa, p. 80.

[102] Mark Harrison, "The Tender Frame of Man": Disease, Climate, and Racial Difference in India and the West Indies, 1760–1860, in: Bulletin of the History of Medicine 70 (1996) 1, p. 68–93, here p. 70.

tropical colonies. They provided commentary on the political choices and constraints of imperialism itself.

REFERENCES

Warwick Anderson, Immunities of Empire: Race, Disease and the New Tropical Medicine, 1900–1920, in: Bulletin of the History of Medicine 70 (1996) 1, p. 94–118.

Warwick Anderson, The Trespass Speaks: White Masculinity and Colonial Breakdown, in: American Historical Review 102 (1997) 5, p. 1343–1370

Hartmut Bartmuss, Alexander Lion. Arzt, Sanitätsoffizier, Pfadfinder, Berlin 2017.

Alison Bashford, Medicine, Gender and Empire, in: Philippa Levine (ed.), Gender and Empire, Oxford 2004, p. 112–133.

James Africanus Beale Horton, Physical and Medical Climate and Meteorology of the West Coast of Africa with Valuable Hints to Europeans for the Preservation of Health in the Tropics, London 1867.

Frank Becker (ed.), Rassenmischehen—Mischlinge—Rassentrennung. Zur Politik der Rasse im deutschen Kolonialreich, Stuttgart 2004.

Ernst Below, Impaludismus, Bakteriologie und Rassenresistenz, in: Archiv für Schiffs- und Tropenhygiene 1 (1897), p. 101–113.

Stephan Besser, Tropenkoller: The Interdiscursive Career of a German Colonial Syndrome, in: George S. Rousseau (ed.), Framing and Imagining Disease in Cultural History, Basingstoke 2003, p. 303–320.

Stephan Besser, Pathographie der Tropen. Literatur, Medizin und Kolonialismus um 1900, Würzburg 2013.

Eva Bischoff, Tropenkoller: Male Self-Control and the Loss of Colonial Rule, in: Maurus Reinkowski/Gregor Thum (eds.), Helpless Imperialists: Imperial Failure, Fear and Radicalization, Göttingen 2013, p. 117–136.

Barbara Busch, Imperialism, Race and Resistance: Africa and Britain 1919–1945, London/New York 1999.

Anna Crozier, What Was Tropical about Tropical Neurasthenia? The Utility of the Diagnosis in the Management of British East Africa, in: Journal of the History of Medicine and Allied Sciences 64 (2009) 4, p. 518–548.

Philip D. Curtin, The Image of Africa: British Ideas and Action, 1780–1850, vol. 1, London 1964.

Philip D. Curtin, The End of the "White Man's Grave"? Nineteenth-Century Mortality in West Africa, in: Journal of Interdisciplinary History 21 (1990), p. 63–88.

Philip D. Curtin, Disease and Empire: The Health of European Troops in the Conquest of Africa, Cambridge 1998.

Anette Dietrich, Weisse Weiblichkeiten. Konstruktionen von "Rasse" und Geschlecht im deutschen Kolonialismus, Bielefeld 2007.

Wolfgang U. Eckart, Medizin und Kolonialimperialismus. Deutschland 1884–1945, Paderborn 1997.

Wolfgang U. Eckart, Nervös in den Untergang. Zu einem medizinisch-kulturellen Diskurs um 1900, in: Zeitschrift für Ideengeschichte 3 (2009) 1, p. 64–79.

Alfred Eckhardt, Häuserbau in Westafrika und die Station Ho, in: Deutsche Kolonialzeitung 4 (1891), p. 43–46.

Alfred Eckhardt, Land, Leute und ärztliche Mission auf der Goldküste, Basel 1894.

Rod Edmond, Returning Fears: Tropical Disease and the Metropolis, in: Felix Driver/Luciana Martins (eds.), Tropical Visions in the Age of Empire, Chicago 2005, p. 175–194.

Georgina H. Endfield/David J. Nash, Missionaries and Morals: Climatic Discourse in Nineteenth-Century Central Southern Africa, in: Annals of the Association of American Geographers 92 (2002) 4, p. 727–742.

Georgina H. Endfield/David J. Nash, "Happy Is The Bride the Rain Falls on": Climate, Health and "the Woman Question" in Nineteenth Century Missionary Documentation, in: Transactions of the Institute of British Geographers 30 (2005) 3, p. 368–386.

Johannes Fabian, Time and the Work of Anthropology. Critical Essays 1971–1991, Chur et al. 1991.

Johannes Fabian, Out of Our Minds. Reason and Madness in the Exploration of Central Africa, Berkley et al. 2000.

Max Fiebig, Über den Einfluss des Alkohols auf den Europäer in den Tropen, in: Archiv für Schiffs- und Tropenhygiene 5 (1901), p. 14–26, 59–66, 92–106.

Max Fiebig, Die Bedeutung der Alkoholfrage für unsere Kolonien, Berlin 1908.

Rudolf Fisch, Die Malaria und ihre Behandlung auf der Goldküste, in: Allgemeine Missionszeitschrift 16 (1889), p. 553–569

Rudolf Fisch, Jahresbericht für 1893, in: An die Freunde des Ärztlichen Zweiges der Basler Mission, Basel 1894, p. 10–13.

Rudolf Fisch, Zur Prophylaxe des Schwarzwasserfiebers, in: Archiv für Schiffs- und Tropenhygiene 6 (1902), p. 10–14.

Rudolf Fisch, Über die Ätiologie der Tuberkulose auf der Goldküste, in: Correspondenz-Blatt für Schweizer Ärzte 34 (1904), p. 761–763.

Rudolf Fisch, Über die Behandlung der Amöbendysentrie und einige andere tropenmedizinische Fragen, in: Archiv für Schiffs- und Tropenhygiene 8 (1904), p. 207–212.

Rudolf Fisch, Über Stoffe zur Moskitosicherung, in: Archiv für Schiffs- und Tropenhygiene 10 (1906), p. 172–175.

Rudolf Fisch, Die Wurmkrankheit auf der Goldküste, in: Die ärztliche Mission 3 (1908), p. 89–90.

Rudolf Fisch, Behandlung der Malaria mit fraktionierten Chinindosen, in: Archiv für Schiffs- und Tropenhygiene 13 (1909), p. 309–312.

Rudolf Fisch, Tropische Krankheiten. Anleitung zu ihrer Verhütung und Behandlung speziell für die Westküste von Afrika, für Missionare, Kaufleute, Pflanzer und Beamte, 1st ed., Basel 1891; 2nd ed., Basel 1894; 3rd ed., Basel 1903; 4th ed., Basel 1912.

Rudolf Fisch, Über Nachteile in der Säuglingsernährung in den Tropen durch homogenisierte Milch und deren Vermeidung, in: Archiv für Schiffs- und Tropenhygiene 16 (1912), p. 220–222.

Harald Fischer-Tiné (ed.), Anxieties, Fear and Panic in Colonial Settings. Empires on the Verge of a Nervous Breakdown, Basingstoke 2016.

Charles Richard Francis, On Opium, Narcotics and Alcohol in the Tropics, in: VIIIème Congrès International d'Hygiène et de démographie, tenu à Budapest du 1er au 9 septembre 1894. Comptes-rendus et mémoires, Budapest 1896, p. 722–729.

Marijke Gijswijt-Hofstra/Roy Porter (eds.), Cultures of Neurasthenia from George Beard to the First World War, Amsterdam/New York 2001.

Andrea Graf, James Africanus Beale Horton, Medizinaltopographien und wissenschaftliche Selbstlegitimierung vor der mikrobiologischen Revolution (ca. 1835–1885), Master Thesis, University of Basel, 2019.

Pascal Grosse, Kolonialismus, Eugenik und bürgerliche Gesellschaft in Deutschland 1850–1918, Frankfurt a. M. 2000.

Pascal Grosse, Turning Native? Anthropology, German Colonialism and the Paradoxes of the "Acclimatization Question", 1885–1914, in: Matti Bunzl/Glenn Penny (eds.), Worldly Provincialism. German Anthropology in the Age of Empire, Ann Arbor 2003, p. 179–197.

Rebekka Habermas, Skandal in Togo. Ein Kapitel deutscher Kolonialherrschaft, Frankfurt a. M. 2016.

Mark Harrison, "The Tender Frame of Man": Disease, Climate, and Racial Difference in India and the West Indies, 1760–1860, in: Bulletin of the History of Medicine 70 (1996) 1, p. 68–93.

Heinrich Hartmann, Tropical Soldiers? New Definitions of Military Strength in the Colonial Context (1884–1914), in: Martin Lengwiler/Nigel Penn/Patrick Harries (eds.), Science, Africa and Europe. Processing Information and Creating Knowledge, London/New York 2019, p. 125–149.

Gottlob Haussleiter, Zur Eingeborenen-Frage in Deutsch-Südwest-Afrika. Erwägungen und Vorschläge, Berlin 1906.

Friedrich Hey, Der Tropenarzt. Ausführlicher Ratgeber für Europäer in den Tropen, sowie für Besitzer von Plantagen und Handelshäusern, Kolonialbehörden und Missionsverwaltungen, 1st ed., Offenbach 1906.

Philipp Horbach, Reichskanzler, Missionare und Herero-Aufstand, Bonn 1904.

Nancy Rose Hunt, A Nervous State: Violence, Remedies and Reverie in Colonial Congo, Durham 2016.

Ronald Hyam, Empire and Sexuality. The British Experience, Manchester 1991.

Will Jackson, Madness and Marginality: The Lives of Kenya's White Insane, Manchester 2013.

Eric C. Jennings, Curing the Colonizers. Hydrotherapy, Climatology, and French Colonial Spas, London 2006.

Ryan Johnson, Commodity Culture. Tropical Health and Hygiene in the British Empire, in: Endeavour 32 (2008) 2, 2008, p. 70–74.

Ryan Johnson, European Clothes and "Tropical" Skin: Clothing Material and British Ideas of Health and Hygiene in Tropical Climates, in: Bulletin of the History of Medicine 83 (2009), p. 530–560.

Dane Kennedy, The Perils of the Midday Sun: Climatic Anxieties in the Colonial Tropics, in: John M. MacKenzie (ed.), Imperialism and the Natural World, Manchester/New York 1990, p. 118–140.

Dane Kennedy, Minds in Crisis: Medico-moral Theories of Disorder in the Late Colonial World, in: Harald Fischer-Tiné (ed.), Anxieties, Fear and Panic in Colonial Settings. Empires on the Verge of a Nervous Breakdown, Basingstoke 2016, p. 27–47.

Ludwig Külz, Zur Hygiene des Trinkens in den Tropen, Flensburg 1904.

Ludwig Külz, Blätter und Briefe eines Arztes aus dem tropischen Deutschafrika, Berlin 1906.

Birthe Kundrus, Moderne Imperialisten. Das Kaiserreich im Spiegel seiner Kolonien, Köln et al. 2003.

Birthe Kundrus, Von Windhoek nach Nürnberg? Koloniale "Mischehenverbote" und die nationalsozialistische Rassengesetzgebung, in: ibid. (ed.), Phantasiereiche. Zur Kulturgeschichte des deutschen Kolonialismus, Frankfurt a. M. 2003, p. 110–131.

Patrick Kury, Der überforderte Mensch. Eine Wissensgeschichte vom Stress zum Burnout, Frankfurt a. M./New York 2012.

Philippa Levine, Sexuality, Gender, and Empire, in: ibid. (ed.), Gender and Empire, Oxford 2004, p. 134–155.

Ulrike Lindner et al. (eds.), Hybrid Cultures—Nervous States. Britain and Germany in a Post(Colonial) World, Amsterdam/New York 2010.

Ulrike Lindner, Koloniale Begegnungen. Deutschland und Grossbritannien als Imperialmächte in Afrika 1880–1914, Frankfurt a. M. 2011.

Alexander Lion, Tropenhygienische Ratschläge, München 1907.

David. N. Livingstone, Tropical Climate and Moral Hygiene: The Anatomy of a Victorian Debate, in: The British Journal for the History of Science 32 (1999) 1, p. 93–110.

David N. Livingstone, Race, Space and Moral Climatology: Notes Toward a Genealogy, in: Journal of Historical Geography 28 (2002) 2, p. 159–180.

Gregory H. Maddox, Disease and Environment in Africa. Imputed Dynamics and Unresolved Issues, in: Karl Ittman/Dennis D. Cordell/Gregory H. Maddox (eds.), The Demographics of Empire. The Colonial Order and the Creation of Knowledge, Athens 2010, p. 198–216.

Patrick Manson, Tropical Research in its Relation to the Missionary Enterprise, Being an Address Delivered at Livingstone College on Commemoration Day, June 29th, 1908, London 1909.

Sandra Mass, Weisse Helden, schwarze Krieger. Zur Geschichte kolonialer Männlichkeit in Deutschland, 1918–1964, Köln 2006.

Sandra Mass, Welcome to the Jungle: Imperial Men, "Inner Africa", and Mental Disorder in Colonial Discourse, in: Maurus Reinkowski/Gregor Thum (eds.), Helpless Imperialists: Imperial Failure, Fear and Radicalization, Göttingen 2013, p. 92–116.

Anne McClintock, Imperial Leather. Race, Gender and Sexuality in the Colonial Contest, New York 1995.

Carl Mense, Tropische Gesundheitslehre und Heilkunde, Berlin 1902.

Carl Mense, Besprechung von Tropische Krankheiten, in: Archiv für Schiffs- und Tropenhygiene 7 (1903), p. 525–526.

Carl Mense, Besprechung von Tropische Krankheiten, in: Archiv für Schiffs- und Tropenhygiene 16 (1913), p. 569.

Jon Miller, Missionary Zeal and Institutional Control. Organizational Contradictions in the Basel Mission on the Gold Coast, 1828–1917, London/New York 2003.

Theodor Müller, Krankheitsbilder von der Goldküste, in: Die ärztliche Mission 7 (1912), p. 131–136.

Theodor Müller, Westafrikanische Krankheiten, in: Die ärztliche Mission 8 (1913), p. 85–89.

Theodor Müller, Über Gelbfieber in Westafrika, in: Die ärztliche Mission 9 (1914), p. 15–22, 40–41.

Gottlieb Olpp (ed.), Tropenhygienische Rundschau, in: Sonderbadruck aus der "Kolonialen Rundschau" (1913) 3, p. 178–184.

Gottlieb Olpp (ed.), Tropenhygienische Rundschau, in: Sonderbadruck aus der "Kolonialen Rundschau" (1913) 6, p. 374–380.

Gottlieb Olpp (ed.), Tropenhygienische Rundschau, in: Sonderbadruck aus der "Kolonialen Rundschau" (1913) 9, p. 551–559.

Gottlieb Olpp (ed.), Tropenhygienische Rundschau, in: Sonderbadruck aus der "Kolonialen Rundschau" (1913) 12, p. 745–753.

Gottlieb Olpp (ed.), Tropenhygienische Rundschau, in: Sonderbadruck aus der "Kolonialen Rundschau" (1914) 3, p. 171–181.

Gottlieb Olpp (ed.), Tropenhygienische Rundschau, in: Sonderbadruck aus der "Kolonialen Rundschau" (1914) 6, p. 359–368.

Hans Paasche, Was ich als Abstinent in den afrikanischen Kolonien erlebte, Reutlingen 1911.

Robert Peckham (ed.), Empires of Panic: Epidemics and Colonial Anxieties, Hong Kong 2015.

Michael Pesek, Vom richtigen Reisen und Beobachten: Ratgeberliteratur für Forschungsreisende nach Übersee im 19. Jahrhundert, in: Berichte zur Wissenschaftsgeschichte 40 (2017) 1, p. 17–38.

Oliver Philips, The "Perils" of Sex and the Panics of Race: The Dangers of Interracial Sex in Colonial Southern Rhodesia, in: Sylvia Tamale (ed.), African Sexualities. A Reader, Cape Town et al. 2011, p. 101–115.

Steven Pierce/Anupama Rao (eds.), Discipline and the Other Body. Correction, Corporeality, Colonialism, Durham 2006.

Albert Plehn, Über Hirnstörungen in den heissen Ländern und ihre Beurteilung, in: Archiv für Schiffs- und Tropenhygiene 10 (1906), p. 220–230.

Albert Plehn, Die Akklimatisationsaussichten der Germanen im tropischen Afrika, in: Verhandlungen des Deutschen Kolonialkongresses 1910, Berlin 1910, p. 888–904.

Friedrich Plehn, Tropenhygiene. Mit spezieller Berücksichtigung der deutschen Kolonien. Ärztliche Ratschläge für Kolonialbeamte, Offiziere, Missionare, Expeditionsführer, Pflanzer und Faktoristen, Jena 1906.

George Basil Price, Discussion on The Causes of Invaliding from the Tropics, in: The British Medical Journal, 15.11.1913, p. 1290–1293.

Joachim Radkau, Das Zeitalter der Nervosität. Deutschland zwischen Bismarck und Hitler, München 1998.

Carina E. Ray, Crossing the Color Line. Race, Sex, and the Contested Politics of Colonialism in Ghana, Athens 2015.

Maurus Reinkowski/Gregor Thum (eds.), Helpless Imperialists: Imperial Failure, Fear and Radicalization, Göttingen 2013.

Philipp Sarasin, Reizbare Maschinen. Eine Geschichte des Körpers, 1765–1914, Frankfurt a. M. 2003.

Ulrike Schaper, Tropenkoller. States of Agitation and Mood Swings in Colonial Jurisdiction in the German Colonies, in: InterDisciplines 6 (2015) 2, p. 75–100.

Heinrich Botho Scheube, Krankheiten der warmen Länder, 1st ed., Jena 1896; 2nd ed., Jena 1900; 3rd ed., Jena 1903; 4th ed., Jena 1910.

Wilhelm Schlatter, Geschichte der Basler Mission 1815–1915, 3 vol., Basel 1916.

Paul Schmidt, Über die Anpassungsfähigkeit der weissen Rasse an das Tropenklima, in: Archiv für Schiffs- und Tropenhygiene 14 (1910), p. 397–417.

Thomas Schwarz, Kolonialer Ekel und die Kultur der Gewalt. Zur strategischen Allianz von Tropen- und Rassenhygiene mit der deutschen Kolonialliteratur, in: Sven Halse (ed.), Worte, Blicke, Träume. Beiträge zum deutschen Kolonialismus in Literatur, Fotografie und Ausbildung, Kopenhagen 2007, p. 23–50.

William John Simpson, The Maintenance of Health in the Tropics, London 1905.

Francesco Spöring, Mission und Sozialhygiene. Schweizer Anti-Alkohol-Aktivismus im Kontext von Internationalismus und Kolonialismus, 1886–1939, Doctoral Thesis, ETH Zurich, 2014.

Nancy Leys Stepan, Picturing Tropical Nature, Ithaca 2001.

Ann Laura Stoler, Race and the Education of Desire. Foucault's History of Sexuality and the Colonial Order of Things, Durham/London 1995.

Ann Laura Stoler, Carnal Knowledge and Imperial Power. Race and the Intimate in Colonial Rule, Berkeley/Los Angeles/London 2002.

Benedict Stuchtey, Die europäische Expansion und ihre Feinde. Kolonialismuskritik vom 18. bis in das 20. Jahrhundert, München 2010.

Helen Tilley, Africa as a Living Laboratory. Empire, Development, and the Problem of Scientific Knowledge, 1870–1950, Chicago 2011.

Megan Vaughan, Curing Their Ills. Colonial Power and African Illness, Cambridge 1991.

Rudolf Virchow, Über Acclimatisation, in: Tageblatt der 58. Versammlung deutscher Naturforscher und Ärzte, Strassburg 1885, p. 540–554.

Frieda von Bülow, Tropenkoller. Episode aus dem deutschen Kolonialleben, Berlin 1896.

Hermann von Wissmann, Afrika. Schilderungen und Rathschläge zur Vorbereitung für den Aufenthalt und Dienst in den Deutschen Schutzgebieten, Berlin 1895.

Hermann Vortisch, Erfahrungen über einige spezifische Krankheiten an der Goldküste, in: Archiv für Schiffs- und Tropenhygiene 10 (1906), p. 537–539.

Hermann Vortisch, Ärztliche Beobachtungen und Erfahrungen auf der Goldküste, in: Deutsche Medizinische Wochenschrift 33 (1907), p. 110–111.

Hermann Vortisch, Über Säuglingsernährung in den Tropen, in: Archiv für Schiffs- und Tropenhygiene 16 (1912), p. 69–77.

Daniel J. Walther, Creating Germans Abroad: Cultural Policies and National Identity in Namibia, Athens 2002.

Luigi Westenra Sambon, Remarks on the Possibility of the Acclimatisation of Europeans in Tropical Regions, in: British Medical Journal 1 (1897), p. 61–66.

Lora Wildenthal, Race, Gender, and Citizenship in the German Colonial Empire, in: Frederick Cooper/Ann Laura Stoler (eds.) Tensions of Empire. Colonial Cultures in a Bourgeois World, Berkeley et al. 1997, p. 263–283.

Lora Wildenthal, German Women for Empire, Durham/London 2001.

Michael Worboys, Germs, Malaria and the Invention of Mansonian Tropical Medicine. From "Diseases in the Tropics" to "Tropical Diseases", in: David Arnold, (ed.) Warm Climates and Western Medicine. The Emergence of Tropical Medicine 1500–1900, Åmsterdam/Atlanta 1996, p. 181–207.

Robert J. C Young, Colonial Desire: Hybridity in Theory, Culture and Race, London 1995.

Hans Ziemann, Wie erobert man Afrika für die weisse und farbige Rasse? in: Beihefte zum Archiv für Schiffs- und Tropenhygiene 11 (1907), p. 235–259.

Hans Ziemann, Hints to Europeans in Tropical Stations, London 1910.

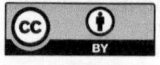

CHAPTER 10

Materialising Hygiene: Remedies, Commodities and Images

Hygiene was more than a metaphor used to encode religious virtues, scientific imperatives, cultural values, social interactions and colonial anxieties. It was a practice that materialised itself in and on individual bodies, and crucially depended on material aids such as drugs, medical equipment, sanitary articles and specific clothing. The Basel Mission actively engaged with these tools of hygiene, from an early interest in natural remedies in West Africa to the establishment of a thriving commodity culture surrounding tropical hygiene around 1900. Remedies and commodities circulating through missionary networks shaped bodily practices, while images produced and propagated by the Basel Mission left a visual legacy that informs our understanding of purity, health and cleanliness to this day. Examined critically, these material and visual sources reveal the profoundly interactive nature of missionary encounters and testify to the conceptual, practical and material exchanges between people in West Africa and Europe.

© The Author(s) 2023   379
L. M. Ratschiller Nasim, *Medical Missionaries and Colonial Knowledge in West Africa and Europe, 1885–1914*,
Cambridge Imperial and Post-Colonial Studies,
https://doi.org/10.1007/978-3-031-27128-1_10

10.1   Materia Medica

From their earliest Christianising efforts overseas, missionaries showed a particular interest in natural remedies, thereby enriching pharmacological knowledge.[1] Due to their prolonged stays abroad, they took a keen interest in finding effective remedies against their frequent health problems. With the help of local experts, they recorded, classified and codified medical plants and the contents of remedies or substances used in their ingredients.[2] The Basel missionaries, who had been on the Gold Coast since 1828, were familiar with African therapeutics and generally supportive of African natural remedies. The arrival of medical missionaries from 1885, however, threatened to devalue these plant-based preparations. The Basel missionary Adolf Mohr addressed a letter to the Committee, in which he expressed his fear over the impending insignificance of remedies used on the Gold Coast and highlighted the importance of their study:

> In my opinion, it is not right to despise this country's medicines ipso facto and to call them 'quackery'. It would certainly not only be worthwhile but also interesting for a doctor to study the local herbs and barks etc. and to examine what they are all about.[3]

Although the Basel missionaries perceived their medical colleagues as being dismissive of medicinal plants, the mission doctors turned out to be rather inquisitive about West African remedies. Fisch, for instance, who created a garden for rare plants, observed that "barks or leaves or roots" usually came from four to eight key plants, which were cooked in a pot of one to three litres of water or palm wine "to extract the active substances."[4] His handbook *Tropische Krankheiten* contained a list of recommended medications, including a wide range of substances and preparations originating from South America, Asia, Oceania, the

---

[1] See, for instance, Renate Wilson, Pious Traders in Medicine: A German Pharmaceutical Network in Eighteenth-Century North America, Philadelphia 2000; Sivasundaram, Natural History Spiritualized.

[2] The Basel missionary Caspar Stolz collected numerous Indian medical plants, which he commented on in his influential publication. See Caspar Stolz, Five Hundred Indian Plants, Their Use in Medicine and the Arts, Mangalore 1881.

[3] Adolf Mohr, Remarks to a letter from R. Fisch, 21.07.1905, BMA, D-1.84.15.

[4] Fisch, Die ärztliche Mission unter den Negern, p. 375.

Americas, Europe and Africa.[5] This illustrates that missionaries played a key role in the connected histories of colonialism, plants and medicine. Their encounters with new medical ingredients overseas fundamentally transformed pharmacology and medical theories at home.[6]

The various substances and preparations used in medical practice and treatment, coined *materia medica*, expanded and diversified rapidly from the seventeenth century. One of the earliest globally traded drugs was the bark of the cinchona tree, which was used as the main remedy against different kinds of fevers.[7] The name of the medicinal tree, which originated in South America, was said to have come from the countess of Chinchon, the wife of a viceroy in Peru, who was cured of a fever by a local physician using the bark of the cinchona tree in 1638, and then supposedly popularised it even before botanists had identified and named the species.[8] Another account assigned the introduction of the cinchona bark into European medical practice to a monk of the Augustinian Order, who had been informed about its medicinal qualities by Peruvians. Cinchona bark was first advertised for sale in England in 1658 and entered the *London Pharmacopoeia* in 1677.[9]

Europeans showed a growing interest in pharmacological plants on the supposed edges of civilisation while most accompanying customs were considered medically and scientifically irrelevant. Studying, classifying and experimenting with tropical plants became an important part of medical training in Europe in the eighteenth century. The Scottish doctor James Lind, an early advocate of naval hygiene, proposed the use of china bark as a malaria prophylaxis in his 1768 *Essay on Diseases Incidental to Europeans in Hot Climates, with the Method of Preventing their Fatal*

---

[5] Fisch, Tropische Krankheiten, 1st ed., p. 189–212; Ibid., Tropische Krankheiten, 2nd ed., p. 195–217; Ibid., Tropische Krankheiten, 3rd ed., p. 181–207; Ibid., Tropische Krankheiten, 4th ed., p. 300–329.

[6] James Beattie, Imperial Landscapes of Health: Place, Plants and People between India and Australia, 1800s–1900s, in: Health & History 14 (2012) 1, p. 100–120.

[7] Stefanie Gänger, A Singular Remedy. Cinchona Across the Atlantic World, 1751–1820, Cambridge 2020; Ibid., Mikrogeschichten des Globalen. Chinarinde, der Andenraum und die Welt während der "globalen Sattelzeit" (1770–1830), in: Boris Barth/Stefanie Gänger/Niels P. Petersson (eds.), Globalgeschichten. Bestandsaufnahme und Perspektiven, Frankfurt a. M 2014, p. 19–40.

[8] Anna E. Winterbottom, Of the China Root: A Case Study of the Early Modern Circulation of Materia Medica, in: Social History of Medicine 28 (2015), p. 22–44.

[9] Chakrabarti, Medicine and Empire, p. 25.

Consequences.[10] In 1820, two French chemists and pharmacists, Joseph-Bienaimé Caventou and Pierre-Joseph Pelletier, identified quinine as the active ingredient of cinchona and started producing quinine from tree bark found in Peruvian and Bolivian forests.[11]

The appropriation and transformation of cinchona into quinine illustrates why the advent of scientific medicine in the 1880s did not put an end to the exploration of colonial and tropical plants, despite marking a new period in medical history. While the Basel missionaries feared that the increasing importance of laboratory medicine and chemical industries would undermine the standing of *materia medica* from the colonies, quite the opposite happened. The chemical and pharmaceutical industries that mushroomed in France, Germany and, most notably, in Basel in the late nineteenth century used active ingredients found in the tropics to manufacture drugs in Europe. The imperial expansion in Africa, therefore, coalesced with the rise of pharmaceutical chemistry in Europe, which started a new era of colonial bioprospection.[12]

Missionaries, botanists and traders, often supported by pharmaceutical companies, now searched for and established commercial monopolies over new and well-known *materia medica*. These were then sent to Europe as industrial raw materials to be converted into drugs through the identification and extraction of their active ingredients, which helped standardise the dosage and manufacture of pills in the laboratory. By transforming medicinal plants from the colonies into factory manufactured drugs, Europeans found a way of appropriating these remedies by putting a supposedly modern and scientific spin on them. *Strophanthus*, a plant that was used by West African healers both as a poison and medicine, offers a fascinating example of the colonial adoption of African *materia medica* into European pharmacological knowledge.[13]

Strophanthin, which people on the Gold Coast used in their poisoned arrows against the British, entered the *British Pharmacopoeia* in 1898, following a complex history of European interest in African medicinal

---

[10] James Lind, Essay on Diseases Incidental to Europeans in Hot Climates, with the Method of Preventing their Fatal Consequences, London 1768.

[11] Chakrabarti, Medicine and Empire, p. 34.

[12] Ibid., p. 191.

[13] Abena Osseo-Asare, Bioprospecting and Resistance: Transforming Poisoned Arrows into Strophantin Pills in Colonial Gold Coast, 1885–1922, in: Social History of Medicine 21 (2008), p. 269–290.

plants. Laboratory experiments on the drug in Edinburgh had led to the discovery of its active ingredient in 1873, which was found to be a particularly effective cardiac drug. Following this discovery, British pharmaceutical companies, such as *Burroughs Wellcome & Co*, procured the plant in large quantities to produce the drug on an industrial scale.[14] In 1905, with the establishment of a British military presence in West Africa, the colonial government outlawed the use of the plant in poisoned arrows. Concurrently, growing international pharmaceutical demand for *Strophanthus* seeds led to an export scheme from the Gold Coast during WWI. This coincided with the marginalisation of its use in African medicine.[15]

One of the remedies recommended in Fisch's *Tropische Krankheiten* was the *simaruba* bark.[16] The Basel missionaries first took notice of *simaruba* when the African pastor Carl Reindorf recommended it to them as a remedy against dysentery.[17] Reindorf later sold his formula containing the ingredient to a missionary of the Bremen Mission for five pounds sterling, who introduced it into Europe. Hermann Gundert, a former Basel missionary in India and grandfather to Herman Hesse, praised the efficacy of the preparation in his diary.[18] In 1904, Fisch also recommended *simaruba* as a therapeutic option for amoebic dysentery in a piece for the *Archiv für Schiffs- und Tropenhygiene*, thereby promoting the use of the African bark in scientific circles.[19] The Basel Mission thus paved a way for medicinal plants from the colonies to enter European medical practice and scientific texts.

The Basel Mission doctor Karl Huppenbauer started a collection of African herbal medicines in 1914, which was lost during the course of

---

[14] Markku Hokkanen, Imperial Networks, Colonial Bioprospecting and Burroughs Wellcome & Co: The Case of *Strophanthus Kombe* from Malawi (1859–1915), in: Social History of Medicine 25 (2012) 3, p. 589–607.

[15] Osseo-Asare, Bioprospecting and Resistance.

[16] Fisch, Tropische Krankheiten, 4th ed., p. 226, 325–326.

[17] Gottlieb Schmid, Letter to Committee, 15.11.1882, BMA, D-1.35.40; Ibid., Letter to Committee, 20.01.1883, BMA, D-1.35.47.

[18] Hermann Gundert, Calwer Tagebuch 1859–1893, ed. by Albrecht Frenz, Stuttgart 1986, p. 499.

[19] Rudolf Fisch, Über die Behandlung der Amöbendysentrie und einige andere tropenmedizinische Fragen, in: Archiv für Schiffs- und Tropenhygiene 8 (1904), p. 207–212.

the First World War.[20] At a time when the study of natural sciences and the practice of medicine in Europe was becoming an increasingly secular pursuit, based on laboratory experiments and chemical drugs, the Basel medical missionaries retained and even revitalised Christian spirituality in the exploration of nature and the art of healing. This enabled them to have closer contact with and insight into the communities with which they worked. The Basel Mission doctors were simultaneously looking for new therapeutic ingredients in West Africa, collecting information about African plants and their medical uses, and introducing new pharmaceuticals and scientific medicine into colonial Africa.

The Basel missionary Adolf Mohr observed in 1905 that "the indigenous possess effective juices of certain leaves, which produce breast milk once applied on the chest."[21] Friedrich Hey became interested in this natural remedy after a number of missionary wives had tried it on themselves. Although he left the Basel Mission in 1902, Hey returned to West Africa in 1904 to work for a German trading company and started examining the remedy for the stimulation of breast milk production more thoroughly. He found out that the plant used in the preparation was *Crassulaceae Kalanchoe,* a type of succulent flowering plant. Because of its scarcity, Hey used unripened fruits of the papaya tree as an alternative, which he had learned, worked in a similar way. He developed a preparation called "Dr. Hey's Lacto-Generator," which was marketed in Germany.[22]

Even though Hey indicated that most physicians were critical of his natural remedy, the product was the first of a whole range of African medical preparations, which he developed and introduced to European consumers.[23] His pharmaceutical products, including a "Syphilis Elixir," "Dr. med. Hey's Regenerator" and "Dr. med. Hey's Cholagogum," were sold to pharmacies and direct to consumers through the companies *Hermann Dahl & Co.* in Hannover and *Dr. Hey's Lacto und Rad-Jo*

---

[20] Karl Huppenbauer, Chirurgische und ophthalmologische Erfahrungen von der Goldküste, in: Archiv für Schiffs- und Tropenhygiene 22 (1918), p. 341–364, here p. 341.

[21] Adolf Mohr, Remarks to a letter from R. Fisch, 21.07.1905, BMA, D-1.84.15.

[22] H. Göring, Dr. Hey's Pflanzenmittel insbesondere zur Erleichterung der Geburt und Muttermilchbeförderung in ihrem Werte für die Volksgesundheit und Sittlichkeit, 1911, p. 24, BMA, G.IV.09; Fischer, Der Missionsarzt Rudolf Fisch, p. 473; Wolters, Dr. Friedrich Hey, p. 346.

[23] Hey, Der Tropenarzt, 1st ed., p. 368.

Versand von Vollrath Wasmuth in Hamburg, of which he owned half. Hey was particularly proud of his "preparation for women's welfare (to facilitate birth)," which he had formulated during his time in West Africa "after many time-consuming and profound studies and experiments."[24]

The founder of the *Archiv für Schiffs- und Tropenhygiene,* Carl Mense, accused Hey of deception and greed for profit, commenting that the composition of his "natural product Lacto-Generator" was not specified and that it was excessively priced at "2 Mark a bottle!"[25] By suggesting that the mission doctor's main objective was personal profit, to such an extent that it distracted from medicine's real purpose, Mense's critique resembled that of European doctors towards African healers. The question of remuneration arose the special interest of scientifically trained physicians, who feared for their economic well-being and professional status both abroad and at home. Competing healthcare providers such as naturopaths, homeopaths and balneologists posed a threat to allopathic practitioners by challenging their exclusive right to professional expertise and subsequent income.[26]

Upon his return to Germany in 1907, Hey gradually moved further away from allopathic medicine and closer to naturopathy, which raised concerns among fellow doctors and political authorities.[27] His intrusive advertising in daily newspapers, leaflets and brochures with slogans such as "Cancer is curable!" alerted the Imperial Heath Department in Berlin. The supervisory authority led a detailed investigation into Hey's preparations in 1913, upon which the former Basel Mission doctor was only allowed to distribute them through pharmacies and had to refrain from advertising his remedies with exaggerated claims. Nonetheless, Hey established his own factory for pharmaceutical preparations in the German

---

[24] Curriculum Vitae Friedrich Hey, BArch, R 86/1768; Dr. med. Hey's "Frauenwohl". Ein aus Pflanzen bereitetes Präparat zur Verhinderung der Beschwerden der Schwangerschaft und zur Erleichterung der Geburt etc., 1907, BMA, G.IV.05.

[25] Carl Mense, Besprechung von Hey Fr., Der Tropenarzt, Wismar 1907, in: Archiv für Schiffs- und Tropenhygiene 12 (1908), p. 204.

[26] Deborah Brunton, The Emergence of a Modern Profession? in: ibid. (ed.), Medicine Transformed. Health, Disease and Society in Europe 1880–1930, Manchester/New York 2004, p. 119–149.

[27] Hey became highly critical of chemically produced drugs as he indicated in his compilation of natural remedies. See Hey, Der Tropenarzt, 1st ed., p. 409–424.

town of Bückeburg in 1920, which he ran until his death forty years later.[28]

Plants were vital commodities for European colonialists, who began venturing overseas in search of exotic spices and tropical plants and later derived great profits from growing these plants in colonial gardens and plantations.[29] However, there was more to this European engagement with tropical flora than the pursuit of commercial profit. The exploration, observation and exploitation of tropical plants and herbs by missionaries, naturalists and businessmen forged a new relationship between the natural world of the tropics and the medical world of Europe.[30] Tropical plants, including cinchona, sarsaparilla and opium, became widely used in European medical practice. Moreover, the rise of botanical and zoological gardens illustrates that tropical nature not only pervaded natural history, science and medicine but also popular culture.[31]

10.2   The Commodification of Hygiene

Tropical hygiene became a busy marketplace around 1900 with handbooks, advertisements and exhibitions promoting commodities for the tropics. Fisch's *Tropische Krankheiten* included a list of suppliers for tropical travel pharmacies since, according to him, most pharmacists were unfamiliar with the climatic peculiarities of the tropics, especially in West Africa where many precautionary measures were required.[32] Fisch thus compiled his own range of tablets together with the owner of the Berlin-based *Oranienapotheke Dr. Kade*, Franz Lutze, who gradually developed his pharmacy into a pharmaceutical factory. The medical chests put together by Fisch and Lutze came in two metal boxes, each weighing 65 pounds—equal to the load of a porter according to Fisch—and could

---

[28] Wolters, Dr. Friedrich Hey, p. 347–350.

[29] Londa Schiebinger, Plants and Empire: Colonial Bioprospecting in the Atlantic World, Cambridge 2004; Julia Angster, Erdbeeren und Piraten. Die Royal Navy und die Ordnung der Welt 1770–1860, Göttingen 2012.

[30] Harries, Butterflies and Barbarians, p. 123–154; Chakrabarti, Medicine and Empire, p. 20–39.

[31] Anderson, Climates of Opinion, p. 136.

[32] Fisch, Tropische Krankheiten, 1st ed., p. 219–225.

be purchased from Dr. Kade's pharmacy directly or, more conveniently, via the order form in Fisch's book.[33]

By endorsing, advertising and selling tropical commodities, the Basel Mission doctors participated in the commodification of the tropics around 1900. Clothes, in particular, played an important role in fashioning the body according to ideas of Christian decency, standards of tropical hygiene and cultural perceptions of civilisation. The medical missionaries offered extensive advice on clothing, including boots, socks, hats, raincoats and underwear, as the adequate protection of the European body in tropical regions became a foremost concern.[34] The type of tropical outfit recommended and advertised by the Basel Mission doctors for women and men is illustrated by two images printed on the inside cover of Friedrich Hey's *Der Tropenarzt* in 1906, showing the mission doctor himself and his wife (Figs. 10.1 and 10.2).[35]

Missionaries, explorers and settlers had long used specific gear that, they hoped, would improve their probability of surviving in the tropics. However, the increasing influence of tropical hygiene around 1900 spawned ever more detailed medical theories and sophisticated technical aids. Researchers in tropical medicine began arguing that actinic radiation, which forms part of the ultraviolet band of the light spectrum, might have adverse physiological effects on white-skinned people in the tropics.[36] In line with this concern, Fisch explained, in *Tropische Krankheiten,* why light-skinned Europeans were much more prone to heat accumulation and sunstroke than Africans with their dark complexion. He concluded: "It is clear that clothing for Europeans in hot zones is not only a matter of civility but also a concern for health in general."[37]

---

[33] Dr. Kade's pharmacy frequently advertised in missionary and colonial publications proclaiming to be the "purveyor to the court of His majesty the Kaiser and King" as well as the supplier to the Imperial Colonial Office and to the High Command of the so-called *Schutztruppe* for all their medical needs in the German colonies. Dr. Kade did not only supply pharmaceuticals, bandages and dressings, but also examination chests, water sterilisers and cooling devices.

[34] See, for example, Hey, Der Tropenarzt, 1st ed., p. 143–157; Fisch, Tropische Krankheiten, 1st ed., p. 19–22; Ibid., Tropische Krankheiten, 4th ed., p. 44–53.

[35] Hey, Der Tropenarzt, 1st ed, Inside Cover.

[36] Johnson, European Clothes and "Tropical" Skin, p. 550–551.

[37] Fisch, Tropische Krankheiten, 1st ed., p. 20.

Fig. 10.1 Friedrich
Hey, Der Tropenarzt.
Ausführlicher Ratgeber
für Europäer in den
Tropen, sowie für
Besitzer von Plantagen
und Handelshäusern,
Kolonialbehörden und
Missionsverwaltungen,
1st ed., Offenbach
1906, Inside Cover

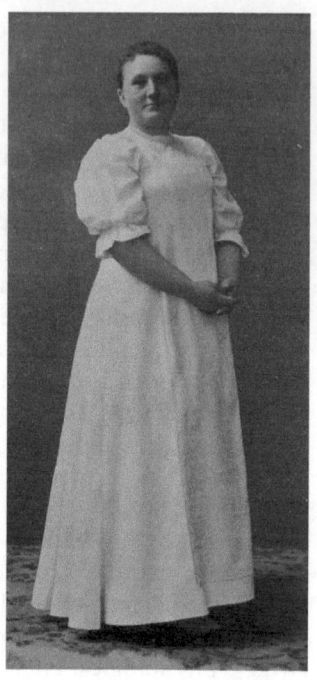

Proper functioning of the skin was one of the key topics in tropical prophylactics.[38] Medical manuals published in the late nineteenth and early twentieth centuries included chapters that focussed on the best type of material for tropical clothing to maintain equilibrium of physiological functions. They advocated the use of special items of dress to protect Europeans from the solar threat such as the flannel binder worn by Hey on the photograph, pith helmets, sunglasses, spine pads and a specially designed red fabric advertised under the trade name "Solaro" to shield the body from actinic rays.[39] By insisting on the need of elaborate equipment and very specific commodities, handbooks on tropical hygiene

[38] Rudolf Fisch, Über Stoffe zur Moskitosicherung, in: Archiv für Schiffs- und Tropenhygiene 10 (1906), p. 172–175.

[39] The "Solaro" was developed by Luigi Westenra Sambon and consisted of a fabric woven of white and coloured thread. Livingstone, Tropical Climate and Moral Hygiene, p. 109; Kennedy, The Perils of the Midday Sun, p. 120.

Fig. 10.2 Friedrich Hey, Der Tropenarzt. Ausführlicher Ratgeber für Europäer in den Tropen, sowie für Besitzer von Plantagen und Handelshäusern, Kolonialbehörden und Missionsverwaltungen, 1st ed., Offenbach 1906, Inside Cover

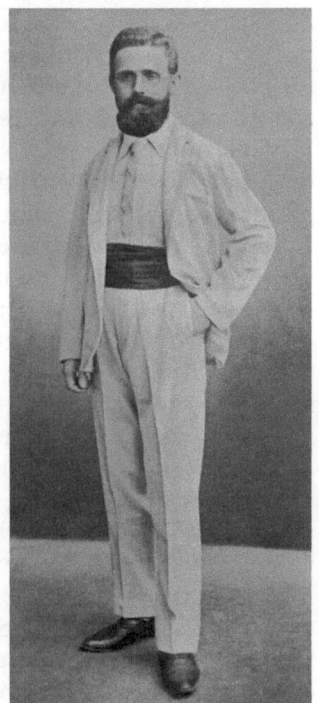

helped maintain climatic fears. They implied that to stay healthy, safe and civilised, Europeans had to consume commodities such as medical books, hygienic accessories and protective clothes.

Ryan Johnson noted that "there are few examples of advances in tropical medicine that do not come bound up with a great clutter of outfits." He argued that it is this "associated paraphernalia that reveals most about how the British saw tropical people, places, health and hygiene."[40] There can be little doubt that tropical commodities shaped and fuelled the imaginary space of the tropics, as Johnson suggested. But they did more than this. They also allowed people to form and express identities along the lines of race, class, gender and religion. Tropical paraphernalia were symbolic expressions of the conviction that social, cultural and racial

[40] Johnson, Commodity Culture, p. 71.

boundaries were essential to the protection, privilege and power of colonial protagonists. With their exclusive and ritualistic use by Europeans, they helped to define and sustain those boundaries, to remind Europeans and Africans alike of the distance between one another.[41]

While most European observers recognised that Africans had their own methods of hygiene, they oftentimes refused to view African bodily practices in the same light as the hygiene guidelines recommended in European medical discourse. Ludwig Külz, for instance, noted that "natural peoples" evinced "an instinctively practised hygiene."[42] By insisting on the need for modern material aids to observe hygiene properly, tropical doctors tried to differentiate themselves from this "instinctively practised hygiene." To avoid being exposed to harmful tropical conditions like the seemingly natural people living in the colonies, Europeans emphasised the importance of medical technologies and equipment.[43]

The British were the first to recognise tropical outfitting as a commercial opportunity, producing a whole range of protective gear from tropical pyjamas and travelling bathtubs to cooling devices and tents, but the German industry soon rose to the challenge. At the 1907 German Army, Marine and Colonial Exhibition in Berlin, an entire section was devoted to the tropical outfitting industry.[44] The commodity culture around tropical hygiene upheld the image of the tropics as an alien space within which a strict attention to daily bodily conduct was essential to the maintenance of white health under the pressure of the sun and humidity. The obsession with protective gear created a clear delineation between European consumers and non-European people, who apparently lacked scientific progress, technological know-how and capitalistic innovation.

In her seminal study on the nexus between commodity culture, imperialism and racism, Anne McClintock assessed "a supplementation of the 'elitist' scientific racism by a popular 'commodity racism'" in late Victorian Britain. She noted that the promotion of tropical products and their colonial contexts, such as teas, biscuits, tobaccos, tins of cocoa

---

[41] Kennedy, The Perils of the Midday Sun, p. 131.

[42] Külz, Grundzüge der kolonialen Eingeborenenhygiene, p. 391.

[43] Patricia Purtschert used the word "techno-colonialism" to describe the importance of technology in forming colonial fantasies and shaping Swiss identity. See Patricia Purtschert, Aviation Skills, Manly Adventures and Imperial Tears. The Dhaulagiri Expedition and Switzerland's Techno-Colonialism, in: National Identities 18 (2016) 1, p. 53–69.

[44] Osayimwese, Colonialism and Modern Architecture in Germany, p. 206–207.

and soaps, stimulated the imagination of consumers to "beach themselves on far-flung shores, tramp through jungles, quell uprisings, restore order and write the inevitable legend of commercial progress across the colonial landscape."[45] The tropical world was a cognitive space, evoking mental images and emotions, used to sell commodities, shape European identities, and promote colonial agendas.[46]

Throughout colonial discourse, the tropics oscillated between the paradisiacal and the pathological, the site of pristine, luscious nature and luxurious abundance alongside primitiveness and danger.[47] Trading companies, colonial enterprises and mission societies used this ambiguous image of the tropical world to advertise and capitalise on tropical commodities. Fisch's 1912 *Tropische Krankheiten* promoted the first colonial cookbook written in the German language, a frequent advertisement in missionary and colonial media of the time. This *Kolonial-Kochbuch*, branded as "indispensable for the stay in the colonies," was published by the German Colonial Economic Committee in 1906. The advertisement read: "Below you will find several highlighted recipes, which best indicate how the conditions in the tropics have been taken into account." The recipes in the colonial cookbook included "antelope pie," "elephant heart," "hippopotamus bacon" and "parrot goulash."[48]

However, the evidence on nutrition practices of both Africans and Europeans in West Africa suggests that these recipes did not reflect the cuisine in the colonies. The diet of the African population consisted mainly of beans, *fufu*—a staple food usually made from cassava—and fish or goat's meat, when means allowed. It is also highly doubtful that these recipes were used by Europeans based in the tropics. Most missionary and

---

[45] McClintock, Imperial Leather, p. 219.

[46] Thomas Richards, The Commodity Culture of Victorian Britain: Advertising and Spectacle, 1851–1914, Stanford 1990; Joanna de Groot, Metropolitan Desires and Colonial Connections. Reflections on Consumption and Empire, in: Catherine Hall/Sonya O. Rose (eds.), At Home with the Empire. Metropolitan Culture and the Imperial World, Cambridge 2006, p. 166–190; Malte Hinrichsen, Racist Trademarks: Slavery, Orient, Colonialism and Commodity Culture, Berlin et al. 2012; Wulf D. Hund/Michael Pickering/Anandi Ramamurthy (eds.), Colonial Advertising and Commodity Racism, Berlin et al. 2013.

[47] Arnold, Inventing Tropicality; Ibid., The Tropics and the Traveling Gaze; Stepan, Picturing Tropical Nature; Endfield/Nash, Missionaries and Morals; Driver/Martins (eds.), Tropical Visions in an Age of Empire.

[48] Kolonialwirtschaftliches Komitee (ed.), Kolonial-Kochbuch, Berlin 1906.

colonial sources from this period describe a very basic diet. As the Basel Mission doctor, Alfred Eckhardt, wrote in referral to the Gold Coast in 1891, the non-existence of cattle, for instance, meant that the missionaries had "to order so-called condensed milk in cans from Europe, while the natives do not know dairy and butter at all."[49]

Similarly, Fisch noted: "Fresh milk can be obtained only in a few places, the strong coffee grown locally is usually drunk with Cham condensed milk."[50] Cham, a town in the Swiss canton of Zug, was home to Europe's first condensed milk factory. The American brothers George and Charles Page founded the Anglo-Swiss Condensed Milk Company in 1866. Farmers from Cham's surrounding regions supplied up to 100,000 litres of milk a day, which was transformed into milk powder. The final product was packed in cans and exported worldwide, mostly to companies in the British Empire. The fast-growing company subsequently established factories all over Europe and eventually merged with Nestlé in 1905.[51] The growing market for global consumer goods illustrates that the Basel Mission, and Switzerland more generally, stood at the heart of transimperial networks.

Next to clothing, advice on nutrition formed another major aspect of tropical hygiene, which was believed to promote both the physical and mental health of Europeans in the tropics.[52] Livingstone College in London, which provided medical training to missionaries from 1893, offered a one-week course on tropical hygiene in March and December of every year, which was open to lay men and women. The course lecture not only dealt with a range of tropical diseases but also prominently addressed

---

[49] Eckhardt, Die Basler Mission auf der Goldküste, p. 9.

[50] Fisch, Tropische Krankheiten, 1st ed., p. 27.

[51] Michael van Orsouw/Judith Stadlin/Monika Imboden, George Page, der Milchpionier: die Anglo-Swiss Condensed Milk Company bis zur Fusion mit Nestlé, Zürich 2005.

[52] Diana M. Natermann, Weisses (Nicht-)Essen im Kongofreistaat und in Deutsch-Ostafrika (1884–1914), in: Norman Aselmeyer/Veronika Settele (eds.), Geschichte des Nicht-Essens. Verzicht, Vermeidung und Verweigerung in der Moderne, Berlin/Boston 2018, p. 237–264; Deborah J. Neill, Of Carnivores and Conquerors: French Nutritional Debates in the Age of Empire, 1890–1914, in: Elizabeth Neswald/David F. Smith/Ulrike Thoms (eds.), Setting Nutritional Standards. Theory, Policies, Practices, Rochester 2017, p. 74–96; Ibid., Finding the "Ideal Diet": Nutrition, Culture and Dietary Practices in France and French Equatorial Africa, c. 1890s to 1920s, in: Food and Foodways 17 (2009) 1, p. 1–28.

subjects such as clothing, food and cookery.[53] The importance attached to the diet of Europeans in tropical colonies is further exemplified by a letter sent by the Inspector of the *Norddeutsche Missionsgesellschaft*, Franz Michael Zahn, to Hermann Prätorius, the Basel Mission's Inspector for Africa, just before Mähly's medical research expedition in 1882–1883:

> I am pleased that you can send out a physician. We will also benefit from this investigation. The tropical climate makes it hard for our brothers to find a suitable diet and the Wurttemberg cuisine, based on spätzli etc., is very unsuitable. A cookbook for African cuisine would be hardly less important than a medical book. Your observant doctor will certainly also look at the kitchen and cellar – i.e. beverages – and find sound advice.[54]

The Basel Mission doctors, who succeeded Mähly in the following three decades, spent considerable time and effort debating the ideal diet for Europeans in tropical colonies.[55] Commodities in the realm of tropical hygiene, including canned milk, travel pharmacies and protective clothing, shaped how Europeans came to see the tropical world and themselves. Although the *Kolonial-Kochbuch* does not give any realistic insights into diet practices in West Africa around 1900, it is a useful source to analyse how a tropical diet, and the tropics more generally, were imagined. It was a commodity that captured the attention of a general public by representing the tropics not only as a dangerous place but also as an exotic and exciting one. The audience for this kind of popular colonial fiction stretched far beyond people who intended to travel or settle in the colonies. Colonial fantasies allowed Europeans to reframe their own identities.

Recipe books, *materia medica*, cacao, medical chests, clothes, Bible translations, condensed milk and many other commodities travelled back

[53] Manson, Tropical Research in its Relation to the Missionary Enterprise, p. 12.

[54] Franz Michael Zahn, Letter to Inspector Prätorious, Bremen, 13.01.1882, BMA, D-1.39.J.4.

[55] Hermann Vortisch, Über Säuglingsernährung in den Tropen, in: Archiv für Schiffs- und Tropenhygiene 16 (1912), p. 69–77; Rudolf Fisch, Über Nachteile in der Säuglingsernährung in den Tropen durch homogenisierte Milch und deren Vermeidung, in: Archiv für Schiffs- und Tropenhygiene 16 (1912), p. 220–222; Ibid., Tropische Krankheiten, 1st ed., p. 26–33; Ibid., Tropische Krankheiten, 4th ed., p. 53–68; Hey, Der Tropenarzt, 1st ed., p. 104–142.

and forth through the Basel Mission's networks.[56] The Basel Mission Trading Company, created in 1859, was the first European trading company to open trading posts in the hinterland of the West African coast in the 1870s, thereby competing with African merchants and their intermediate trade. The company, which supplied the Basel Mission stations with European goods and, in return, exported palm oil, cacao, rubber, cotton and other commodities from the colonies, employed 4304 people in West Africa and India, of which only 74 were European, in 1911.[57] Worldly matters mattered much more to missions than their rhetoric was prepared to acknowledge, as Birgit Meyer showed for the nineteenth-century Gold Coast.[58] This is especially true for the Basel Mission, whose influential patrician supporters had direct interest in the West African trade.

The history of the Basel Mission shows that despite Protestantism's emphasis on the Word, material matters were not simply outward things subordinate to inward faith.[59] The civilising mission fundamentally relied on material culture and had consequences that were both cosmological and worldly. This becomes particularly evident when looking at the history of hygiene. In the name of improving purity, health and cleanliness in West Africa, the Basel Mission doctors introduced new medical equipment, chloroform, bicycles, protective clothing, quinine,

---

[56] It was not unusual for the Basel missionaries to transport over 1,000 kilos of goods from abroad back home, as a regulation on baggage allowance shows, in which the Inspector felt compelled to warn them that the mission society only covered transport costs up to 500 kilos. Amtsblatt 17 (1905) 378, p. 3, in: Verordnungen und Mitteilungen für die Missionare der Basler Mission ("Amtsblatt"), herausgegeben vom Missionskomitee, XIII.–XX. (1901–1909), Basel 1909, BMA, Q-9,1a.

[57] Haller, Transithandel, p. 95–96.

[58] Birgit Meyer, Christian Mind and Worldly Matters. Religion and Materiality in Nineteenth-Century Gold Coast, in: Journal of Material Culture 2 (1997) 3, p. 311–337. See further Dick Houtman/Birgit Meyer (eds.), Things: Religion and the Question of Materiality, New York 2012.

[59] Ratschiller, Material Matters; Kirsten Rüther, The Power Beyond. Mission Strategies, African Conversion and the Development of a Christian Culture in the Transvaal, Hamburg 2001, ch. 8; Comaroff/Comaroff, Of Revelation and Revolution, vol. 2, ch. 4; Ballantyne, Entanglements of Empire, ch. 3; David Morgan, Introduction: The Matter of Belief, in: ibid. (ed.), Religion and Material Culture: The Matter of Belief, New York 2010, p. 1–12; Dick Houtman/Birgit Meyer, Introduction: Material Religion—How Things Matter, in: ibid. (eds.), Things: Religion and the Question of Materiality, New York 2012, p. 1–23.

handbooks, mosquito nets and architecture styles to both Europeans and Africans, thereby shaping the meaning of hygiene.

The Basel missionaries' commodities, objects and technical novelties aroused considerable interest in West Africa. Brigit Meyer argued that in the nineteenth century on the Gold Coast, "Christian identity itself" was "to a large extent produced through the consumption of Western commodities."[60] The Basel Mission's trading posts offered a steadily expanding range of consumer goods to the population in West Africa around 1900. Household items, including tablecloths, cutlery, bed linen, towels, pillows and irons carried great weight as symbols and instruments of Christian domesticity. Other commodities for personal hygiene such as clothes, hand mirrors, umbrellas, toiletries and soap were seen as tools for remaking the body and the self in the Protestant image.[61]

By focussing on soap especially, Timothy Burke demonstrated that missionaries in Zimbabwe carved out a market for industrially produced care products.[62] Soap represented not just a cleaning product but the superiority of industrial production over natural products, Christianity over African beliefs and whiteness over blackness. Moreover, Anne McClintock argued that the marketing of British-manufactured soap and the spread of cleanliness through the promotion of routines of personal hygiene was a means of imposing social order and control in newly colonised areas.[63] Studies analysing soap advertisements suggest that there was a widespread penetration of manufactured toiletry products into colonial Africa, which was achieved through advertising campaigns that associated cleanliness with whiteness and civilisation.[64]

However, a closer look at sanitary practices in West Africa reveals a more nuanced picture than the one promoted through soap advertising.

[60] Meyer, Christian Mind and Worldly Matters, p. 311.

[61] Jean Comaroff, The Empire's Old Clothes: Fashioning the Colonial Subject, in: David Howes (ed.), Cross-Cultural Consumption: Global Markets, Local Realities, New York 1996, p. 19–38.

[62] Burke, Lifebuoy Men, Lux Women; Ibid., "Sunlight Soap Has Changed My Life": Hygiene, Commodification, and the Body in Colonial Zimbabwe, in: Hildi Hendrickson (ed.), Clothing and Difference: Embodied Identities in Colonial and Postcolonial Africa, Durham 1996, p. 189–212.

[63] McClintock, Imperial Leather, p. 207–231.

[64] Anandi Ramamurthy, Imperial Persuaders. Images of Africa and Asia in British Advertising, Manchester 2003, p. 24–62; Ciarlo, Advertising Empire, p. 108–113, 135–138, 240–245, 259–265.

Reports in the Basel Mission archives suggest that both Africans and Europeans oftentimes used soap made from mimosa or *anago samina*— "black soap." Originating in West Africa, this kind of soap was usually made by women using ash of locally harvested plants and dried peels, which gave the soap its characteristic dark colour. Although the Basel Mission imported soap from a factory in the Black Forest and thus contributed to the expansion of the European care product market in colonial Africa, it appears that many West Africans and missionaries continued to use natural, locally produced soap well into the twentieth century.[65]

As the example of soap advertisement shows, colonial imagery not only shaped perceptions of race and cleanliness in the age of High Imperialism, but has also obstructed historical research into bodily practices during the colonial period. The power of colonial images is particularly tangible in the representation of African bodies, which have anchored perceptions of purity, health and cleanliness in public memory. As one of the oldest and most prolific organisations to print and distribute photographs from the colonial world, the Basel Mission crucially moulded these images of hygiene.[66]

10.3   BEYOND THE COLONIAL GAZE

The Basel Mission doctors used diverse visual languages to document their medical mission in West Africa for various interest groups at home. Their photographs served different purposes; some were taken as private souvenirs, sent to family and friends, and never published. Others were used in the Basel Mission seminary to illustrate lessons and familiarise pupils with the natural and human environments of their future mission fields. Others again became highly publicised images, reproduced as post-cards or displayed in popular exhibitions in order to generate attention and donations. These types of images have impacted our ways of seeing and persist in the visual language of many aid campaigns. The images taken by the medical missionaries and the diverse contexts in which they

---

[65] Reports by the Mission Trading Company from India and Africa, 1883–1911, BMA, BHG-14.13.02. The reports show that the Basel Mission also operated soap factories in India.

[66] Jenkins, The Earliest Generation of Missionary Photographers in West Africa.

appeared make it possible to analyse the different strategies that were used in the visualisation of Africa and its people during the colonial period.[67]

From as early as the 1880s, the Basel Mission doctors contributed to the creation of a colonial gaze of African bodies in European media. Their photographs appeared in scientific journals where they contributed to the visual representation of tropical diseases and African bodies as objects of investigation. Photography helped to expand the systematic documentation and scientific cataloguing of places and people around the world, which had been a preoccupation of Europeans ever since their earliest explorations. In 1909, the *Archiv für Schiffs- und Tropenhygiene* published an image of a leg affected by a filaria tumour. The corresponding article explained that the mission doctor Rudolf Fisch had removed the tumour from a woman on the Gold Coast and sent it to the *Institut für Schiffs- und Tropenkrankheiten* in Hamburg, where it was analysed and compared to filaria worms from other samples extracted on people in tropical Africa.[68]

The Basel Mission doctors not only engaged with medical science, they also published anthropological papers, which contained photographs of the people they studied.[69] The end of the nineteenth century saw the emergence of anthropological images, such as the engraving printed in Alfred Eckhardt's 1894 monograph *Land, Leute und ärztliche Mission auf der Goldküste*, captioned "Negro types from the Gold Coast"

[67] On missionary photography in Africa more generally, see Marianne Gullestad, Picturing Pity: Pitfalls and Pleasures in Cross-Cultural Communication. Image and Word in a North Cameroon Mission, New York/Oxford 2007; Rainer Alsheimer, Bilder erzählen Geschichte. Eine Fotoanthropologie der Norddeutschen Mission in Westafrika, Berlin 2010; Gesine Krüger, Schrift und Bild. Missionsfotografie im südlichen Afrika, in: Historische Anthropologie 19 (2011) 1, p. 123–143; T. Jack Thompson, Light on Darkness? Missionary Photography of Africa in the Nineteenth and Early Twentieth Centuries, Grand Rapids/Cambridge 2013; Adam Jones, Through a Glass, Darkly. Photographs of the Leipzig Mission from East Africa, 1896–1939, Leipzig 2013.

[68] Ernst Rodenwaldt, Filarien-Tumor, von Herrn Missionsarzt Dr. R. Fisch eingesandt an das Institut für Schiffs- und Tropenkrankheiten, in: Archiv für Schiffs- und Tropenhygiene 13 (1909), p. 332.

[69] Ernst Mähly, Zur Geographie und Ethnographie der Goldküste, in: Verhandlungen der Naturforschenden Gesellschaft in Basel 7 (1885) 3, p. 809–852; Hermann Vortisch, Die Neger der Goldküste, in: Globus 89 (1906), p. 277–283, 293–297; Rudolf Fisch, Die Dagbamba. Eine ethnographische Skizze, in: Baessler-Archiv 3 (1912) 2/3, p. 132–164.

(Fig. 10.3).[70] People in the colonies were photographed as representatives of their assigned ethnic groups, described according to their physical features, ascribed certain characteristics and catalogued as ethnographic types in encyclopaedias. These images not only quenched scientific thirst but they also gradually found their way into everyday imagery through their widespread distribution. By printing postcards depicting "native types" publishers realised that they could "profitably appeal to the desire for exoticism, and often eroticism, under the guise of scientific knowledge," as David MacDougall showed.[71]

In the name of medical research and scientific progress, the Basel Mission doctors photographed their patients, often naked, documenting the diseases affecting them. The fourth edition of Rudolf Fisch's *Tropische Krankheiten* in 1912 contained 37 figures including statistical tables,

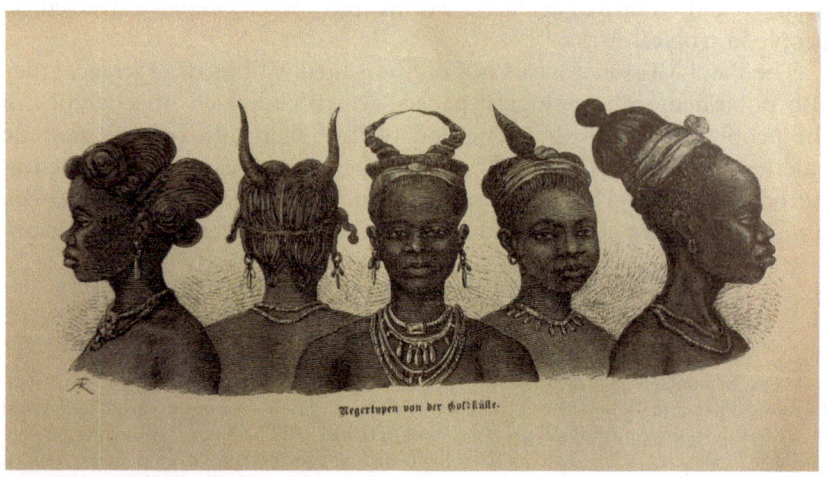

Fig. 10.3 Alfred Eckhardt, Land, Leute und ärztliche Mission auf der Goldküste, Basel 1894, p. 11

---

[70] Eckhardt, Land, Leute und ärztliche Mission, p. 11. Engravings were based on photographs and cheaper to reproduce. Although the techniques by which a photographic image can be transferred mechanically into print became a practicable prospect for the Basel Mission around 1890, engravings continued to be printed widely well after that.

[71] David MacDougall, The Corporeal Image: Film, Ethnography, and the Senses, Princeton 2006, p. 178.

magnified photographs of parasites under the microscope, drawings of disease vectors and, most prominently, photographs of patients in West Africa suffering from a range of illnesses. Some conditions such as elephantiasis, framboesia and yaws, which the medical missionaries had mistaken for syphilis for many years, led to severe physical changes and were thus particularly well suited for visual display. These images not only served as scientific documentation, but also satisfied the insatiable desire of the European public for curiosities from the colonies. The myth of the "Dark Continent," already well established in Europe by this time, was further cemented through the constant representation of pathological bodies.[72]

A major challenge in working with photographic sources is that their conditions of production are hard, or sometimes even impossible, to retrieve. Simultaneously, their fluid and equivocal nature means that these images were able to absorb different, partly contradictory, meanings depending on the settings in which they appeared. Visual sources comprise amalgamations and ambiguities, which disclose the fundamentally interactive fabric of missionary entanglements. By tracing these changing meanings, historians can expose inconsistencies in the dominant colonial and racist visual narrative. The visual language emerging in the colonial period left ample room for mixed messages and contradicting interpretations. Image captions offer one way of exposing photographs as cultural artefacts rather than truthful representations of Africa.

The Basel Mission's popular exhibition touring through Switzerland, Germany and Alsace in 1912 contained an image of a "priest of the deities with amulets," as the caption stated.[73] However, when Rudolf Fisch sent the photograph to Basel three years earlier, he wrote that it depicted an "African medicine man carrying his pharmacy on his head" (Fig. 10.4).[74] Fisch clearly identified the man in the picture as a medical man, acknowledging that he possessed certain medical knowledge, authority and

[72] John Bale, Foreign Bodies. Representing the African and the European in an Early Twentieth Century 'Contact Zone', in: Geography 84 (1999), p. 25–34; Ratschiller, Kranke Körper.

[73] Rudolf Fisch, Priest of the deities with amulets, 1885/1911, BMA, QD-34.001.0043.

[74] Ibid. African medicine man carrying his pharmacy on his head, 1885/1911, BMA, D-30.63.099.

remedies. Yet in the exhibition, the curators transformed him into a spiritual figure with charms, thereby entirely omitting his medical expertise and drawing the visitors' attention to their campaign against superstitious practices instead. The Basel Mission's publicity work focussed on conveying a clear and unequivocal message to supporters at home, often at the expense of the more informative and nuanced annotations of the medical missionaries in West Africa.[75]

The images appearing in evangelical media offered seemingly clear-cut evidence for the positive impact of missionary work by juxtaposing pictures of what missionaries branded as traditional African society with pictures symbolising transformation in the Christian image. Thus, photographs of "witch doctors" appeared next to images of medical assistants, as was the case in the 1912 exhibition. The picture contrasting the

Fig. 10.4 Rudolf Fisch, African medicine man carrying his pharmacy on his head, 1885/1911, BMA, D-30.63.099

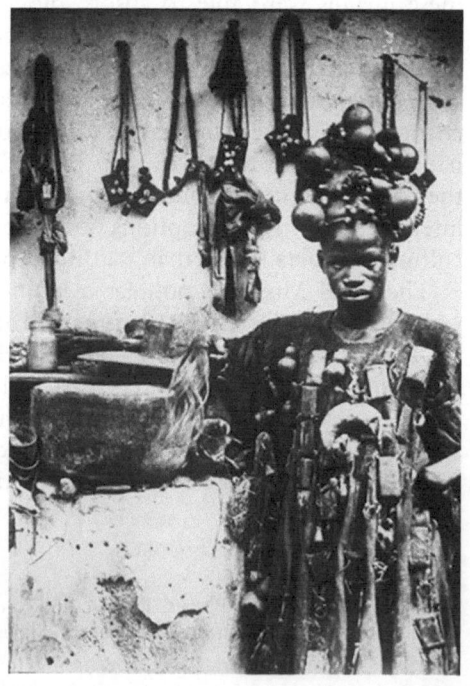

---

[75] Ratschiller, "Die Zauberei spielt in Kamerun eine böse Rolle!".

"priest of the deities with amulets" showed "Dr. Fisch's African assistants" (Fig. 10.5).[76] Although Fisch had identified them as Robert Asare and Henry Owusu in his original annotation, the popular display turned them into nameless auxiliaries who testified to the apparent success of the medical mission in West Africa. With their suits, white shirts, ties and a wedding ring, they embodied religious, medical and cultural change all at once. This two-fold narrative operated on a time-scale demarcating the old and new ways in which West Africans dealt with disease, dirt and deity.

Medical assistants were a popular motif in the Basel Mission's publicity work. They symbolised not only the possibility for individual change but also promised profound societal change, ranging from spiritual to material issues. Beyond their role as poster children for the medical mission, however, the medical assistants held considerable power over the medical missionaries, who heavily relied on their cooperation not only in administrating medical care but also in promoting the medical mission among

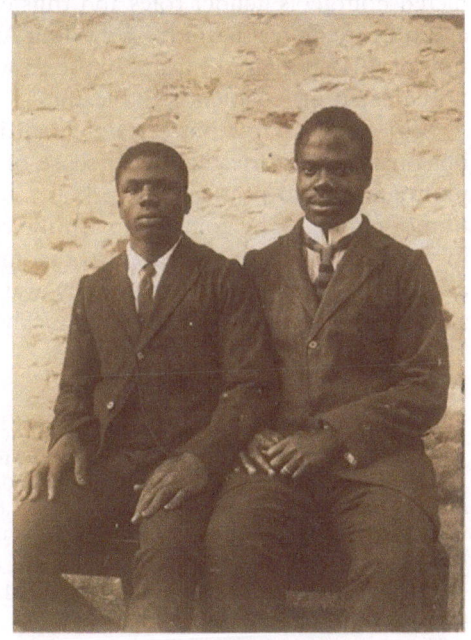

Fig. 10.5 Rudolf Fisch, Dr. Fisch's African assistants, 1885/1911, BMA, D-30.10.25

[76] Rudolf Fisch, Dr. Fisch's African assistants, 1885/1911, BMA, D-30.10.25.

402 L. M. RATSCHILLER NASIM

the general population.[77] Some assistants sourced and sold their own medications, while others used their training to look for better employment opportunities, which angered the mission doctors.[78] Robert Asare and Henry Owusu, for example, left in 1905 and 1908 respectively for positions in the mining industry.[79]

A recurring theme within the Basel Mission's photographs published in colonial magazines showed Africans doing dishes and laundry. Some of these washing scenes took place within the mission setting, under the supervision of a missionary wife on the mission compound for example, and reinforced the message that the mission was responsible for cleanliness in the colonies. Others showed African washing practices and thus indicated that attention to cleanliness was to be found across the globe, regardless of missionary activities. Moreover, many pictures, such as the one taken by the Basel missionary Otto Schkölziger in Cameroon, indicated that washing was not the sole responsibility of women (Fig. 10.6).[80] Photographs depicting African men washing clothes and dishes contradicted bourgeois gender roles and thus emasculated them, adding to the ambivalent colonial narrative regarding African masculinity. The feminisation of African men in European media was contradicted by depictions of unregulated male violence and laziness.

Although photographs certainly contributed to cementing Europeans' imaginations of Africa and their sense of superiority over African people, photography did not simply work as a tool of empire. While the invention of photography coincided with the consolidation of colonial empires in Africa, this medium was not the monopoly of Europeans. Unlike any other technology, photography was appropriated across the world almost simultaneously.[81] Africans quickly picked up the new technology,

---

[77] Ibid., Annual report for 1905, 02.02.1906, BMA, D-1.84a.19.

[78] See for example, Alfred Eckhardt, Letter to Committee, 02.09.1890, BMA, D-1.52.93; Hermann Vortisch, Annual report for 1903, 08.04.1904, BMA, D-1.79.14; Ibid., Annual report for 1904, 20.01.1905, BMA, D-1.81.35; Rudolf Fisch, Annual report for 1908, 13.01.1909, BMA, D-1.90.20; Ibid., Annual report for 1909, 31.12.1909, BMA, D-1.93.24.

[79] Rudolf Fisch, Annual report for 1906, 26.02.1907, BMA, D-1.86.11; Ibid., Annual report for 1908, 13.01.1909, BMA, D-1.90.20.

[80] Otto Schkölziger, Laundry work in Cameroon, 1891/1909, BMA QE-32.030.0003.

[81] Pascal Martin Saint-Léon/N'Goné Fall/Frédérique Chapuis (eds.), Anthology of African and Indian Ocean Photography, Paris 1999.

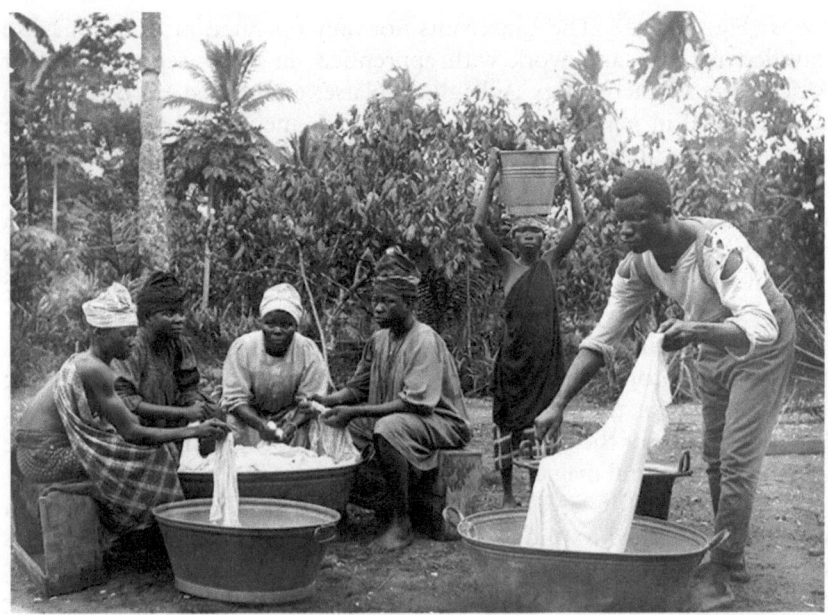

Fig. 10.6 Otto Schkölziger, Laundry work in Cameroon, 1891/1909, BMA QE-32.030.0003

which circulated and flourished through local and global networks of exchange. Photographers, clients and images moved across West Africa often crossing political and cultural boundaries.[82] Two of the first West Africans to operate a photography studio were George and his son Albert Lutterodt, who opened their business in Accra in 1876.[83]

In one of the oldest portraits in the Met collection, dating from the early 1880s, the Lutterodts carefully staged the importance of their client with four men surrounding him striking a pose and displaying elaborate

[82] Jürg Schneider, The Topography of the Early History of African Photography, in: History of Photography 34 (2010) 2, p. 134–146; Erin Haney, Photography and Africa, London 2010, p. 3–34.

[83] Erin Haney, Lutterodt Family Studios and the Changing Face of Early Portrait Photographs from the Gold Coast, in: John Peffer/Elisabeth L. Cameron (eds.), Portraiture and Photography in Africa, Bloomington 2013, p. 67–101.

props (Fig. 10.7).[84] The Lutterodts not only operated in Accra but also travelled to train and work with apprentices in other regions of West Africa. One of them, Alex Agbaglo Acolatse, established his own studio around 1900 in neighbouring Togo. Like his mentors, he specialised in portraits of the upper class and documented the social and political life of the African elite in the German colony.[85] These photographers, their clients and the images they produced testify to the complexity of African societies during the colonial period. The history of photography shows that any simplifying assumptions contrasting modern, rational and science based Europeans to backward, superstitious Africans are inadequate.[86]

In the late nineteenth and early twentieth centuries, most Europeans associated photography, which many of them encountered in magic lantern shows for the first time, with supernatural phenomena. After all, Fox Talbot, one of the prominent pioneers of photography, had called the technology "natural magic," identifying in it "the character of the marvellous."[87] Aware of its awe-inspiring appeal, the Basel Mission doctors in West Africa resorted to photography alongside other technologies, such as surgery, to demonstrate that a higher power was on their side. However, photography seems to have enriched African beliefs and cultures rather than devaluing them. Heike Behrend and Tobias Wendl pointed out that in many African languages the word for "photographic negative" was the same as for "ghost or dead spirit" and that photographs were commonly incorporated into ancestor veneration.[88]

The Basel Mission doctors' visual legacy demonstrates that their images adopted multiple layers of meaning that went beyond their own intentions and goals. Their images not only acquired new connotations in evangelical, scientific and colonial contexts but were, at their origin, products of

---

[84] George Lutterodt/Albert George Lutterodt, Five men, 1880/1885, The Metropolitan Museum of Art, 1999.184.1, https://www.metmuseum.org/art/collection/search/512837 (last access: 22.07.2022).

[85] Giulia Paoletti/Yaëlle Biro, Photographic Portraiture in West Africa: Notes from "In and Out of the Studio", in: Metropolitan Museum Journal 51 (2016), p. 183–199.

[86] Landau, Introduction: An Amazing Distance, p. 24.

[87] Cited in: Don Slater, Photography and Modern Vision: The Spectacle of "Natural Magic", in: Chris Jencks (ed.), Visual Culture, London/New York 1995, p. 218–237, here p. 227.

[88] Heike Behrend/Tobias Wendl, Social Aspects of Photography in Africa, in: John Middleton (ed.), The Encyclopedia of Subsaharan Africa, vol. 3, New York 1997, p. 409–415, here p. 411.

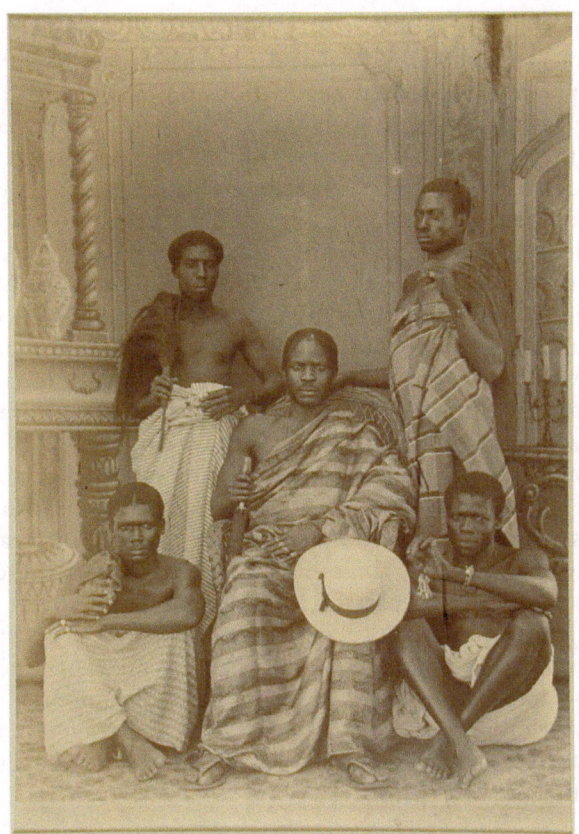

Fig. 10.7 George Lutterodt/Albert George Lutterodt, Five men, 1880/1885, The Metropolitan Museum of Art, 1999.184.1, https://www.metmuseum.org/art/collection/search/512837 (last access: 22.07.2022)

negotiations, cooperation and, at times, violence in West Africa. By paying attention to the very creation of these photographs as material sources and taking seriously the notion that African people were active participants in this process, historians can both reconstruct and fragment the colonial gaze. The image of Fisch's medical assistants, for example, shows that clothing was a feature of Christian culture that provided Africans with a tool to claim social status, as Kirsten Rüther has argued.[89]

Clothes played a key role in negotiations on purity, health and cleanliness. They were central in fashioning Christian identity, an imperial market for tropical hygiene and the civilising mission. At the same time, clothes were also products of entanglements on the ground in West Africa, disclosing intimate and revealing details. They testify to the prolonged and tangible exchanges between the Basel missionaries and the people with whom they lived. Clothes are communicative symbols that are used to maintain religious purity, indicate social roles, display cleanliness, express cultural identity, denote economic status and serve as emblems for political power. West Africans attached great importance to clothing as a form of communication, which is reflected in this West African proverb: "A person without clothes is a person without language."[90]

The photograph of the Basel missionaries Jakob Keller and Gottlieb Spellenberg was taken by their fellow missionary Eugen Schuler in Bali-Nyonga, a state in the Cameroon Grasslands, in 1902 and reached Basel in 1911 (Fig. 10.8).[91] The three Basel missionaries visited the Kingdom in November of 1902 as part of an exploration trip to the area. This image is part of a series of twelve pictures that show Basel missionaries wearing the clothes of the Bali people. To fully understand the value of these photographs, it is essential to keep in mind the importance attached to protective clothing for Europeans in tropical colonies as well as the pre-eminent role of missionaries in trying to reform the dress of the individuals they wished to convert.[92]

[89] Rüther, The Power Beyond, p. 213.

[90] On the importance of clothes for colonial and African history, see Hildi Hendrickson (ed.), Clothing and Difference: Embodied Identities in Colonial and Post-colonial Africa, Durham 1996; Leslie W. Rabine, The Global Circulation of African Fashion, Oxford 2002; Jean Allman (ed.), Fashioning Africa: Power and the Politics of Dress, Bloomington 2004; Colleen E. Kriger, Cloth in West African History, Lanham 2006; Pedro Machado/Sarah Fee/Gwyn Campbell (eds.), Textile Trades, Consumer Cultures, and the Material Worlds of the Indian Ocean: An Ocean of Cloth, Cham 2018.

[91] Gottlieb Spellenberg, Missionar Keller und Spellenberg im Baligewand, 1902/1911, BMA, E–30.25.039.

[92] Kenneth Scott/Gareth Griffiths (eds.), Mixed Messages: Materiality, Textuality, Missions, New York 2005; Comaroff/Comaroff, Of Revelation and Revolution, vol. 2, p. 233–235.

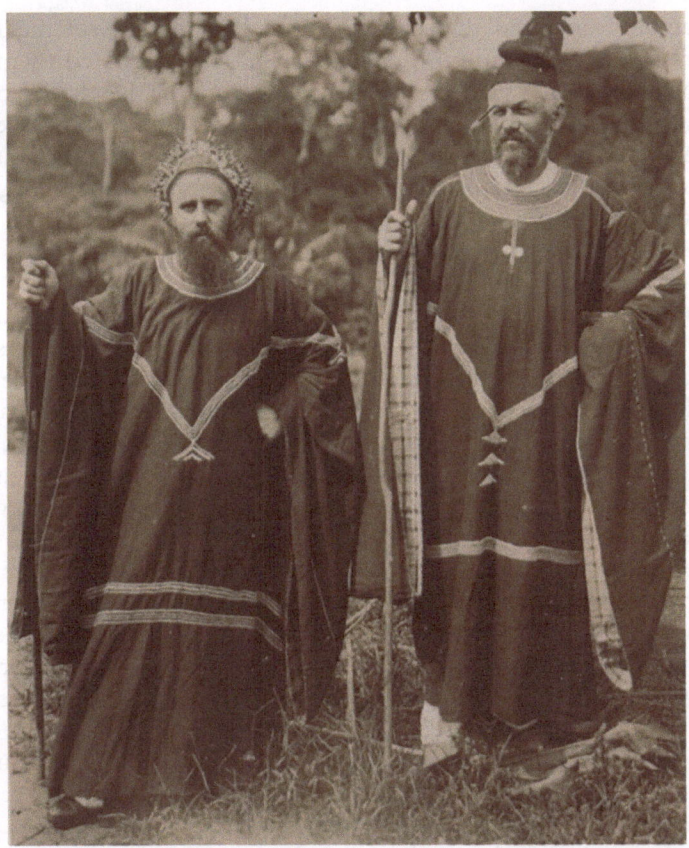

Fig. 10.8 Eugen Schuler, The missionaries Keller and G. Spellenberg in Bali robes, 1902/1911, BMA, E–30.25.039

By covering their bodies in African cloth, the missionaries pushed the boundaries of purity, health and cleanliness. Historians have generally assumed that clothing worn by Europeans in the tropical world served the purpose of marking strict boundaries between colonisers and colonised, expressing and legitimising the rule of a few over many.[93] Ryan Johnson,

[93] Comaroff, The Empire's Old Clothes: Fashioning the Colonial Subject; Comaroff/ Comaroff, Of Revelation and Revolution, vol. 2, ch. 5.

for example, suggested that tropical attire did not only set the British apart from the population in the colonies but also separated them from their own locality.[94] Conversely, the pictures of the Basel missionaries wearing Bali clothes indicate that rather than sealing themselves off, they engaged with their social and material surroundings. By doing so, they not only breached medical recommendations but also transgressed cultural and racial norms.

The photographs of the Basel missionaries wearing African clothing originated from complex interactions and were highly polyvalent, symbolising intimacy, on the one hand, and arousing fears of too much assimilation or "going native" on the other. The fact that these pictures were held back by the missionaries in Cameroon and only arrived in Basel years after they were taken suggests that the missionaries recognised that they had broken a taboo by transgressing metropolitan sensibilities. At the same time, it underlines the value of photographic sources, which offer unique insights into social interactions, cultural exchanges and political negotiations on the ground in West Africa.

The clothes visible in the image of Keller and Spellenberg were given to them by Fonyonga II, the *fon*—ruler—of Bali-Nyonga. They were part of a mutual exchange of gifts, a diplomatic rapprochement between the Basel missionaries and Fonyonga II. In 1903, Eugen Schuler reported in the *Evangelisches Missionsmagazin* that towards the end of their stay in Bali-Nyonga, the *fon* had sent them local dresses with the royal badge via his spokesperson and had requested them to appear on the market square wearing them. The missionaries complied with the *fon's* request, who, according to Schuler, seemed "very pleased" to see the missionaries in Bali clothes: "With the royal garment he wanted to honour us and was proud that he could present us to all the people present in this attire."[95]

While the missionaries perceived Fonyonga II's presents as tribute to their presence in Bali-Nyonga, the *fon* pursued a long-term plan to strengthen his position vis-à-vis the colonial power by building a strategic partnership with the Basel Mission. The garments he had given to the missionaries were not ordinary clothes, but rather regalia of high office and status that could only be awarded by people of the same or

---

[94] Johnson, Commodity Culture, p. 73.

[95] Eugen Schuler, Im Lande der Bali. Eine Kundschaftsreise der Basler Missionare ins Hinterland von Nordkamerun, in: Evangelisches Missionsmagazin 47 (1903), p. 191–214, here p. 212.

higher status.[96] To be walking through the market square in this attire was considered an adequate inauguration into political office in Bali-Nyonga. Fonyonga II integrated the missionaries in his system of rule by dressing them in political clothes, accommodating them in his palace and presenting them to his people and foreign visitors.[97]

The Basel Mission opened a station in Bali in May of 1903 and campaigned on behalf of Fonyonga II, helping him to gain political authority in the eyes of the German colonial authorities. Their negotiations with the German military assured that the Bali region was spared from raids by the *Schutztruppe*. The Basel Mission's support of Fonyonga II eventually led to his official approval as *Oberhäuptling*—"big chief"—of the whole Bali region by the German colonial government in 1905.[98] In exchange, the *fon* supported the Basel missionaries by providing them with food, helping them with infrastructure and construction, commandeering porters for their expeditions and children for the mission schools. In Fonyonga II, the Basel Mission had an influential ally, who was now officially in charge of a considerable territory.[99]

The *fon*'s dominant position in the Cameroon Grasslands, however, became increasingly problematic for the German authorities, who accused him of harbouring imperialist desires. The ruler of Bali-Nyonga had become too influential in the eyes of the colonial government and they began to curtail his power.[100] Disappointed by this development, the *fon* eventually ended his cooperation with the Basel Mission. Fonyonga II's authority, his diplomatic skills and political strategy, which are often concealed in colonial accounts, are embodied in the clothes he gave to the

[96] Paul Jenkins, Warum tragen die Missionare Kostüme? Forschungsmöglichkeiten im Bildarchiv der Basler Mission, in: Historische Anthropologie 4 (1996) 2, p. 292–392.

[97] Andreas Merz/Thomas Meyer, "You be good so, you be king." Allianzbildung zwischen Bali-Nyonga (Kamerun) und der Basler Mission, in: Beat Sottas/Thomas Hammer/Lilo Roost Vischer/Anne Mayor (eds.), Werkschau Afrikastudien—Le forum suisse des africanistes, vol. 1, Hamburg 1997, p. 110–127.

[98] Ferdinand Ernst, Die öffentliche Anerkennung Fonyongas als Oberhäuptling, Kamerun 1905, BMA, E-10.3, Nr. 11.

[99] Ratschiller, Material Matters, p. 126–132.

[100] Elisabeth M. Chilver, Paramountcy and Protection in the Cameroons: The Bali and the Germans, 1889–1913, in: Prosser Gifford/William Roger Louis (eds.), Britain and Germany in Africa: Imperial Rivalry and Colonial Rule, New Haven/London 1967, p. 479–511, here p. 498.

Basel missionaries. Material and visual sources facilitate a better understanding of African experiences and actions during the colonial period. They form valuable sources for questioning hegemonic colonial narratives and testify to processes of entanglement between West Africa and Europe.

REFERENCES

Jean Allman (ed.), Fashioning Africa: Power and the Politics of Dress, Bloomington 2004.

Rainer Alsheimer, Bilder erzählen Geschichte. Eine Fotoanthropologie der Norddeutschen Mission in Westafrika, Berlin 2010.

Warwick Anderson, Climates of Opinion. Acclimatization in Nineteenth-Century France and England, in: Victorian Studies 35 (1992) 2, p. 135–157.

Julia Angster, Erdbeeren und Piraten. Die Royal Navy und die Ordnung der Welt 1770–1860, Göttingen 2012.

David Arnold, Inventing Tropicality, in: ibid. (ed.), The Problem of Nature. Environment, Culture, and European Expansion, London 1996, p. 141–168.

David Arnold, The Tropics and the Traveling Gaze: India, Landscape, and Science, 1800–1856, Seattle 2006.

John Bale, Foreign Bodies. Representing the African and the European in an Early Twentieth Century 'Contact Zone', in: Geography 84 (1999), p. 25–34.

Tony Ballantyne, Entanglements of Empire. Missionaries, Māori, and the Question of the Body, Durham/London 2014.

James Beattie, Imperial Landscapes of Health: Place, Plants and People between India and Australia, 1800s–1900s, in: Health & History 14 (2012) 1, p. 100–120.

Heike Behrend/Tobias Wendl, Social Aspects of Photography in Africa, in: John Middleton (ed.), The Encyclopedia of Subsaharan Africa, vol. 3, New York 1997, p. 409–415.

Deborah Brunton, The Emergence of a Modern Profession? in: ibid. (ed.), Medicine Transformed. Health, Disease and Society in Europe 1880–1930, Manchester/New York 2004, p. 119–149.

Timothy Burke, Lifebuoy Men, Lux Women. Commodification, Consumption and Cleanliness in Modern Zimbabwe, Durham/London 1996.

Timothy Burke, "Sunlight Soap Has Changed My Life": Hygiene, Commodification, and the Body in Colonial Zimbabwe, in: Hildi Hendrickson (ed.), Clothing and Difference: Embodied Identities in Colonial and Postcolonial Africa, Durham 1996, p. 189–212.

Pratik Chakrabarti, Medicine and Empire, 1600–1960, Basingstoke 2014.

Elisabeth M. Chilver, Paramountcy and Protection in the Cameroons: The Bali and the Germans, 1889–1913, in: Prosser Gifford/William Roger Louis (eds.), Britain and Germany in Africa: Imperial Rivalry and Colonial Rule, New Haven/London 1967, p. 479–511.

David Ciarlo, Advertising Empire. Race and Visual Culture in Imperial Germany, London 2011.

Jean Comaroff, The Empire's Old Clothes: Fashioning the Colonial Subject, in: David Howes (ed.), Cross-Cultural Consumption: Global Markets, Local Realities, New York 1996, p. 19–38.

John Comaroff/Jean Comaroff, Of Revelation and Revolution, vol. 2: The Dialectics of Modernity on a South African Frontier, Chicago 1997.

Jonas N. Dah, Missionary Motivations and Methods. A Critical Examination of the Basel Mission in Cameroon 1886–1914, Basel 1983.

Felix Driver/Luciana Martins (eds.), Tropical Visions in an Age of Empire, Chicago/London 2005.

Alfred Eckhardt, Die Basler Mission auf der Goldküste, in: O. Frick (ed.), Geschichten und Bilder aus der Mission, vol. 10, Halle 1891, p. 3–19.

Alfred Eckhardt, Land, Leute und ärztliche Mission auf der Goldküste, Basel 1894.

Georgina H. Endfield/David J. Nash, Missionaries and Morals: Climatic Discourse in Nineteenth-Century Central Southern Africa, in: Annals of the Association of American Geographers 92 (2002) 4, p. 727–742.

Rudolf Fisch, Die ärztliche Mission unter den Negern. Ansprache am Jahresfest der Basler Mission am 3. Juli 1895, in: Evangelisches Missionsmagazin 39 (1895), p. 371–377.

Rudolf Fisch, Über die Behandlung der Amöbendysentrie und einige andere tropenmedizinische Fragen, in: Archiv für Schiffs- und Tropenhygiene 8 (1904), p. 207–212.

Rudolf Fisch, Über Stoffe zur Moskitosicherung, in: Archiv für Schiffs- und Tropenhygiene 10 (1906), p. 172–175.

Rudolf Fisch, Tropische Krankheiten. Anleitung zu ihrer Verhütung und Behandlung speziell für die Westküste von Afrika, für Missionare, Kaufleute, Pflanzer und Beamte, 1st ed., Basel 1891; 2nd ed., Basel 1894; 3rd ed., Basel 1903; 4th ed., Basel 1912.

Rudolf Fisch, Über Nachteile in der Säuglingsernährung in den Tropen durch homogenisierte Milch und deren Vermeidung, in: Archiv für Schiffs- und Tropenhygiene 16 (1912), p. 220–222.

Rudolf Fisch, Die Dagbamba. Eine ethnographische Skizze, in: Baessler-Archiv 3 (1912) 2/3, p. 132–164.

Friedrich Hermann Fischer, Der Missionsarzt Rudolf Fisch und die Anfänge medizinischer Arbeit der Basler Mission an der Goldküste (Ghana), Herzogenrath 1991.

Stefanie Gänger, Mikrogeschichten des Globalen. Chinarinde, der Andenraum und die Welt während der "globalen Sattelzeit" (1770–1830), in: Boris Barth/Stefanie Gänger/Niels P. Petersson (eds.), Globalgeschichten. Bestandsaufnahme und Perspektiven, Frankfurt a. M 2014, p. 19–40.

Stefanie Gänger, A Singular Remedy. Cinchona Across the Atlantic World, 1751–1820, Cambridge 2020.

Joanna de Groot, Metropolitan Desires and Colonial Connections. Reflections on Consumption and Empire, in: Catherine Hall/Sonya O. Rose (eds.), At Home with the Empire. Metropolitan Culture and the Imperial World, Cambridge 2006, p. 166–190.

Marianne Gullestad, Picturing Pity: Pitfalls and Pleasures in Cross-Cultural Communication. Image and Word in a North Cameroon Mission, New York/ Oxford 2007.

Hermann Gundert, Calwer Tagebuch 1859–1893, ed. by Albrecht Frenz, Stuttgart 1986.

Lea Haller, Transithandel. Geld- und Warenströme im globalen Kapitalismus, Berlin 2019.

Erin Haney, Lutterodt Family Studios and the Changing Face of Early Portrait Photographs from the Gold Coast, in: John Peffer/Elisabeth L. Cameron (eds.), Portraiture and Photography in Africa, Bloomington 2013, p. 67–101.

Erin Haney, Photography and Africa, London 2010.

Patrick Harries, Butterflies and Barbarians. Swiss Missionaries and Systems of Knowledge in South-East Africa, Oxford 2007.

Sandip Hazareesingh/Harro Maat (eds.), Local Subversions of Colonial Cultures. Commodities and Anti-Commodities in Global History, London 2016.

Hildi Hendrickson (ed.), Clothing and Difference: Embodied Identities in Colonial and Post-colonial Africa, Durham 1996.

Friedrich Hey, Der Tropenarzt. Ausführlicher Ratgeber für Europäer in den Tropen, sowie für Besitzer von Plantagen und Handelshäusern, Kolonialbehörden und Missionsverwaltungen, 1st ed., Offenbach 1906.

Malte Hinrichsen, Racist Trademarks: Slavery, Orient, Colonialism and Commodity Culture, Berlin et al. 2012.

Markku Hokkanen, Imperial Networks, Colonial Bioprospecting and Burroughs Wellcome & Co: The Case of Strophanthus Kombe from Malawi (1859–1915), in: Social History of Medicine 25 (2012) 3, p. 589–607.

Dick Houtman/Birgit Meyer (eds.), Things: Religion and the Question of Materiality, New York 2012.

Dick Houtman/Birgit Meyer, Introduction: Material Religion—How Things Matter, in: ibid. (eds.), Things: Religion and the Question of Materiality, New York 2012, p. 1–23.

Wulf D. Hund/Michael Pickering/Anandi Ramamurthy (eds.), Colonial Advertising and Commodity Racism, Berlin et al. 2013.

Karl Huppenbauer, Chirurgische und ophthalmologische Erfahrungen von der Goldküste, in: Archiv für Schiffs- und Tropenhygiene 22 (1918), p. 341–364.

Paul Jenkins, The Earliest Generation of Missionary Photographers in West Africa and the Portrayal of Indigenous People and Culture, in: History of Africa 20 (1993), p. 89–118.

Paul Jenkins, Warum tragen die Missionare Kostüme? Forschungsmöglichkeiten im Bildarchiv der Basler Mission, in: Historische Anthropologie 4 (1996) 2, p. 292–392.

Ryan Johnson, Commodity Culture. Tropical Health and Hygiene in the British Empire, in: Endeavour 32 (2008) 2, 2008, p. 70–74.

Ryan Johnson, European Clothes and "Tropical" Skin: Clothing Material and British Ideas of Health and Hygiene in Tropical Climates, in: Bulletin of the History of Medicine 83 (2009), p. 530–560.

Adam Jones, Through a Glass, Darkly. Photographs of the Leipzig Mission from East Africa, 1896–1939, Leipzig 2013.

Dane Kennedy, The Perils of the Midday Sun: Climatic Anxieties in the Colonial Tropics, in: John M. MacKenzie (ed.), Imperialism and the Natural World, Manchester/New York 1990, p. 118–140.

Kolonialwirtschaftliches Komitee (ed.), Kolonial-Kochbuch, Berlin 1906.

Colleen E. Kriger, Cloth in West African History, Lanham 2006.

Gesine Krüger, Schrift und Bild. Missionsfotografie im südlichen Afrika, in: Historische Anthropologie 19 (2011) 1, p. 123–143.

Ludwig Külz, Grundzüge der kolonialen Eingeborenenhygiene, in: Beihefte zum Archiv für Schiffs- und Tropenhygiene 15 (1911) 8, Leipzig 1911, p. 387–480.

Paul S. Landau, Introduction. An Amazing Distance. Pictures and People in Africa, in: ibid./Deborah D. Kaspin (eds.), Images and Empires. Visuality in Colonial and Postcolonial Africa, Berkeley/Los Angeles/London 2002, p. 1–40.

James Lind, Essay on Diseases Incidental to Europeans in Hot Climates, with the Method of Preventing their Fatal Consequences, London 1768.

David. N. Livingstone, Tropical Climate and Moral Hygiene: The Anatomy of a Victorian Debate, in: The British Journal for the History of Science 32 (1999) 1, p. 93–110.

David MacDougall, The Corporeal Image: Film, Ethnography, and the Senses, Princeton 2006.

Pedro Machado/Sarah Fee/Gwyn Campbell (eds.), Textile Trades, Consumer Cultures, and the Material Worlds of the Indian Ocean: An Ocean of Cloth, Cham 2018.

Ernst Mähly, Zur Geographie und Ethnographie der Goldküste, in: Verhandlungen der Naturforschenden Gesellschaft in Basel 7 (1885) 3, p. 809–852.

Patrick Manson, Tropical Research in its Relation to the Missionary Enterprise, Being an Address Delivered at Livingstone College on Commemoration Day, June 29th, 1908, London 1909.

Anne McClintock, Imperial Leather. Race, Gender and Sexuality in the Colonial Contest, New York 1995.

Carl Mense, Besprechung von Hey Fr., Der Tropenarzt, Wismar 1907, in: Archiv für Schiffs- und Tropenhygiene 12 (1908), p. 204.

Andreas Merz/Thomas Meyer, "You Be Good So, You Be King." Allianzbildung zwischen Bali-Nyonga (Kamerun) und der Basler Mission, in: Beat Sottas/Thomas Hammer/Lilo Roost Vischer/Anne Mayor (eds.), Werkschau Afrikastudien—Le forum suisse des africanistes, vol. 1, Hamburg 1997, p. 110–127.

Birgit Meyer, Christian Mind and Worldly Matters. Religion and Materiality in Nineteenth-Century Gold Coast, in: Journal of Material Culture 2 (1997) 3, p. 311–337.

David Morgan, Introduction: The Matter of Belief, in: ibid. (ed.), Religion and Material Culture: The Matter of Belief, New York 2010, p. 1–12.

Diana M. Natermann, Weisses (Nicht-)Essen im Kongofreistaat und in Deutsch-Ostafrika (1884–1914), in: Norman Aselmeyer/Veronika Settele (eds.), Geschichte des Nicht-Essens. Verzicht, Vermeidung und Verweigerung in der Moderne, Berlin/Boston 2018, p. 237–264.

Deborah J. Neill, Finding the "Ideal Diet": Nutrition, Culture and Dietary Practices in France and French Equatorial Africa, c. 1890s to 1920s, in: Food and Foodways 17 (2009) 1, p. 1–28.

Deborah J. Neill, Of Carnivores and Conquerors: French Nutritional Debates in the Age of Empire, 1890–1914, in: Elizabeth Neswald/David F. Smith/Ulrike Thoms (eds.), Setting Nutritional Standards. Theory, Policies, Practices, Rochester 2017, p. 74–96

Abena Osseo-Asare, Bioprospecting and Resistance: Transforming Poisoned Arrows into Strophantin Pills in Colonial Gold Coast, 1885–1922, in: Social History of Medicine 21 (2008), p. 269–290.

Giulia Paoletti/Yaëlle Biro, Photographic Portraiture in West Africa: Notes from "In and Out of the Studio", in: Metropolitan Museum Journal 51 (2016), p. 183–199.

Patricia Purtschert, Aviation Skills, Manly Adventures and Imperial Tears. The Dhaulagiri Expedition and Switzerland's Techno-Colonialism, in: National Identities 18 (2016) 1, p. 53–69.

Leslie W. Rabine, The Global Circulation of African Fashion, Oxford 2002.

Anandi Ramamurthy, Imperial Persuaders. Images of Africa and Asia in British Advertising, Manchester 2003.

Linda Ratschiller, "Die Zauberei spielt in Kamerun eine böse Rolle!" Die ethnografischen Ausstellungen der Basler Mission (1908–1912), in: Rebekka Habermas/Richard Hölzl (eds.), Mission global. Eine Verflechtungs-geschichte seit dem 19. Jahrhundert, Köln/Weimar/Wien 2014, p. 241–264.

Linda Ratschiller, Kranke Körper. Mission, Medizin und Fotografie zwischen der Goldküste und Basel 1885–1914, in: ibid./Siegfried Weichlein (eds.), Der schwarze Körper als Missionsgebiet. Medizin, Ethnologie, Theologie in Afrika und Europa 1880–1960, Köln/Weimar/Wien 2016, p. 41–72.

Linda Ratschiller, Material Matters: The Basel Mission in West Africa and Commodity Culture around 1900, in: ibid./Karolin Wetjen (eds.), Verflochtene Mission. Perspektiven auf eine neue Missionsgeschichte, Köln/Weimar/Wien 2018, p. 117–139.

Thomas Richards, The Commodity Culture of Victorian Britain: Advertising and Spectacle, 1851–1914, Stanford 1990.

Ernst Rodenwaldt, Filarien-Tumor, von Herrn Missionsarzt Dr. R. Fisch einge-sandt an das Institut für Schiffs- und Tropenkrankheiten, in: Archiv für Schiffs-und Tropenhygiene 13 (1909), p. 332.

Kirsten Rüther, The Power Beyond. Mission Strategies, African Conversion and the Development of a Christian Culture in the Transvaal, Hamburg 2001.

Pascal Martin Saint-Léon/N'Goné Fall/Frédérique Chapuis (eds.), Anthology of African and Indian Ocean Photography, Paris 1999.

Londa Schiebinger, Plants and Empire: Colonial Bioprospecting in the Atlantic World, Cambridge 2004.

Jürg Schneider, The Topography of the Early History of African Photography, in: History of Photography 34 (2010) 2, p. 134–146.

Eugen Schuler, Im Lande der Bali. Eine Kundschaftsreise der Basler Missionare ins Hinterland von Nordkamerun, in: Evangelisches Missionsmagazin 47 (1903), p. 191–214.

Kenneth Scott/Gareth Griffiths (eds.), Mixed Messages: Materiality, Textuality, Missions, New York 2005.

Sujit Sivasundaram, Natural History Spiritualized. Civilizing Islanders, Culti-vating Breadfruit, and Collecting Souls, in: History of Science 39 (2001), p. 417–443.

Don Slater, Photography and Modern Vision: The Spectacle of "Natural Magic", in: Chris Jencks (ed.), Visual Culture, London/New York 1995, p. 218–237.

Nancy Leys Stepan, Picturing Tropical Nature, Ithaca 2001.

Caspar Stolz, Five Hundred Indian Plants, Their Use in Medicine and the Arts, Mangalore 1881.

T. Jack Thompson, Light on Darkness? Missionary Photography of Africa in the Nineteenth and Early Twentieth Centuries, Grand Rapids/Cambridge 2013.

Michael van Orsouw/Judith Stadlin/Monika Imboden, George Page, der Milch-pionier: die Anglo-Swiss Condensed Milk Company bis zur Fusion mit Nestlé, Zürich 2005.

Hermann Vortisch, Die Neger der Goldküste, in: Globus 89 (1906), p. 277–283, 293–297.

Hermann Vortisch, Über Säuglingsernährung in den Tropen, in: Archiv für Schiffs- und Tropenhygiene 16 (1912), p. 69–77.

Renate Wilson, Pious Traders in Medicine: A German Pharmaceutical Network in Eighteenth-Century North America, Philadelphia 2000.

Anna E. Winterbottom, Of the China Root: A Case Study of the Early Modern Circulation of Materia Medica, in: Social History of Medicine 28 (2015), p. 22–44.

Christine Wolters, Dr. Friedrich Hey (1864–1960), Missionsarzt und Bücke-burger Unternehmer, in: Hubert Höing (ed.), Strukturen und Konjunkturen. Faktoren in der schaumburgischen Wirtschaftsgeschichte, Bielefeld 2004, p. 328–366.

CHAPTER 11

Conclusion

11.1   METROPOLITAN REFLECTIONS

The history of tropical medicine and hygiene demonstrates how knowledge acquired in colonial encounters gave rise to a new scientific discipline and shaped metropolitan approaches to public health. As Europeans ventured overseas, doctors developed theories and practices of sanitation to enhance health on ships, colonial stations and in military and naval quarters.[1] Their hygiene measures, such as promoting cleanliness, ventilation and the disposal of waste, were adopted by social reformers in European societies, where the hygiene movement reached full blossom right at the time that heralded the high imperial phase. Experience derived from dealing with frail health and illness abroad boosted the rise of preventive medicine at home, where hygiene began to be integrated into state policy in the late nineteenth century. Mission societies and missionaries were key protagonists of this dialogical history of hygiene during the colonial period, a fact that has been widely overlooked by historians of mission, science and colonialism.

---

[1] Roberto Zaugg, Guerre, maladie, empire. Les services de santé militaires en situation coloniale pendant le long XIXe siècle, in: ibid. (ed.), Histoire, Médecine et Santé 10 (2016), p. 9–16; Chakrabarti, Medicine and Empire, ch. 3 and ch. 5.

© The Author(s) 2023   417
L. M. Ratschiller Nasim, *Medical Missionaries and Colonial Knowledge in West Africa and Europe, 1885–1914*,
Cambridge Imperial and Post-Colonial Studies,
https://doi.org/10.1007/978-3-031-27128-1_11

Inversely, tropical colonies also served as a magnifying glass for social developments and scientific controversies that had their origins in Europe. Medical discussions and their social importance were illuminated from a different perspective gained abroad, reinforcing metropolitan ambitions and fears. The Basel missionary Jakob Stutz, who attended to the sick in Sakbayeme in Cameroon, published an article in the journal of the Society for Medical Mission in Stuttgart, in which he claimed: "There are more sick people at home than out here." He explained that there were "a whole range of diseases linked to over-civilisation, culture, technology and its operations" that did not occur in Cameroon at all or only very rarely.[2] These reflections produced in the colonies were altered not only by various geographical locations, social environments, political contexts, professional networks and institutional dynamics but also through confrontation with unexpected observations.[3]

Hygiene activists utilised Africa as a mirror image through which to advance the reform of the lower classes in European societies. The German navy officer Hans Paasche, a prominent life reformer, teetotaller and opponent to vaccines, crafted a popular novel in which he mocked the poor health of Europeans, especially their smoking, alcohol abuse and urban life, by putting his satirical remarks into the mouth of Lukanga Mukara, a fictional explorer sent by his African king to report on life in Germany.[4] The popularity of colonial novels and medical handbooks highlights that knowledge of tropical hygiene reached a far greater audience than the limited number of Europeans in the tropics that were directly concerned with these preventive measures.

The preoccupation with environmental factors for human health was not exclusive to the tropics; it was part of a larger pathologisation of space.[5] Hygiene campaigners mapped out topographies of dirt and disease

---

[2] Jakob Stutz, Aus meiner ärztlichen Praxis, in: Verein für ärztliche Mission in Stuttgart (ed.), Mitteilungen aus der ärztlichen Mission 10 (1911), p. 4–7, here p. 4.

[3] Heather J. Sharkey, Introduction: The Unexpected Consequences of Christian Missionary Encounters, in: ibid. (ed.), Cultural Conversions. Unexpected Consequences of Christian Missionary Encounters in the Middle East, Africa, and South Africa, New York 2013, p. 1–26.

[4] Hans Paasche, Die Forschungsreisen des Afrikaners Lukanga Mukara ins Innerste Deutschlands, Hamburg 1921.

[5] Rob Shields, Places on the Margin. Alternative Geographies of Modernity, London 1991.

in European cities to disentangle what they perceived as a dangerous amalgamation of bodies in space. Luigi Westenra Sambon, a physician who was decorated by the French and Italian governments for his work during the cholera epidemic of 1884, argued that in many ways urban life in the "major European centres of civilisation" was far more conducive to physical deterioration than life in the tropics through the "herding together of dense masses of population" and "a more strenuous struggle for existence, alcoholism, and immorality."[6] Sambon, who had recently visited Central Africa, addressed the Royal Geographical Society in London on the "Acclimatization of Europeans in Tropical Lands" in 1898:

> The problem of tropical colonisation is one of the most important and pressing issues with which European states have to deal. Civilisation has favoured unlimited multiplication, and thereby intensified the struggle for existence, the limitation of which seemed to be its very object. [...] I know full well that the question of emigration is beset with a variety of moral, social, political, and economic difficulties; but it is the law of nature, and civilisation has no better remedy for the evils caused by overcrowding.[7]

Sambon regarded Africa as a kind of overflow basin for the societies in industrialised Europe, portraying colonialism as an inevitable consequence of European development. Demographic arguments played an important role in the formal colonisation of Africa in the 1880s, and even before in forging arguments for the necessity of European imperial endeavours. Similarly, Hans Ziemann, medical advisor to the German colonial government in Cameroon, declared at the 14th International Congress for Hygiene and Demography in 1907 that "the population mass continues to swell in Europe" and thus urgently argued for "the

---

[6] Luigi Westenra Sambon, Acclimatization of Europeans in Tropical Lands, in: Geographical Journal 12 (1898) 6, p. 589–606, here p. 591.

[7] Ibid., p. 589.

need to find new land for this teeming population."[8] Fears about over-population kept questions of acclimatisation and tropical hygiene on the political agendas of European colonial powers.[9]

Hygiene touched on fundamental religious, scientific and political questions of human nature and coexistence. Johannes Fabian highlighted the role of hygiene in his 1990 essay on *Religious and Secular Colonization*, arguing that "aside from connecting secular and religious colonial ideology," it also had the "metaphorical function of transporting special concerns to a universal plane."[10] The question of whether Europeans could acclimatise to a supposedly hostile environment evolved into a major anthropological debate about the origins and future of mankind. Much of the literature on tropical medicine and hygiene used a strategy that imbued a problem, defined as being caused specifically by the tropics, with universal significance, endangering the very core of human civilisation.

The Basel Mission doctors occupied the front lines of tropical hygiene and exemplified that the only way for Europeans to successfully hold their ground in the colonies was through asceticism, self-discipline and temperance. They argued that these virtues, derived from Pietist purity ideals, not only protected white men and women against physical harms and mental breakdowns in the tropics but also formed the basis of colonial rule. The perceived danger of the tropics called for moral steadfastness, allowing the Basel Mission doctors to promote their precepts of hygiene to white settlers, medical colleagues, imperial policy-makers, colonial stakeholders and a general public at home concerned with tropical medicine and hygiene. Many Europeans valued their holistic approach, which promised both prevention from physical suffering and alleviation of their cultural and political anxieties.

---

[8] Ziemann, Wie erobert man Afrika, p. 247.

[9] Heinrich Hartmann has offered a reading of demographics as colonial history, arguing that colonial contexts led to a reconfiguration of the scientific criteria used to examine fitness and the social practices associated with them. Hartmann, Tropical Soldiers?

[10] Fabian, Time and the Work of Anthropology, p. 162.

The Basel Mission's hygiene mission in West Africa came to an abrupt end at the outbreak of the First World War.[11] After losing many of their German staff in combat, their Swiss missionaries were expelled from the Gold Coast and Cameroon. By the end of the war, the Basel Mission had been forced to leave all territories under British and French control, despite the fact that, as a Swiss organisation, they should have legally been treated as neutral and protected by colonial governments.[12] They were readmitted to the colonies after the Great War, restarting their medical mission on the Gold Coast and in Cameroon in the mid-1920s, after recovering from their lack of personnel and funds.[13] Despite the sudden cessation of their operations in West Africa, the Basel Mission doctors and their negotiations of hygiene had lasting effects on religious, scientific and colonial bodies of knowledge.

Firstly, the Basel Mission doctors re-established the Pietist unity between body and soul by modern scientific means, taking back control over bodily matters from worldly protagonists. Building on their religious socialisation and medical training, they appropriated and developed postulates from the hygiene movement, legitimising evangelical goals to a wider public. They leveraged the spread of religious ideas, practices and images of purity by operating as polyvalent brokers of knowledge in multiple markets. Hygiene allowed them to recodify Pietist purity, which in turn affected the values and norms of hygiene more broadly. The popularity of their medical handbooks, scientific articles and colonial accounts shows that hygienic knowledge between 1885 and 1914 was infused with puritan notions linking physical dirt to moral filth. By promoting individual responsibility for health and moral improvement, their postulates provided a source of inspiration for social reformers and policy-makers, shaping public health debates well into the twentieth century.

Secondly, the Basel Mission doctors both facilitated and challenged the formation of tropical medicine and hygiene as an institutionalised

---

[11] Felicity Jensz, "Als der Krieg ausbrach": Die persönlichen Erinnerungen deutscher Missionare in Kamerun um 1914, in: Michael Eckardt (ed.), Mission Afrika: Geschichtsschreibung über Grenzen hinweg. Festschrift für Ulrich van der Heyden, Stuttgart 2019, p. 87–103.

[12] Jenkins, Short History, p. 16.

[13] Schmid, Medicine, Faith and Politics in Agogo, p. 31–37; Eckart, Medizin und Kolonialimperialismus, p. 254.

medical speciality around 1900. They continued to be valued as in-the-field observers after the turn of the century but were gradually excluded from developments taking place in metropolitan laboratories since their emphasis lay on evangelical activism and hands-on medical aid. In the colonies, however, tropical medicine and hygiene remained a practical form of knowledge, combining scientific theories with environmental experiences and moral imperatives. The Basel medical missionaries' wealth of experience in tropical regions continued to shape medical practice abroad while their influence on the academic discipline at home decreased.

Thirdly, the Basel medical missionaries contributed to the formation of colonial knowledge by circulating texts, images and commodities to urban and rural populations at home. Hygiene held a special place in the imagination of Africa, which continues to shape conceptions of the other and the self in European societies to this day. The Basel Mission doctors gained particular significance as brokers of colonial knowledg in the Swiss context since Switzerland lacked formal colonies. Swiss constructions of purity, health and cleanliness became an effective political, cultural and social tool for the exclusion of minorities and the assertion of a national identity in the twentieth century.[14] These ideas and practices of civic cleansing and political purification were based on categories of difference along racial, social and gender lines, originating in nineteenth-century colonial entanglements and negotiations of hygiene.

Tropical medicine and hygiene continued to preoccupy German and Swiss audiences well after 1914, when German colonies ceased to exist and the Basel Mission temporarily lost their mission fields. Wolfgang Eckart has shown that in Germany the field of tropical medicine became a sphere of vigorous colonial revisionism after the end of colonial rule.[15] The First World War damaged the transnational networks among specialists in tropical medicine, which was particularly difficult for German

---

[14] Just recently, an expert commission published their final report on administrative detention in twentieth century Switzerland, analysing the imprisonment of people deemed a threat to the public order because of their apparent self-neglect, indolence and immorality. See Unabhängige Expertenkommission Administrative Versorgungen (eds.), Organisierte Willkür. Administrative Versorgungen in der Schweiz 1930–1981, Schlussbericht, Zürich 2019.

[15] Eckart, Medizin und Kolonialimperialismus, p. 505–540.

scientists whose research depended on access to African and other tropical colonies.[16] In Switzerland, the growing animosity between European nations caused researchers to reorient their efforts towards the creation of their own institution. The Swiss Tropical Institute in Basel—fondly referred to as the *Tropeli* by the Swiss—was founded in 1943. Situated on officially neutral territory, the institution became a hub for scientific and colonial networks.[17]

11.2 Lines of Hygiene

Scientists, colonial authorities and the Basel Mission doctors shared notions of European superiority across professional, national and imperial networks, convinced of the benefits scientific medicine would bring to the African population.[18] The presence of Europeans in the tropics, however, caused endless self-questioning. There was a growing sense of anxiety in both physical and moral terms as imperial powers expanded into Africa and the implications that this held for European bodies and souls. Despite new evidence on the development cycles and transmission paths of disease pathogens, the colonial community remained divided on the best way to combat them. Knowledge of tropical hygiene was controversial, ambivalent and volatile, forcefully illustrating the paradox of colonial rule, based on contradictory feelings of superiority and fear.[19]

The making of hygiene between 1885 and 1914 shows that purity, health and cleanliness were not clearly defined, solid concepts but explicit and implicit efforts to draw lines of difference. As Europeans familiarised themselves with what appeared to them as the new world, they developed

---

[16] Neill, Science and Civilizing Missions.

[17] Lukas Meier, Swiss Science, African Decolonization and the Rise of Global Health, 1940–2010, Basel 2014.

[18] Neill, Networks in Tropical Medicine; Manuela Bauche, Race, Class or Culture? The Construction of the European in Colonial Malaria Control, in: Comparativ 25 (2015) 5/6, p. 116–136.

[19] Manuela Bauche, Von der Unmöglichkeit, klare Grenzen zu ziehen. Rassismus und Medizin in den deutschen Kolonien, in: Naika Foroutan et al. (eds.), Das Phantom "Rasse". Zur Geschichte und Wirkungsmacht von Rassismus, Köln 2018, p. 115–130; Stoler, Cultivating Bourgeois Bodies and Racial Selves.

increasingly elaborate theories to conceptualise difference between themselves and the people they encountered.[20] The codification of difference saw a gradual shift from an early emphasis on civilisation, which could be spread by education economics and religion, to more rigid physical criteria. By 1900, arguments about fundamental biological differences between races had taken deep root in European societies, aided by the scientific systematisation of the body in the nineteenth century.[21]

Historiographical questions have been raised about the extent to which missionary thinking correlated with theories of race in the late nineteenth and early twentieth centuries.[22] The Basel missionaries produced numerous anthropological accounts on the people in West Africa, not only examining their languages and cultural customs, but also commenting on their bodily practices and physical appearance. The Committee used these reports to develop new conversion strategies and presented them to the pupils in the seminary in Basel. Jakob Stutz and Friedrich Ebding, for instance, compiled a range of studies on the hygiene, diet and daily life of the population in Cameroon, which was used as teaching material.[23] Missionaries also recognised the growing scientific kudos attached to the study of non-European cultures and

[20] Roxann Wheeler, The Complexion of Race: Categories of Difference in Eighteenth-Century British Culture, Pennsylvania 2000; Londa Schiebinger, The Anatomy of Difference: Race and Sex in Eighteenth-Century Science, in: Eighteenth-Century Studies 23 (1990) 4, p. 387–405.

[21] Christian Geulen, Der Rassenbegriff. Ein kurzer Abschnitt seiner Geschichte, in: Naika Foroutan et al. (eds.), Das Phantom "Rasse". Zur Geschichte und Wirkungsmacht von Rassismus, Köln 2018, p. 23–34; Damon Salesa, Race, in: Philippa Levine/John Marriott (eds.), The Ashgate Research Companion to Modern Imperial Histories, Oxon/New York 2012, p. 429–448; Waltraud Ernst/Bernard Harris (eds.), Race, Science and Medicine, 1700–1960, London/New York 1999.

[22] Thomas Altena, "Etwas für das Wohl der schwarzen Neger beitragen" – Überlegungen zum "Rassenbegriff" der evangelischen Missionsgesellschaften, in: Frank Becker (ed.), Rassenmischehen—Mischlinge—Rassentrennung. Zur Politik der Rasse im deutschen Kolonialreich, Stuttgart 2004, p. 54–81; Cleall, Missionary Discourses of Difference; Richard Hölzl, Rassismus, Ethnogenese und Kultur. Afrikaner im Blickwinkel der deutschen katholischen Mission im 19. und frühen 20. Jahrhundert, in: WerkstattGeschichte 59 (2012), p. 7–34.

[23] Friedrich Ebding, Hygienisches aus Kamerun, BMA, Box containing teaching material on ethnography, without signature; Ibid., On Nutritional Practices in Cameroon, BMA, E-10.022.16d; Jakob Stutz, Ethnographie von Kamerun, BMA, Box containing teaching material on ethnography, without signature.

contributed to anthropological knowledge both in public debates and academic deliberations.[24]

The Basel Mission doctor Alfred Eckhardt devoted a whole chapter to the physiology of the people on the Gold Coast in his 1894 monograph, writing that "anyone who is used to the black or rather dark brown faces, actually finds most of them pretty" and that "particularly children often have very cute curly heads." While he conceded that "old heathens" and "fetish priests" were an exception, he appealed to his readers that "if you could look into the peaceful face of the dear pastor Asare, you would have no choice but to grow fond of him."[25] Eckhardt's depiction certainly contributed to the objectification and generalisation of African people but his writings also show that he believed in an innate equality between Europeans and Africans. In one of his articles for the Basel Mission's medical journal he expressed "a special love" for the Krobo people, admiring their diligence and their "sense for a clean, nice home," stating that "nowhere are the houses nicer than in Krobo."[26]

At the same time, the Basel Mission doctors contributed to scientific processes that codified biological difference. Their examination reports of African patients, parishioners and school children, published in scientific journals like the *Archiv für Schiffs- und Tropenhygiene*, claimed alarmingly high infection rates of diseases such as hookworm, tuberculosis, yellow fever and syphilis.[27] Whereas their medical mission in West Africa had limited impact on African ideas and practices of health due

---

[24] Harries, Anthropology; Ibid., From the Alps to Africa; Maxwell, The Soul of the Luba; Przyrembel, Wissen auf Wanderschaft.

[25] Eckhardt, Land, Leute und Ärztliche Mission auf der Goldküste, p. 10.

[26] Eckhardt, Ein Arbeitsjahr in Odumase (Goldküste), p. 10.

[27] Hermann Vortisch, Statistik und Bericht über das erste Halbjahr 1904 der ärztlichen Mission auf der Goldküste, in: Archiv für Schiffs- und Tropenhygiene 9 (1905), p. 346–354; Ibid. Erfahrungen über einige spezifische Krankheiten an der Goldküste, in: Archiv für Schiffs- und Tropenhygiene 10 (1906), p. 537–539; Ibid., Ärztliche Beobachtungen und Erfahrungen auf der Goldküste, in: Deutsche Medizinische Wochenschrift 33 (1907), p. 110–111; Ibid., Aus der Arbeit eines Missionsarztes, in: Schweizerische Rundschau für Medizin 38 (1912), p. 1025–1036; Rudolf Fisch, Über die Ätiologie der Tuberkulose auf der Goldküste, in: Correspondenz-Blatt für Schweizer Ärzte 34 (1904), p. 761–763; Ibid., Die Wurmkrankheit auf der Goldküste, in: Die ärztliche Mission 3 (1908), p. 89–90; Ibid., Über die Darmparasiten der Goldküstenneger, in: Archiv für Schiffs- und Tropenhygiene 12 (1908), p. 711–718; Ibid., Filarientumor, eigesandt an das Institut für Schiffs- und Tropenkrankheiten, in: Archiv für Schiffs- und Tropenhygiene 13 (1909), p. 332; Theodor Müller, Krankheitsbilder von der Goldküste, in: Die ärztliche Mission

to intricate patterns of rejection and appropriation, their pathological representations of black bodies contributed to scientific theories of racial difference. Although the Basel medical missionaries rarely spoke about race directly, their medical studies were rooted in a logic of biological difference, whatever proclamations they may also have made about human universalism.

During his medical studies, Friedrich Hey had been a student of Julius Kollmann at the University of Basel, a renowned scientist of his time whose controversial legacy involved research into racial anthropology.[28] Kollmann frequently used people exhibited in *Völkerschauen*—human zoos—for anatomical examinations during their stay in Switzerland.[29] Hey assisted Kollmann in his surveys and attended a series of anthropological displays held at the Zoological Garden in Basel during his studies.[30] Over the following two decades, the mission doctor repeatedly boasted that he had been a student of Kollman, who in turn

7 (1912), p. 131–136; Ibid., Über Gelbfieber in Westafrika, in: Die ärztliche Mission 9 (1914), p. 15–22, 40–41.

[28] Kollmann studied medicine in Munich, Berlin, Paris and London. From 1878 to 1913, he was Professor for Comparative Anatomy at the University of Basel. See Balthasar Staehlin, Völkerschauen im Zoologischen Garten Basel 1879–1935, Basel 1993, p. 116–122; Schär, Tropenliebe, p. 122–124. Recently, Pascal German has argued that Switzerland played a key role in the formation of racial science in the early twentieth century. See Pascal Germann, Race in the Making. Colonial Encounters, Body Measurements and the Global Dimensions of Swiss Racial Science, 1900–1950, in: Patricia Purtschert/Harald Fischer-Tiné (eds.), Colonial Switzerland. Rethinking Colonialism from the Margins, Basingstoke 2015, p. 50–72; Ibid., Laboratorien der Vererbung: Rassenforschung und Humangenetik in der Schweiz, 1900–1970, Göttingen 2016.

[29] Historians have shown that the performers in these displays were not merely passive objects, but on the contrary, took up the roles assigned to them actively and often even subversively. Rea Brändle, Nayo Bruce. Geschichte einer afrikanischen Familie in Europa, Zürich 2007; Andrew Zimmerman, Anthropology and Antihumanism in Imperial Germany, Chicago/London 2001, p. 15–37.

[30] Initially, the most important organisers of *Völkerschauen* had been German animal traders, such as Carl Hagenbeck from Hamburg. From the early 1880s, Swiss amusement parks and zoological gardens displayed people, particularly originating from Asia and Africa. During Hey's medical studies, the Basel zoo saw the performance of an "East African caravan" and a "wild Africa" group in 1889, a "Somali" caravan in 1891, as well as people from the Upper Nile and a "Dinka Negro caravane" from Sudan in 1892. Staehlin, Völkerschauen im Zoologischen Garten Basel 1879–1935. See also Rea Brändle, Wildfremd, hautnah. Zürcher Völkerschauen und ihre Schauplätze 1835–1964, 2nd ed., Zürich 2013.

asserted that Hey had completed his studies with "great diligence and understanding."[31]

In 1896, Friedrich Hey commented on the effects of alcoholism in West Africa in a private letter, later published in the Basel Mission's medical journal: "As is well known, the people native to the tropics have less moral strength than the ones of the North and this is why the Negroes pounce on this palate-irritating drink and thus perish in body and spirit."[32] Hey's citation illustrates that the Basel medical missionaries held deep-seated assumptions about the weak moral constitution of West Africans. However, while the Basel Mission doctors mapped out and propagated boundaries of difference, these were premised on moral rather than genetic terms. The full range of Social Darwinist ideas, including fundamental hereditary differences and the inevitability of competition and extinction, never appears in their writings. These ideas ran directly counter to their strenuous attempts to introduce purity, health and cleanliness to the population in West Africa.

By combining statements of difference with assertions of human unity, the Basel Mission doctors highlighted the capacity of their work to bring individual salvation and cultural progress. Reflecting the activities of city missionaries, deaconesses and fervent evangelicals at home, they thought that working-class and colonial subjects could, by means of hygiene education, be uplifted to the realms of the civilised. While they were certainly not immune to offensive caricatures of Africans, they did not draw lines of hygiene along fixed physical characteristics such as skin colour and disease immunity but rather considered cultural markers such as housing and clothing as powerful indicators of otherness. They aspired to create pure spaces by transforming people's material environment, believing that modestly clothed Christians belonged in proper houses that could protect them from the sullied environment.

The Basel Mission's whole endeavour in West Africa was based on the premise that their missionaries would find and tackle filth in both physical and moral terms. However, many accounts in the Basel Mission archives disrupt this uniform picture, questioning the dominant assumption that Africans lacked notions of purity, health and cleanliness, and breaching

---

[31] Curriculum Vitae Friedrich Hey, BArch, R 86/1768.

[32] Friedrich Hey, Auszug aus einem privaten Brief aus Odumase, in: Unsere ärztliche Mission. Bericht vom Jahr 1896, Basel 1897, p. 7–12, here p. 10.

commonly held racial stereotypes among the European public. Theodor Müller's wife, Elisabeth, dedicated a whole article to "Peter, my chef," who was not a Christian but what she classified as an "African heathen," in a popular missionary magazine after her return home:

> Another estimable quality, which is still far from being found amongst all Christians, was his cleanliness. He was particularly meticulous with himself and with his own things. How clean his room looked! On the walls he had hung, next to a few pictures, a whole gallery of shoes. His bed was covered by a big, white mosquito net. A few boxes containing his toiletries, an 'Easy-Chair', a mirror and a whole range of medicine bottles constituted the remaining inventory of the small room.[33]

This citation illustrates how missionaries used Africa as a mirror to reflect on the possibility of change at home. If Africans, who had to deal with difficult climates and a lack of Christian civilisation, could adopt knowledge of hygiene and climb the ladder of civilisation, so might the European poor in working-class neighbourhoods. The example of Peter, who embraced scientific and cultural progress, condemned those Christians at home who seemed to spurn cleanliness and civilisation on their doorstep. Elisabeth Müller's account also shows how contradictory the panoply of missionary sources dealing with the cleanliness of African people was. The inconsistent and fragmented nature of the Basel Mission's knowledge production is particularly striking in this case because Peter is described as not following Christian faith yet still employing an extraordinary number of hygienic measures and commodities.

The ambivalent observations in missionary accounts were part of the Basel Mission's binary advertising strategy, emphasising both the pressing necessity and present achievements of their work to donors and supporters at home. However, they were also expressions of the Basel missionaries' professional and personal dilemmas. While they took hierarchical differences between Africans and Europeans for granted, as it was this disparity that justified their civilising mission, they had to overcome these supposed differences to reach the people they wished to convert. Their belief in the

---

[33] Elisabeth Müller, Skizzen aus meinen afrikanischen Missionserlebnissen, in: Fliegende Missions-Blätter 4 (1917), p. 3–6, here p. 4.

transformative power of individual conversion implied that boundaries of race, class and gender could be transcended.

11.3   SHIFTS OF MEANINGS

The fact that the Basel Mission doctors enjoyed approval in religious, scientific and colonial spaces of knowledge highlights the interdiscursive and multi-relational character of hygiene. Hygiene was a portmanteau term that combined pre-existing and new bodies of knowledge. These included changing conceptions of religious purity, scientific assumptions of health ranging from environmental to bacteriological theories, and colonial views of cleanliness expressed in the fields of social and racial hygiene. The overriding concern for hygiene both abroad and at home in the late nineteenth and early twentieth centuries enabled the Basel Mission doctors to situate themselves at the interface of these three spaces of knowledge—a concept used in this study as a method to disentangle some of the different threads of theory and practice that were interwoven in the making of hygiene in this period.

Simultaneously, the position of the Basel Mission doctors as protagonists in religious, scientific and colonial spaces of knowledge illustrates the complex interplay between these domains. The history of hygiene exposes the religious fabric of both scientific and colonial knowledge. Seemingly scientific and secular notions of hygiene emerging in the nineteenth century were based on concepts originating from religious tenets of purity and morality. The interactions between the religious, scientific and colonial spaces of knowledge shifted between 1885 and 1914, affecting the relevance of the Basel Mission doctors. While their knowledge became less significant for the laboratory-based scientific space of knowledge, it gained meaning for colonial knowledge on acclimatisation and tropical hygiene due to its strong practical focus and moral dimension.

The Basel medical missionaries participated in the hygienic operation of creating different spaces of knowledge by drawing lines between different types of knowledge. They labelled ideas and practices as "rational vs irrational," "religious vs superstitious" and "European vs African" for example. Their studies were used by metropolitan researchers and helped to establish new disciplines such as social anthropology and tropical medicine. Yet the Basel Mission doctors were gradually excluded from academic networks, which grew tighter and more impermeable,

increasingly sealing themselves off in the name of disciplinary specialisation and professionalisation. Paradoxically, the Basel Mission doctors'
scientific contributions fell victim to these processes of differentiation and
secularisation, "practices of purification" they had themselves contributed
to.

The synergy between the religious, scientific and colonial spaces of
knowledge is certainly not unique to the history of hygiene. However,
hygiene is unique in the sense that it addresses an anthropological dimension of human existence. It comprises a biological instinct, a medical
necessity, a social behaviour, a technical process, a cultural code of
conduct, an aesthetic ideal and a moral belief. Beyond its discursive function, hygiene is in many cases tacit knowledge, entailing emotions such as
disgust and fear and materialising in and on individual bodies in the form
of body language, everyday practices and habitus. Notions and behaviours
of purity and cleanliness transcend geographical locations, historical situ-
ations, social environments and political conditions. The Basel Mission
doctors used hygiene as an entry point to the conceptual and material
worlds of both Africans and Europeans. While many of their theological
concepts were not met by a receptive audience, questions of purity, health
and cleanliness addressed a matter of concern to literally everyone.

Knowledge of hygiene emerged from ongoing negotiations between
people, networks and institutions on different continents. The Basel
Mission doctors were particularly interactive actors in the making of
hygiene from 1885 to 1914 due to their global scope, practical approach
and material resources, both in their popular appeal to a general public in
Europe and in their engagement with people in West Africa. They heavily
relied on African medical assistants, parishioners, teachers and patients for
their knowledge production. However, in the circulation of knowledge
between West Africa and Europe, the contributions of these protagonists
were often concealed. Aware of metropolitan expectations and conventions, the Basel Mission doctors reclassified the data and information
provided by Africans, reframed their interpretations and amended their
knowledge to serve their own purposes.

The question as to what extent African ideas and practices of purity,
health and cleanliness moulded European knowledge of hygiene remains
a thorny one, given the grave disparity in archival source material, the
discrepancies within both the African and European canon of knowledge, and the complex exchanges and mutual appropriations between
the two. Nonetheless, notions and behaviours of hygiene between 1885

and 1914 clearly arose from demarcation processes both at home and abroad, which are easily misunderstood when the imperial context in which they played out is not taken into account. In their introduction to the volume on *Engaging Colonial Knowledge*, Ricardo Roque and Kim A. Wagner argued that colonial knowledge "was the expression of worlds and visions brought into contact; a formation of stories and words that, rather than simply coalescing, could bind indigenous and European images and understandings to each other."[34]

Despite their triumphal accounts for audiences at home, the Basel Mission doctors faced constant challenges abroad, forcing them to adapt their strategies and compromise their ideals. Their experience in West Africa was shaped by the varying expectations and reactions of African protagonists, the unpredictability of colonial officials, the competition of rival missions, interpersonal strife with fellow missionaries, devastating illness and the loss of family members and friends. Failures, conflicts and frustrations were part and parcel of their everyday lives, highlighting both the fragility of their existence and the interactive nature of their knowledge production. Texts, images and commodities of hygiene between 1885 and 1914 were products of complex colonial entanglements and protracted negotiations surrounding key distinctions underlying and shaping the human condition: purity and impurity, health and disease, cleanliness and dirt.

REFERENCES

Thomas Altena, "Etwas für das Wohl der schwarzen Neger beitragen"—Überlegungen zum "Rassenbegriff" der evangelischen Missionsgesellschaften, in: Frank Becker (ed.), Rassenmischehen—Mischlinge—Rassentrennung. Zur Politik der Rasse im deutschen Kolonialreich, Stuttgart 2004, p. 54–81.

Manuela Bauche, Race, Class or Culture? The Construction of the European in Colonial Malaria Control, in: Comparativ 25 (2015) 5/6, p. 116–136.

Manuela Bauche, Von der Unmöglichkeit, klare Grenzen zu ziehen. Rassismus und Medizin in den deutschen Kolonien, in: Naika Foroutan et al. (eds.), Das Phantom "Rasse". Zur Geschichte und Wirkungsmacht von Rassismus, Köln 2018, p. 115–130.

Rea Brändle, Nayo Bruce. Geschichte einer afrikanischen Familie in Europa, Zürich 2007.

[34] Ricardo Roque/Kim A. Wagner, Introduction: Engaging Colonial Knowledge, p. 4.

Rea Brändle, Wildfremd, hautnah. Zürcher Völkerschauen und ihre Schauplätze 1835–1964, 2nd ed., Zürich 2013.

Pratik Chakrabarti, Medicine and Empire, 1600–1960, Basingstoke 2014.

Esme Cleall, Missionary Discourses of Difference. Negotiating Otherness in the British Empire, Basingstoke 2012.

Wolfgang U. Eckart, Medizin und Kolonialimperialismus. Deutschland 1884–1945, Paderborn 1997.

Alfred Eckhardt, Ein Arbeitsjahr in Odumase (Goldküste), in: An die Freunde des Ärztlichen Zweiges der Basler Mission, Basel 1893, p. 5–11.

Alfred Eckhardt, Land, Leute und ärztliche Mission auf der Goldküste, Basel 1894.

Waltraud Ernst/Bernard Harris (eds.), Race, Science and Medicine, 1700–1960, London/New York 1999.

Johannes Fabian, Time and the Work of Anthropology. Critical Essays 1971–1991, Chur et al. 1991.

Rudolf Fisch, Über die Ätiologie der Tuberkulose auf der Goldküste, in: Correspondenz-Blatt für Schweizer Ärzte 34 (1904), p. 761–763.

Rudolf Fisch, Die Wurmkrankheit auf der Goldküste, in: Die ärztliche Mission 3 (1908), p. 89–90.

Rudolf Fisch, Über die Darmparasiten der Goldküstenneger, in: Archiv für Schiffs- und Tropenhygiene 12 (1908), p. 711–718.

Rudolf Fisch, Filarientumor, eigesandt an das Institut für Schiffs- und Tropenkrankheiten, in: Archiv für Schiffs- und Tropenhygiene 13 (1909), p. 332.

Pascal Germann, Race in the Making. Colonial Encounters, Body Measurements and the Global Dimensions of Swiss Racial Science, 1900–1950, in: Patricia Purtschert/Harald Fischer-Tiné (eds.), Colonial Switzerland. Rethinking Colonialism from the Margins, Basingstoke 2015, p. 50–72.

Pascal Germann, Laboratorien der Vererbung: Rassenforschung und Humangenetik in der Schweiz, 1900–1970, Göttingen 2016.

Christian Geulen, Der Rassenbegriff. Ein kurzer Abschnitt seiner Geschichte, in: Naika Foroutan et al. (eds.), Das Phantom "Rasse". Zur Geschichte und Wirkungsmacht von Rassismus, Köln 2018, p. 23–34.

Patrick Harries, Anthropology, in: Norman Etherington (ed.), Missions and Empire, Oxford 2005, p. 238–260.

Patrick Harries, From the Alps to Africa: Swiss Missionaries and the Rise of Anthropology, in: Helen L. Tilley/Robert J. Gordon (eds.), Ordering Africa. Anthropology, European Imperialism and the Politics of Knowledge, Manchester 2007, p. 201–224.

Heinrich Hartmann, Tropical Soldiers? New Definitions of Military Strength in the Colonial Context (1884–1914), in: Martin Lengwiler/Nigel Penn/

Patrick Harries (eds.), Science, Africa and Europe. Processing Information and Creating Knowledge, London/New York 2019, p. 125–149.

Friedrich Hey, Auszug aus einem privaten Brief aus Odumase, in: Unsere ärztliche Mission. Bericht vom Jahr 1896, Basel 1897, p. 7–12.

Richard Hölzl, Rassismus, Ethnogenese und Kultur. Afrikaner im Blickwinkel der deutschen katholischen Mission im 19. und frühen 20. Jahrhundert, in: WerkstattGeschichte 59 (2012), p. 7–34.

Paul Jenkins, Short History of the Basel Mission, Basel 1989.

Felicity Jensz, "Als der Krieg ausbrach": Die persönlichen Erinnerungen deutscher Missionare in Kamerun um 1914, in: Michael Eckardt (ed.), Mission Afrika: Geschichtsschreibung über Grenzen hinweg. Festschrift für Ulrich van der Heyden, Stuttgart 2019, p. 87–103.

David Maxwell, The Soul of the Luba. W.F.P. Burton, Missionary Ethnography and Belgian Colonial Science, in: History and Anthropology 19 (2008) 4, p. 325–351.

Lukas Meier, Swiss Science, African Decolonization and the Rise of Global Health, 1940–2010, Basel 2014.

Elisabeth Müller, Skizzen aus meinen afrikanischen Missionserlebnissen, in: Fliegende Missions-Blätter 4 (1917), p. 3–6.

Theodor Müller, Krankheitsbilder von der Goldküste, in: Die ärztliche Mission 7 (1912), p. 131–136.

Theodor Müller, Über Gelbfieber in Westafrika, in: Die ärztliche Mission 9 (1914), p. 15–22, 40–41.

Deborah J. Neill, Networks in Tropical Medicine. Internationalism, Colonialism, and the Rise of a Medical Specialty, 1890–1930, Stanford 2012.

Deborah J. Neill, Science and Civilizing Missions. Germans and the Transnational Community of Tropical Medicine, in: Bradley Naranch/Geoff Eley (eds.), German Colonialism in a Global Age, Durham/London 2014, p. 74–92.

Hans Paasche, Die Forschungsreisen des Afrikaners Lukanga Mukara ins Innerste Deutschlands, Hamburg 1921.

Alexandra Przyrembel, Wissen auf Wanderschaft. Britische Missionare, ethologisches Wissen und die Thematisierung religiöser Selbstgefühle um 1830, in: Historische Anthropologie 19 (2011) 1, p. 31–53.

Ricardo Roque/Kim A. Wagner, Introduction: Engaging Colonial Knowledge, in: ibid. (eds.), Engaging Colonial Knowledge. Reading European Archives in World History, Basingstoke/New York 2012, p. 1–32.

Damon Salesa, Race, in: Philippa Levine/John Marriott (eds.), The Ashgate Research Companion to Modern Imperial Histories, Oxon/New York 2012, p. 429–448.

Luigi Westenra Sambon, Acclimatization of Europeans in Tropical Lands, in: Geographical Journal 12 (1898) 6, p. 589–606.

Bernhard C. Schär, Tropenliebe. Schweizer Naturforscher und niederländischer Imperialismus in Südostasien um 1900, Frankfurt a. M./New York 2015.

Londa Schiebinger, The Anatomy of Difference: Race and Sex in Eighteenth-Century Science, in: Eighteenth-Century Studies 23 (1990) 4, p. 387–405.

Pascal Schmid, Medicine, Faith and Politics in Agogo: A History of Health Care Delivery in Rural Ghana, ca. 1925 to 1980, Wien/Zürich 2018.

Heather J. Sharkey, Introduction: The Unexpected Consequences of Christian Missionary Encounters, in: ibid. (ed.), Cultural Conversions. Unexpected Consequences of Christian Missionary Encounters in the Middle East, Africa, and South Africa, New York 2013, p. 1–26.

Rob Shields, Places on the Margin. Alternative Geographies of Modernity, London 1991.

Staehlin, Völkerschauen im Zoologischen Garten Basel 1879–1935, Basel 1993.

Ann Laura Stoler, Cultivating Bourgeois Bodies and Racial Selves, in: Catherine Hall (ed.), Cultures of Empire. A Reader: Colonizers in Britain and the Empire in the Nineteenth and Twentieth Centuries, New York 2000, p. 87–119.

Jakob Stutz, Aus meiner ärztlichen Praxis, in: Verein für ärztliche Mission in Stuttgart (ed.), Mitteilungen aus der ärztlichen Mission 10 (1911), p. 4–7.

Unabhängige Expertenkommission Administrative Versorgungen (eds.), Organisierte Willkür. Administrative Versorgungen in der Schweiz 1930–1981, Schlussbericht, Zürich 2019.

Hermann Vortisch, Statistik und Bericht über das erste Halbjahr 1904 der ärztlichen Mission auf der Goldküste, in: Archiv für Schiffs- und Tropenhygiene 9 (1905), p. 346–354.

Hermann Vortisch, Erfahrungen über einige spezifische Krankheiten an der Goldküste, in: Archiv für Schiffs- und Tropenhygiene 10 (1906), p. 537–539.

Hermann Vortisch, Ärztliche Beobachtungen und Erfahrungen auf der Goldküste, in: Deutsche Medizinische Wochenschrift 33 (1907), p. 110–111.

Hermann Vortisch, Aus der Arbeit eines Missionsarztes, in: Schweizerische Rundschau für Medizin 38 (1912), p. 1025–1036.

Roxann Wheeler, The Complexion of Race: Categories of Difference in Eighteenth-Century British Culture, Pennsylvania 2000.

Roberto Zaugg, Guerre, maladie, empire. Les services de santé militaires en situation coloniale pendant le long XIXe siècle, in: ibid. (ed.), Histoire, Médecine et Santé 10 (2016), p. 9–16.

Hans Ziemann, Wie erobert man Afrika für die weisse und farbige Rasse? in: Beihefte zum Archiv für Schiffs- und Tropenhygiene 11 (1907), p. 235–259.

Andrew Zimmerman, Anthropology and Antihumanism in Imperial Germany, Chicago/London 2001.

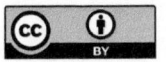

APPENDIX

SHORT BIOGRAPHIES

Alfred Eckhardt (BV 1139)

Date and place of birth: 22.01.1859 in Grosshesselohe, Munich

Admission to the BM as a medical student: 27.04.1883
Ordination: 30.06.1887 in Münster

Studies: Theology in Tubingen 1878–1880
Medicine in Tubingen, Basel and Berlin 1880–1887

Stays on the Gold Coast: Aburi 1887–1888
Christiansborg 1888–1891
Odumase 1891–1893

Day and place of death: 24.04.1893 in Aburi due to a liver abscess

Rudolf Fisch (BV 985)

Date and place of birth: 19.11.1856 in Aarau, Switzerland

Studies: Medicine in Basel 1880–1884

Admission to the BM: 12.08.1875
Previous occupation: Saddler

© The Editor(s) (if applicable) and The Author(s) 2023
L. M. Ratschiller Nasim, *Medical Missionaries and Colonial Knowledge in West Africa and Europe, 1885–1914*,
Cambridge Imperial and Post-Colonial Studies,
https://doi.org/10.1007/978-3-031-27128-1

Ordination: 17.08.1884 in Berne

Stays on the Gold Coast: Aburi 1885–1911

From 1911: Chaplain in Wädenswil and later Horgen (Switzerland)
1911–1914: Publications and lecture tours for the BM
1912–1913: At the service of the Evangelical Society in the Canton of Aargau
1914–1931: At the service of the Evangelical Society in the Canton of Zurich

Day and place of death: 02.12.1946 in Wädenswil, Switzerland

Arthur Häberlin (BV 1674)

Date and place of birth: 09.04.1878 in Mauren bei Berg, Switzerland

Previous occupation: Medical doctor
1907–1910: Contracted as medical doctor by the BM

Stays in Cameroon: Bonaku 1907–1910

End of service for the BM: no contract renewal

Physician in Zurich

Day and place of death: 15.03.1940 due to suicide in the penitentiary Regensberg, Canton of Zurich

Friedrich Hey (BV 1261)

Date and place of birth: 14.11.1864 in Dörrenbach, Palatinate

Admission to the BM: 01.09.1888
Previous occupation: Orderly (*Krankenwärter*)
Ordination: 09.02.1895 in Betsaal

Studies: Medicine in Basel 1880–1894

Stays on the Gold Coast: Aburi 1895
Odumase 1896–1899
Kumase 1899

Stays in Cameroon: Bonaku 1900–1902

Expulsion from the BM in July of 1903

1902–1904: Medical practitioner in Netstal, Canton of Glarus
1904–1908: Physician for trading companies on the Gold Coast
1906: British government physician
1908–1910: Director of the sanatorium in Bas Eilsen, Germany
From 1910: Medical practitioner in Bückeburg, Germany
From 1920: Manufacturer of pharmaceutical preparations in Bückeburg

Day and place of death: 30.12.1960 in Bückeburg

Karl Huppenbauer (BV 2090)

Date and place of birth: 05.04.1884 in Akropong, Gold Coast

Studies: Medicine in Tubingen and Kiel 1904–1910

1911–1913: Resident physician in Schwäbisch Hall, Tubingen and Stuttgart

1914–1917: Contracted as medical doctor by the BM in Aburi, Gold Coast

1918: Internment in London for 3 months
1918–1919: Military doctor in Freudenstadt
1919–1931: Physician (from 1926 Directing Senior Physician) at the *Tropengenesungsheim*—Tropical Convalescent Home—in Tubingen

1931–1934: BM doctor in Agogo, Gold Coast

1935–1937: British government physician in Ghana and additional work for the BM in Togo

Day and place of death: 15.04.1959 in Leonberg, Baden-Wurttemberg

Ernst Mähly

Date and place of birth: 23.04.1856 in Basel, Switzerland

Studies: Medicine in Basel, Leipzig, Tubingen

1878–1889: General practitioner in Basel

1882: Studies at Max von Pettenkofer's Hygiene Institute in Munich for four months and travels to Edinburgh to study English publications and meet British doctors who had practised in the tropics

1882–1883: Medical research expedition to the Gold Coast, contracted by the BM

1889: Accompanies Friedrich Nietzsche to Jena and another patient to India

1890–1894: Further training as a psychiatrist and resident physician at the clinics Königsfelden and St. Pirminsberg in Pfäfers, Switzerland

Date and place of death: 30.05.1894, due to suicide at the clinic in Pfäfers

Theodor Müller (BV 1808b)

Date and place of birth: 31.07.1880 in Crailsheim, Wurttemberg

Admission to the BM: 04.10.1898
Ordination: 19.09.1909 in Heidelberg, 01.07.1909 in Münster

Studies: Medicine in Marburg, Munich and Heidelberg 1901–1906

1906–1908: Resident physician in Karlsruhe
1908: Military doctor

Stays on the Gold Coast: Aburi 1909–1914

From 1916: At the service of the Evangelical Synod of North America
1916–1927: Pastor in North Tonawanda, USA
1922–1924: Doctor at the Adams-Memorial-Hospital, Perrysburg, USA
1924–1941: Doctor at the Deaconess Hospital in Buffalo, USA
From 1927: Representative of the BM in the USA

Day and place of death: 17.12.1941 in North Tonawanda near Buffalo, New York State, USA

Hermann Vortisch (BV 1537)

Date and place of birth: 18.06.1874 in Lörrach, Baden

Studies: Medicine in Basel, Tubingen, Munich, Greifswald 1896–1901

1901–1903: Resident physician in Berne, doctor at the Women's Hospital in Basel

Admission to the BM: 17.12.1902

Stays on the Gold Coast: Aburi 1903–1905

Stays in Cameroon: Bonaku 1905

Transfer to China due to health reasons
1906–1913: Basel Mission doctor in Honyen in China
1914–1928: Director of the hospital for epileptics in Kork, Baden
1928–1938: Writer for the BM

Day and place of death: 02.05.1944 in Lörrach, Baden

BIBLIOGRAPHY

ARCHIVAL SOURCES

BASEL MISSION ARCHIVES (BMA)

Annual Reports
Circular Letters
Committee Protocols
Correspondences
Curricula
Decrees
Personal Files
Quarterly Reports

FEDERAL ARCHIVES, BERLIN-LICHTERFELDE (BARCH)

R 86/1768 Reichsgesundheitsamt: Akte zu Friedrich Hey, 1913–1938
R 86/2747 Sitzungen des Reichs-Gesundheitsrats, 1908–1911
R 86/4593 Reichsgesundheitsamt: Geschlechtskrankheiten, vol. 5, 1908–1929
R 1001/3900a Missionstätigkeit in Kamerun, 1904–1908
R 1001/3900/1 Auswärtiges Amt, Kolonialabteilung, Akten betreffend Mission-stätigkeit in Kamerun, Kirchen- und Schulsachen, 1904–1928
R 1001/3900j vol. 1, 1886–1890
R 1001/3901 vol. 2, 1891–1896
R 1001/3902 vol. 3, 1897–1900
R 1001/3903 vol. 4, 1900–1903

© The Editor(s) (if applicable) and The Author(s) 2023   443
L. M. Ratschiller Nasim, *Medical Missionaries and Colonial Knowledge in West Africa and Europe, 1885–1914*,
Cambridge Imperial and Post-Colonial Studies,
https://doi.org/10.1007/978-3-031-27128-1

R 1001/3904 vol. 5, 1904–1909

R 1001/3905 vol. 6, 1910–1918

R 1001/3921 Reichskolonialamt, Akten betreffend: Abgrenzung der evangelischen und katholischen Missionsgebiete in Kamerun, 1890–1895

R 1001/4427 Enteignung in Duala, vol. 1, 1910–1913

R 1001/4428 Enteignung in Duala, vol. 2, 1913

R 1001/4429 Enteignung in Duala, vol. 3, 1913–1914

R 1001/5764 Enteignung in Duala, vol. 8, 1913–1914

R 1001/5834 Malaria und Schwarzwasserfieber, vol. 1, 1890–1894

R 1001/5863 Einführung einer obligatorischen Chinin-Prophylaxe gegen Malaria, 1901–1902

R 1001/5865 Einführung einer obligatorischen Chinin-Prophylaxe gegen Malaria, vol. 3, 1903–1904

R 1001/5965 Expeditionen und Wissenschaft: Gesundheitswesen, 1906–1910

R 1001/6043 Reichs-Kolonialamt, Akten betreffend: Internationale Hygiene-Ausstellung, vol. 1, 1909–1910

R 1001/6044 Reichs-Kolonialamt, Akten betreffend: Internationale Hygiene-Ausstellung, vol. 2, 1910–1924

R 5101/23107 Evangelische Missionsgesellschaft in Basel, 1882–1940

R 8023 Deutsche Kolonialgesellschaft: Tropenhygiene, 1887–1934

R 8023/1002 vol. 1, 1887–1890

R 8023/1003 vol. 2, 1890–1891

R 8023/1004 vol. 3, 1891–1892

R 8023/1005 vol. 4, 1893–1895

R 8023/1006 vol. 5, 1895–1908

R 8023/1007 vol. 6, 1909–1910

R 8023/1008 vol. 7, 1911–1934

R 8023/1011 Bearbeitung in den Feldern, 1893–1895

R 8023/1013 Westafrikanische Küste, 1890–1893

R 8023/1020 Tropenausrüstungen. Apotheken in den deutschen Kolonien, 1891–1894

R 8023/1022 Sanitätswesen in den deutschen Kolonien, vol. 1, 1896–1908

R 8023/1023 Sanitätswesen in den deutschen Kolonien, vol. 2, 1908–1910

R 8023/1024 Sanitätswesen in den deutschen Kolonien, vol. 3, 1911–1926

R 8023/1028 Untersuchungen über die Akklimatisationsfähigkeit der Deutschen und ihrer Nachkommen in tropischen Gebieten, 1912

SOAS Archives

CBMS/03/X/4/1/1 Basel Mission 1912–1918

CWM/LMS/07/02/04 London Missionary Society, Incoming Correspondence: Switzerland, 1798–1843

IMC-CBMS/01 International Missionary Council and Conference of British
Missionary Societies Archive, Africa, 1910–1945
MMS/Special Series/Biographical/West Africa/FBN 4

SECRET STATE ARCHIVES PRUSSIAN CULTURAL HERITAGE (GStA PK)

I. HA Rep 89 32507 Missionen, vol. 1, 1886–1904
I. HA Rep 89 32508 Missionen, vol. 2, 1905–1919
I. HA Rep 89 32512 Krankenhäuser, Krankenansiedlungen und Gesundheitssta-
tionen, 1889–1906
I. HA Rep 89 32513 Deutsches Institut für ärztliche Mission, 1901–1910

STATE ARCHIVES OF THE CANTON BASEL-STADT (StABS)

PA 878 Archiv der Basler Höhenklinik Davos, 1896–1992

JOURNALS & SERIES

Allgemeine Missionszeitschrift 1874–1914
An die Freunde des Ärztlichen Zweiges der Basler Mission 1891–1894
Archiv für Schiffs- und Tropenhygiene 1897–1914
Correspondenzblatt der Basler Missionare 1885–1914
Der Evangelische Heidenbote 1828–1914
Deutsche Kolonialzeitung 1884–1914
Deutsches Kolonialblatt 1890–1914
Die ärztliche Mission 1906–1914
Evangelisches Missionsmagazin 1815–1914
Journal of Tropical Medicine 1898–1914
Medical Missions at Home and Abroad 1880–1910
Reichskolonialamt (ed.), Medizinal-Berichte über die Deutschen Schutzgebiete,
Berlin 1903–1914
Tropenhygienische Rundschau 1913–1914
Unsere ärztliche Mission 1895–1898
Verband der deutschen Vereine für ärztliche Mission (ed.), Jahrbücher der
Ärztlichen Mission, Gütersloh 1910–1914
Verein für ärztliche Mission (ed.), Jahresberichte, Stuttgart 1898–1914

WO OPAC "01 International Missionary Council and Conference of British
Missionary Societies archive, MICA, 1910–1945
d Baptist in Public Proceedings New Asian docs +

STATE ARCHIVES MICHIGAN CULTURAL HERITAGE (1850 JR.)

HA Rep 80 25102 Direction vol. 1 1856–1908
and HA Rep 80 25203 Mission vol. 2 1905–1917
d. HA Rep 80 25233 Kirchenbücher, Konfirmationen und Vermittlung
nahen 1880–1906
HA Rep 85 25251 Deutscher in Übersee Kirche Abteilung 1921–1938

STATE ARCHIVES THE ... DELOW Basel Staat 101A85

PP 78 an der Inländer Völkerbund Dr. 9, 1690 1922

BIBLIOGRAPHY

Allgemeine Missions- nachrichten 1874–1918
Beitrag ... die Ausserung ... der Gesellschaft 1907 1929
Archiv für Missionswissenschaft Gütersloh 1913–1914
Der Evangelische Heidenbote Basel ...
der deutsche evangelischen Kirche Deutsche 1875 1929
Mission Chronicle 1881 1922
Beiträge ... Missionskunde 1903 1914
Der christliche Hausfreund 1919
Protestantische Monatsschrift 1930 1938
Jahrbuch ... Deutschen Evangelischen 1895–1924
Nachrichten aus der ... Missionsland 1880–1910
Barmer Missions ... Missionsarbeit ... Rheinische Mission 1828
... 1830

Das ... Rheinischen Mission 1913–1914
Mission africaine Mission 1895 1899
Verband der Deutschen Vereine ... im Ausland 1917 1940
Reichskolonialamt Archiv Gütersloh 1917 1936
Neue Allgemeine Mission (ed.) Jahresberichte Stuttgart 1895 1914

INDEX